# AI and IoT Technology and Applications for Smart Healthcare Systems

In recent years, the application of Artificial Intelligence (AI) and Internet of Things (IoT) technologies in smart healthcare has been increasing. We are approaching a world where connected smart devices tell people when they need to visit a doctor because these devices will be able to detect health problems and discover symptoms of illness that may need medical care. AI-collaborative IoT technologies can help medical professionals with decision-making. These technologies can also help develop a sustainable and smart healthcare system.

***AI and IoT Technology and Applications for Smart Healthcare Systems*** helps readers understand complex scientific topics in a simple and accessible way. It introduces the world of AI-collaborative IoT physics, explaining how this technology behaves at the smallest level and how this can revolutionize healthcare. The book shows how IoT technology and AI can work together to make computers more powerful and capable of solving complex problems in the healthcare sector. Exploring the effect of AI-collaborative technology on IoT technologies, the book discusses how IoT can benefit from AI algorithms to enable machines to learn, make decisions, and process information more efficiently. Because smart machines create more perceptive devices and systems, the application of this technology raises important ethical questions about privacy, security, and the responsible development of healthcare IoT technology, which this book covers. The book also provides insight into the potential applications of these technologies not only in the healthcare industry but also in related fields, such as smart transportation, smart manufacturing, and smart cities.

## ADVANCES IN COMPUTATIONAL COLLECTIVE INTELLIGENCE

**Edited by**
**Dr. Subhendu Kumar Pani**
**Principal, Krupajal Group of Institutions, India**

**Published**

**Social Media and Crowdsourcing**
*By Sujoy Chatterjee, Thipendra P Singh, Sunghoon Lim, and Anirban Mukhopadhyay*
ISBN: 978-1-032-38687-4

**Edge Computational Intelligence for AI-Enabled IoT Systems**
*By Shrikaant Kulkarni, Jaiprakash Narain Dwivedi, Dinda Pramanta, and Yuichiro Tanaka*
ISBN: 978-1-032-20766-7

**AI and IoT Technology and Applications for Smart Healthcare Systems**
*By Alex Khang*
ISBN: 978-1-032-68490-1

**Forthcoming**

**Artificial Intelligence and Machine Learning for Risk Management of Natural Hazards and Disasters**
*By Cees van Westen, Romulus Costache, Dimitrios A. Karras, R. S. Ajin, and Sekhar L. Kuriakose*
ISBN: 978-1-032-23276-8

**Computational Intelligence in Industry 4.0 and 5.0 Applications: Challenges and Future Prospects**
*Joseph Bamidele Awotunde, Kamalakanta Muduli, and Biswajit Brahma*
ISBN: 978-1-032-53922-5

**Deep Learning for Smart Healthcare: Trends, Challenges and Applications**
*K. Murugeswari, B. Sundaravadivazhagan, S. Poonkuntran, and Thendral Puyalnithi*
ISBN: 978-1-032-45581-5

**Explainable AI and Cybersecurity**
*By Mohammad Tabrez Quasim, Abdullah Alharthi, Ali Alqazzaz, Mohammed Mujib Alshahrani, Ali Falh Alshahrani, and Mohammad Ayoub Khan*
ISBN: 978-1-032-42221-3

**Machine Learning in Applied Sciences**
*By M. A. Jabbar, Shankru Guggari, Kingsley Okoye, and Houneida Sakly*
ISBN: 978-1-032-25172-1

For more information about this series, please visit: https://www.routledge.com/Advances-in-Computational-Collective-Intelligence/book-series/ACCICRC

# AI and IoT Technology and Applications for Smart Healthcare Systems

Edited by Alex Khang

CRC Press
Taylor & Francis Group
Boca Raton London New York

CRC Press is an imprint of the
Taylor & Francis Group, an **informa** business
AN AUERBACH BOOK

First edition published 2024
by CRC Press
2385 Executive Center Drive, Suite 320, Boca Raton, FL 33431

and by CRC Press
4 Park Square, Milton Park, Abingdon, Oxon, OX14 4RN

*CRC Press is an imprint of Taylor & Francis Group, LLC*



ISBN: 978-1-032-68490-1 (hbk)
ISBN: 978-1-032-67964-8 (pbk)
ISBN: 978-1-032-68674-5 (ebk)

DOI: 10.1201/9781032686745

Typeset in Times LT Std
by Apex CoVantage, LLC

# Contents

# Preface

In recent years, the scope of application of AI and IoT technologies in smart healthcare has increased. It seems humans are approaching a world where connected smart devices tell people when they need to visit their doctor because they are aware of a health problem and have discovered symptoms that might be concerning. The goal of using AI-collaborative IoT technologies is to constantly help hand to medical professionals in the decision-making of sustainable development in a smart healthcare system to serve better for the life of citizens.

To complete the objectives of designing and implementing the core components of the medical ecosystem is effective management of the development of emerging IoT technologies and applications, starting with strategy and investing the complex models and diversity of frameworks into a healthcare industry, especially the core infrastructure elements are including activities of the public and private healthcare services as well as innovative AI-collaborative IoT technologies and other intelligent devices for supporting continuous operating in the smart healthcare sector.

This book will share and contribute new ideas, methodologies, technologies, approaches, models, frameworks, theories, and practices to develop, improve, and resolve the challenging issues associated with the leveraging of the advanced solutions of AI-collaborative IoT Technology and Machine Vision in designing and implementing advanced infrastructure for the smart healthcare services. This book targets a mixed audience of students, engineers, scholars, researchers, academics, doctors, and professionals who are learning, researching, and working in the healthcare industry in different countries.

Happy reading!

# Acknowledgments

The book ***AI and IoT Technology and Applications for Smart Healthcare Systems*** is based on the design and implementation of Artificial Intelligence (AI), Internet of Things (IoT), Healthcare Internet of Things (IoHT), Computer Vision, and Applications for various activities in the smart healthcare industry.

Preparing and designing a book outline to introduce these concepts to readers around the world is the passion and noble mission of the editorial team. To make this idea a reality and contribute to the success of this book, the greatest thanks belong to the efforts, experiences, enthusiasm, and trust of the contributors.

To all the reviewers with whom we have had the opportunity to collaborate and remotely monitor their hard work, we acknowledge their tremendous support and valuable comments not only for the book but also for future book projects.

We also express our deep gratitude for all the pieces of advice, support, motivation, sharing, collaboration, and inspiration we received from our faculty, contributors, educators, professors, scientists, scholars, engineers, and academic colleagues.

Last but not least, we are really grateful to our publisher, CRC Press (Taylor & Francis Group), for their wonderful support in ensuring the timely processing of the manuscript and bringing this book to the readers as soon as possible.

Thank you, everyone.

**Editor: Alex Khang**

# About the Editor

**Alex Khang** is a professor in information technology, D.Sc. D.Litt., AI and a data scientist, software industry expert, and the Chief of Technology Officer (AI and Data Science Research Center) at the Global Research Institute of Technology and Engineering, North Carolina, United States. He has over 28 years of teaching and research experience in information technology at the Universities of Science and Technology in Vietnam, India, and the United States. He has published 74 documents indexed in Scopus, 52 authored books (in computer science 2000–2010 in Vietnam), two authored books (software development), and 50 book chapters. He has published 18 edited books and calling for chapters for 13 edited books in the fields of AI ecosystem (AI, ML, DL, IoT, robotics, data science, big data, and quantum computing), smart city ecosystem, healthcare ecosystem, Fintech technology, and blockchain technology (since 2020). He has over 28 years of working experience as a software product manager, data engineer, AI engineer, cloud computing architect, solution architect, software architect, and database expert in the foreign corporations of Germany, Sweden, the United States, Singapore, and multinationals (former CEO, former CTO, former engineering director, product manager, and senior software production consultant).

# Contributors

**Arulmurugan A.**
Assistant Professor
Department of Computing Technologies
SRM Institute of Science and Technology, Kattankulathur Campus
Chennai, Tamil Nadu, India

**Gobinath A.**
Assistant Professor
Department of Information Technology
Velammal College of Engineering and Technology
Madurai, Tamil Nadu, India

**Ragimova Nazila Ali**
Associate Professor
Azerbaijan State Oil and Industry University
Baku, Azerbaijan

**Abuzarova Vusala Alyar**
Educated Information Technologies
Azerbaijan State Oil and Industry University
Baku, Azerbaijan

**Nageswara Rao A.V.**
Associate Professor
Department of Electronics & Communication Engineering
Narasaraopeta Engineering College
Narasaraopeta, Andhra Pradesh, India

**Mammadova Bilqeyis Azer**
Azerbaijan State Oil and Industry University
Baku, Azerbaijan

**Maheswari B.**
Assistant Professor
Department of Computer Science and Engineering
R.M.K Engineering College
Kavaraipettai, Tamil Nadu, India

**Narendra Kumar Rao B.**
Professor and Program Head
AIML, School of Computing
MB University
Tirupati, Andhra Padesh, India

**Shaik Bajidvali**
Associate Professor
Department of Electronics & Communication Engineering
Narasaraopeta Engineering College
Narasaraopeta, Andhra Pradesh, India

**Ayush Kumar Bar**
UG, Computer Science and Engineering
Techno Engineering College
Banipur, West Bengal, India

**Dheerdhwaj Barak**
Assistant Professor
Department of Computer Science
Vaish College of Engineering, MDU Rohtak
Rohtak, Haryana, India

**Debanjan Basu**
School of Sciences
CHRIST (Deemed to be University)
Bangalore, Karnataka, India

**Sachin Chaudhary**
Assistant Professor
School of Computer Science and Application
IIMT University Meerut
Meerut, Uttar Pradesh, India

**Avijit Kumar Chaudhuri**
Assistant Professor
Computer Science and Engineering
Techno Engineering College
Banipur, West Bengal, India

**Puspraj Singh Chauhan**
ECE Department
Pranveer Singh Institute of Technology
Kanpur, Uttar Pradesh, India

**Ayushya Chongder**
School of Sciences
CHRIST (Deemed to be University)
Bangalore, Karnataka, India

**Nobhonil Roy Choudhury**
M. Tech
Department of Computer Science
Brainware University
Barasat, Kolkata, West Bengal, India

**Svetlana Chumachenko**
Doctor of Science, Professor
Head of Design Automation Department
Kharkiv, National University of Radio Electronics
Kharkiv, Ukraine

**Mukesh Patil D.**
Department of Electronics & Telecommunication Engineering
Ramrao Adik Institute of Technology
DY Patil Deemed to be University
Navi-Mumbai, Maharashtra, India

**Supratim Dasgupta**
Numpy Ninja
Delaware, US

**Namrata Dhanda**
Department of Computer Science and Engineering
Amity University Uttar Pradesh
Lucknow Campus
Lucknow, Uttar Pradesh, India

**Pooja E.**
Assistant Professor
Department of Computer Science and Engineering
Rajalakshmi Institute of Technology
Chembarambakkam, Tamil Nadu, India.

**Ushaa Eswaran**
Principal and Professor
Indira Institute of Technology and Sciences
Markapur, Andhra Pradesh, India

**Sailaja G.**
Research Scholar
School of Computing
MB University
Tirupati, Andhra Padesh, India

**Shivnath Ghosh**
Ph.D.
Department of Computer Science
Brainware University
Barasat, Kolkata, West Bengal, India

**Sonam Gour**
Department of Computer Engineering
Poornima College of Engineering
Jaipur, Rajasthan, India

**Tanmay Gupta**
Pranveer Singh Institute of Technology
Kanpur, Uttar Pradesh, India

**Vladimir Hahanov**
Doctor of Science
Professor of Computer Engineering Faculty
Design Automation Department
Kharkiv National University of Radio Electronics
Kharkiv, Ukraine

**Vugar Abdullayev Hajimahmud**
Doctor of Technical Sciences
Associate Professor
Azerbaijan State Oil and Industry University
Baku, Azerbaijan

**Shahistha Jabeen Hashim**
Numpy Ninja
Dover, Delaware

**Rashad Ismibeyli**
Associate Professor
Azerbaijan University of Architecture and Construction
Baku, Azerbaijan

**Ankit Jain**
ECE Department
Pranveer Singh Institute of Technology
Kanpur, Uttar Pradesh, India

**Roohum Jegan**
Department of Electronics & Communication Engineering
BMS College of Engineering
Bangalore, Karnataka, India

**Anusha K.**
Narasimha Reddy Engineering College
Hyderabad, Telangana, India

**Gajanan Birajdar K.**
Department of Electronics Engineering
Ramrao Adik Institute of Technology
DY Patil Deemed to be University
Navi-Mumbai, Maharashtra, India

**Sudha K.**
Assistant Professor
Department of Computer Science and Business Systems
R.M.D Engineering College
Kavaraipettai, Tamil Nadu, India

**Ana Kadarningsih**
Department of Management
University of Dian Nuswantoro
Semarang, Indonesia

**Bhakti Kaushal**
Department of Electronics & Telecommunication Engineering
Ramrao Adik Institute of Technology
DY Patil Deemed to be University
Navi-Mumbai, Maharashtra, India

**Imran Ullah Khan**
ECE Department
Integral University
Lucknow, Uttar Pradesh, India

**Mrunalini Kulkarni H.**
Assistant Professor
Department of Pharmaceutical Chemistry
School of Pharmacy
Vishwakarma University
Pune, Maharashtra, India

**Dinesh Kumar**
Harrisburg University of Science & Technology
Harrisburg, Pennsylvania

**Eugenia Litvinova**
Doctor of Science
Professor of Computer Engineering Faculty
Design Automation Department
Kharkov National University of Radio Electronics
Kharkiv, Ukraine

**Anandan M.**
Associate Professor
Department of Electronics and Communication Engineering
Vel Tech Rangarajan Dr. Sagunthala R&D Institute of Science and Technology
Chennai, Tamil Nadu, India

**Sirish Kumar M.**
Associate Professor
School of Computing
MohanBabu University
Tirupati, Andhra Padesh, India

**Qaffarova Zeynab Mehman**
Azerbaijan State Oil and Industry University
Baku, Azerbaijan

**Kenneth John Menezes**
School of Sciences
CHRIST (Deemed to be University)
Bangalore, Karnataka, India

**Nidhya M. S.**
Associate Professor
Department of Computer Science and IT
Jain Deemed-to-be University
Bangalore Murthal, India

**Suresh Kumar N.**
Professor
Civil Engineering
Kalasalingam Academy of Research and Education
Krishankoil, Tamil Nadu, India

**Girija P.**
Assistant Professor
Department of Computer Science and Engineering
Vel Tech Rangarajan Dr. Sagunthala R&D Institute of Science and Technology
Chennai, Tamil Nadu, India

**Harikrishna P.**
Associate Professor
Department of Computational Intelligence
Malla Reddy College of Engineering and Technology
Hyderabad, Telangana, India

**Pashmina Doshi P.**
Assistant Professor
Faculty of Commerce and Management
Vishwakarma University
Pune, Maharashtra, India

**Rajeswari P.**
Professor
Department of Electronics and Communication Engineering
Velammal College of Engineering and Technology
Madurai, Tamil Nadu, India

**Rajneesh Panwar**
Assistant Professor
School of Computer Science and Application
IIMT University Meerut
Meerut, Uttar Pradesh, India

**Purvi Parmar**
Dwarkadas J. Sanghvi College of Engineering
Mumbai, Maharashtra, India

**Baishali Patra**
Numpy Ninja
Dover, Delaware

**Anh P. T. N.**
Doctor
Master of Medicine
Ho Chi Minh City University of Medicine and Pharmacy Hospital
Ho Chi Minh City, Vietnam

**Kalaiyarasan R.**
Assistant Professor
Department of ECE
Sri Manakula Vinayagar College of Engineering and Technology
Puducherry, India

**Kaviarasan R.**
Associate Professor
Department of Computer Science and Engineering
Rajeev Gandhi Memorial College of Engineering and Technology
Nandyal, Andhra Pradesh, India

**Poonam Inamdar R.**
Assistant Professor
Department of Pharmaceutical Chemistry, School of Pharmacy
Vishwakarma University
Pune, Maharashtra, India

**Siva Subramanian R.**
Associate Professor
Department of Computer Science and Engineering
R.M.K College of Engineering and Tech
Puduvoyal, Tamil Nadu, India

**Seenu Raj**
Numpy Ninja
Dover, Delaware

**Kavitha Rajamohan**
School of Sciences
CHRIST (Deemed to be University)
Bangalore, Karnataka, India

**Harsh Rana**
Thakur College of Engineering and Technology
Kandivali East
Mumbai, Maharashtra, India

**Sangeetha Rangasamy**
School of Business and Management
CHRIST (Deemed to be University)
Bangalore, Karnataka, India

**Smitha Raveendran**
Department of Electronics Engineering
Ramrao Adik Institute of Technology
DY Patil Deemed-to-be-University
Navi-Mumbai, Maharashtra, India

**Akankshya Rout**
UG
Computer Science and Engineering
Techno Engineering College
Banipur, West Bengal, India

**Javeed Md. S.**
Associate Professor
Department of Electronics & Communication Engineering
Narasaraopeta Engineering College
Narasaraopeta, Andhra Pradesh, India

**Sanamreddy Sandhya**
School of Computing
MohanBabu University
Tirupati, Andhra Pradesh, India

**Rahul Sarkar**
UG
Computer Science Engineering
Cooch Behar Government Engineering College
Cooch Behar, West Bengal, India

**Miloni Shah**
Dwarkadas J. Sanghvi College of Engineering
Mumbai, Maharashtra, India

**Stavan Shah**
Dwarkadas J. Sanghvi College of Engineering
Mumbai, Maharashtra, India

**Vrushank Shah**
Assistant Professor
Head of Department Electronics & Communication Engineering
Indus Institute of Technology & Engineering
Indus University
Ahmedabad, Gujarat, India

**Kewal Krishan Sharma**
Professor
School of Computer Science and Application
IIMT University Meerut
Meerut, Uttar Pradesh, India

**Reena Sharma**
Department of Computer Engineering
Poornima College of Engineering
Jaipur, Rajasthan, India

**Vikas Sharma**
Assistant Professor
School of Computer Science and Application
IIMT University Meerut
Meerut, Uttar Pradesh, India

**Anita Shukla**
BSH Department
Pranveer Singh Institute of Technology
Kanpur, Uttar Pradesh, India

**Khushwant Singh**
Research Scholar
Department of Computer Science
University Institute of Engineering and Technology
MDU Rohtak
Rohtak, Haryana, India

**Yudhvir Singh**
Professor
Department of Computer Science
University Institute of Engineering and Technology
MDU Rohtak
Rohtak, Haryana, India

**Triwiyanto**
Department of Medical Electronics Technology
Poltekkes Kemenkes Surabaya, Indonesia

**Abhishek Vaghela**
Indus University
Ahmedabad, Gujarat, India

**Ponnala Vaishnavi**
School of Computing
MohanBabu University
Tirupati, Andhra Padesh, India

**Tarun Kumar Vashishth**
Associate Professor
School of Computer Science and Application
IIMT University Meerut
Meerut, Uttar Pradesh, India

**Anil Vasoya**
Thakur College of Engineering and Technology
Mumbai, Maharashtra, India

**Rajat Verma**
Department of Computer Science and Engineering
Pranveer Singh Institute of Technology
Kanpur, Uttar Pradesh, India

**Mohit Yadav**
Assistant Professor
Department of Mathematics
University Institute of Sciences
Chandigarh University
Gharuan, Mohali, India

**Tarun Kasida Zahoor**
Department of Mathematics with Applications in Computer Science
MSCMACS, School of Sciences Indira Gandhi National Open University (IGNOU)
Kolkata, West Bengal, India

# 1 The Era of the Digital Healthcare System and Its Impact on Human Psychology

*Alex Khang, Vladimir Hahanov, Eugenia Litvinova, Svetlana Chumachenko, Triwiyanto, Ragimova Nazila Ali, Ana Kadarningsih, Rashad İsmibeyli, Vugar Abdullayev Hajimahmud, Abuzarova Vusala Alyar, Qaffarova Zeynab Mehman, Mammadova Bilqeyis Azer, and Anh P. T. N.*

## 1.1 INTRODUCTION

The current era is called the "digital era" and includes the widespread application of information and communication technologies (ICT) in every sector – from daily life to huge industries. The primary concept that forms the basis of the digital era, as well as ICT, is the concept of "information". With digitalization, it became possible to process, use and transmit information in a virtual environment – in other words, in a computer environment – through communication technologies, which in turn brought the era of digitalization together with ICT (Khang & Rana et al., 2023).

Along with the "Data Age" of the period, an extreme increase in information in all fields was also observed. On the other hand, it is more convenient to access this information now than it was in the last century. Data overload has both positive and negative aspects. The main disadvantage is which information is true or false. At this point, three concepts stand out: Data, Information and Knowledge. Although, at first glance, they seem like similar concepts, the fundamental differences between them make them the most important tools of the current era.

- **Data**: These are raw values obtained from various sources using various methods. In other words, it is a collection of values obtained from the original source but not yet processed. Access to such a set of values in any sector is quite easy, and the number is overwhelming.
- **Information**: The second concept after data is a set of data obtained by processing, interpreting or structuring data within a specific content or field. In other words, information is a set of processed data.

DOI: 10.1201/9781032686745-1

- **Knowledge**: The last and most important concept is the collection of information derived and personalized from information – what we know. Basically, knowledge with a more specific purpose is directed in a specific direction. It is basically a direction that requires concrete action with an end goal, such as decision-making, etc.

The relationship between these concepts can be shown as follows: Data → Information → Knowledge. Be it data, information or knowledge, each has always existed in various sectors and has grown tremendously with this era. One of these sectors is healthcare.

## 1.2 THE DATA FACTOR IN HEALTH

The human factor at the core of healthcare has evolved over time into a data set with the integration of Information Technology (IT). In other words, a person is a whole set of data that exists together with both physiological functions and behaviors. The main issue was the correct processing of this data set. This became possible with the help of IT. In general, if we look at the history of healthcare, the view of the human being as a set of data began from the moment when the study of the human body began. The human body remains the most complex creature in the world. There is more information about man that is still not fully studied than in previous centuries. This is related to the development of technology, especially smart technology. The illustration in Figure 1.1 shows a person's transition to a digital data set.

The data obtained about this entity, which has been studied since ancient times, has never been enough to fully understand it. Data obtained before technological development was stored on various paper carriers or simply in oral speech still exists and formed the basic database for the development of healthcare today. Today, along with having more data about the human body, the correct processing of this data has also become possible due to the digital era. On the other hand, human learning has become possible in the virtual environment in addition to the concrete-real environment (Gole et al., 2017).

Currently, the information available in healthcare is obtained from different signals as well as in the real environment – as the human body stores data mainly in signals. This includes electroencephalogram (EEG), electrocardiogram (ECG), electrooculography (EOQ), etc. On the other hand, 80% of data in healthcare is mainly

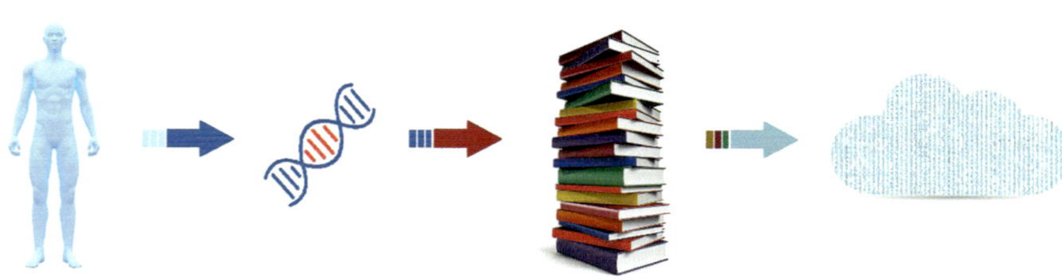

**FIGURE 1.1** Human as the main source of data.

descriptive data, which is data derived from signals. Proper management of data sets – data collection, storage, processing, proper use, etc. – ultimately enables the development of healthcare.

## 1.3 DIGITAL HEALTHCARE

### 1.3.1 Healthcare in the Digital Environment

The healthcare sector can be divided into two parts: Classic Healthcare[1] and Modern Healthcare. Classic Healthcare can mean the period that lasted until the last century (the integration of smart technology into the healthcare sector). Modern Healthcare is the era that began with the integration of Artificial Intelligence-based technologies into the healthcare sector. The relationship between these two distinct eras of healthcare, known as pre- and post-technology, manifests itself in a variety of areas.

#### 1.3.1.1 Data Management

As mentioned, data is one of the most important elements for the healthcare sector. The main goal here is the correct management of this data. Data management refers to all operations performed on data. On the other hand, this process differs in Classical and Modern Healthcare. Data storage, transmission, and processing were limited in terms of time in classical healthcare. As such, each of these data was mostly stored on different paper carriers, and when it was necessary to review them later, it took some time to find each one. In terms of security, it had both positive and negative aspects (Khang & Hahanov et al., 2022).

Keeping them in paper or local carriers had the positive effect of keeping them safe for a long time as long as no accident occurred. And there were no cases of these data being stolen or distorted by a third party. On the other hand, in Modern Healthcare, data management is preferred in terms of time and cost. Most recently, data storage from cloud technologies offers a more convenient environment to work with them. The main problem here is related to security, but it is possible to solve this problem as a result of the right security policy of companies offering cloud services (Khang & Ragimova et al., 2022).

#### 1.3.1.2 Contact with Patients

Remote patient monitoring, remote doctor contact and remote personalized treatment became possible with the integration of Artificial Intelligence technologies in healthcare. Unlike traditional treatment methods, remote treatment also shows its positive aspects. Unlike hospital treatment, home treatment is more beneficial for the patient from a psychological point of view (Rath et al., 2024). On the other hand, remote communication is more advantageous for people living in remote areas. However, healthcare can be accessed in any area where the internet is available. Another advantage of this is the time limit. Coming to the hospital and waiting in line is a waste of time, so remote treatment is useful. Also, making an online appointment while coming to the hospital is another advantage. These are the advantages available to the sick (Rowe, 2008).

On the part of the hospital – i.e., for the staff – assigning shifts, transferring the patient's information directly to the doctor and performing all internal processes without the need for time loss and physical effort are more easily implemented thanks to robotic process automation technologies (Khang, Abdullayev & Litvinova et al., 2024). In general, in addition, improving the quality of service in healthcare, conducting treatments, testing new drugs, predicting diseases, conducting training operations in a virtual environment for medical candidates, saving both costs and time by automating continuous processes and increasing efficiency and effectiveness has become possible and convenient with the integration of Artificial Intelligence-based technologies into the healthcare environment (Anh et al., 2024).

### 1.3.2 World Health Organization – Global Strategy for Digital Health

The World Health Organization has presented a Global Strategy for Digital Health covering the years 2020–2025. The World Health Organization's Global Strategy for Digital Health aims to support countries in strengthening their health systems and achieving the vision of health for all through the application of digital health technologies (WHO, 2021) as shown in Figure 1.2.

### 1.3.3 Technology Examples in Digital Health

Technology examples in digital health include improving quality of life, improving well-being, disease prediction and prevention, the healthy living of the elderly,

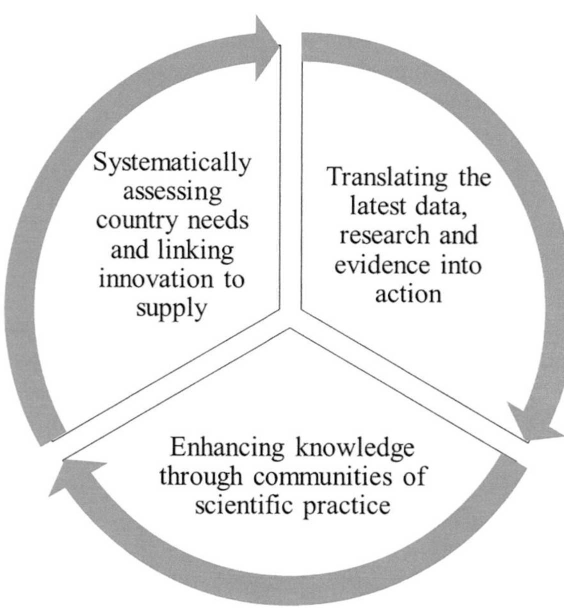


**FIGURE 1.2** The main goals of the Global Strategy (Khang, 2021).

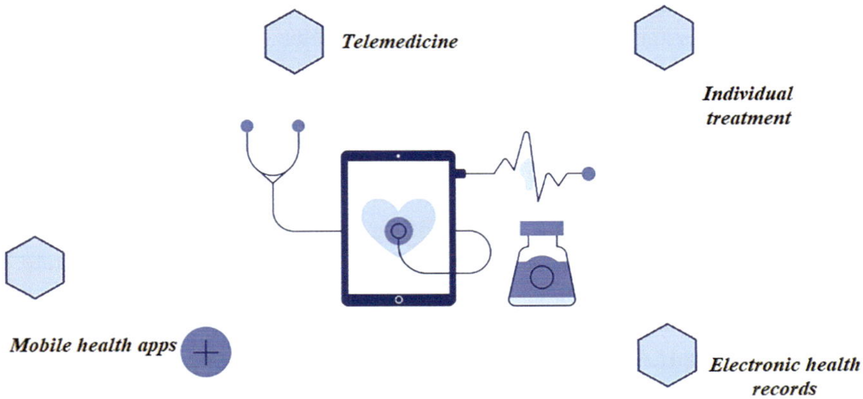


**FIGURE 1.3** Digital healthcare services.

prevention of child mortality related to the provision of proper, high-quality services to people in poverty without racial discrimination, as well as increasing efficiency and effectiveness and decreasing time and costs in healthcare. Digital development has an important place in the healthcare environment in order to save money and solve similar problems. The integration of AI-based technologies in healthcare is the main helper in solving the current problems.

Artificial Intelligence (AI) technology and other technologies related to it, including the Internet of Things (IoT), Computer Vision, Big Data, Virtual and Augmented Reality, Blockchain, Robotic Processing Automation (RPA), etc., have an important role in the development of healthcare. With their integration into healthcare, various medical services, personalized medical services and various digital devices have been created in the field of medicine as shown in Figure 1.3. Digital health technologies can be viewed in two parts: Services and Devices (Khang, Abdullayev & Hrybiuk et al., 2024).

#### 1.3.3.1 Services

- **Telemedicine:** Telemedicine is a service in itself and involves the distribution of other medical services and medical information through communication and information technologies. Telemedicine is the provision of medical services at a distance. Thus, it includes remote communication between the patient and the doctor, remote monitoring of the patients, notification related to the taking of medicines, etc.
- **Individualized treatment:** This is a high-quality type of service, and the main issue is a complete analysis of the patient and preparation of an individual treatment plan. Various capabilities of Artificial Intelligence, data analytics – especially Big Data Analytics – are used here.
- **Electronic health records:** This includes patient information histories and digital versions of records previously stored on paper carriers. All reports about the patient's treatments, progress, medications, etc., are kept here.

- **Mobile health apps:** These smart apps based on artificial intelligence help people understand what disease they have without consulting a doctor by having real symptoms databases. Still, for the current period, such applications are somewhat unable to make a complete and real diagnosis, but it is possible to encounter a completely different situation in the future.

#### 1.3.3.2 Devices

- **Wearable devices:** These are one of the key innovations for healthcare. Through wearable devices, it is possible to measure heart rate, pulse rate, step count, monitor sleep patterns, remind patients of medication time, exercise time, meal time, etc.
- **AI ecosystem:** Artificial Intelligence, Internet of Things and Big Data technologies are used in providing these services.

## 1.4 SOCIAL PSYCHOLOGICAL ASPECTS OF DIGITAL HEALTHCARE

Humans are social beings, and they constantly interact with each other. The social psychology of a person is how his inner world, behavior and thoughts affect himself and others. In other words, it is understood as the influence of a person's thoughts and behavior on others. Man, as a social being, constantly affects and is affected (Divvela & Ritik et al., 2023). The role of Social Psychology in human life is important. It manifests itself in various areas of human life and health behaviors. While the human factor plays an important role in classical and modern healthcare, the influence of human will and human behavior on medical services is great. On the other hand, digital healthcare, in turn, affects human behavior (Jang et al., 2011).

Social psychology has the potential to make valuable contributions to important medical issues, including the etiology, prevention, management and treatment of disease and issues of healthcare delivery (Taylor, 1978). Digital health services identify three social influence factors that influence users' health behaviors: social capital, social support and social value (Lee & Kim, 2021).

First, social capital can be defined as tangible or intangible capital accumulated by an individual or group (Jang et al., 2011). Second, social support refers to the various types of resources that an individual receives in social relationships, including love, recognition, information and material and support from family, relatives, friends, supervisors or peers within the organization (Cohen & Hoberman, 1983). Third, social value contributes to public welfare and community development in all areas, including society, economy, environment and culture. Such value is given by society and shared with others. Thus, the whole society aims to realize desirable and rightly promoted values (Balliet et al., 2009).

The impact of digital health services on patients' behavior can be appreciated from a psychological point of view. The main issue is related to the trust of the user-patient in the service. Another concept of social psychology in medicine is health psychology. It is possible to look at the impact of digital healthcare on patients in the direction of health psychology: health psychology, health promotion and protection and disease prevention; understanding how people react, cope with illness and recover; personalization of treatment and interventions; health systems development and health policy (Practicalhealthpsychology, 2017).

Among the services offered by digital health services are early identification (prediction) of diseases, their prevention and personalization of services provided to patients. Services offered with the help of technologies in digital healthcare are related to areas covered by health psychology. A high level of psychology, especially motivation, plays an important role in the healing of diseases. The patient can get more effective results in a place where he feels more comfortable (this is mainly at home) with correct treatment (this is mainly possible with personalized treatment). Through personalized treatment, the patient begins the process of getting rid of the disease with a correct treatment method that is necessary for him and affects his body and psychology (Cohen & Hoberman, 1983).

Basically, creating personalized rooms for the hospital patient is also an advantage because the human brain is always looking for a place where it can feel comfortable. For this purpose, personalized rooms (a room similar to the patient's own room) or even treatment in the patient's own home are more appropriate. The services offered by digital healthcare are mainly aimed at improving the patient's quality of life. On the other hand, for healthcare, a number of previously mentioned social aspects are important, which is reflected in digital healthcare and healthcare services (Balliet et al., 2009).

## 1.5 CONCLUSION

The new era change that started with the integration of smart technologies in various sectors is also manifested in the healthcare sector. Unlike Classical Healthcare, Modern Healthcare tries to incorporate many possibilities of ICT and integrates many technological capabilities such as Artificial Intelligence, Internet of Things, big data, computer vision, machine learning, deep learning, virtual and augmented reality, etc. With this, the development of healthcare in the digital era continues (Vrushank & Vidhi et al., 2023).

In the digital age, with the help of IT in healthcare, a person becomes a database. The information obtained from them is analyzed and improved, and the internal and external environment of a person is studied. In addition to being a source of information, people are an important capital for healthcare. One of the main goals of healthcare is to improve the quality of life of a person and to provide the right service in this direction. This is where digital health and smart technologies come to the rescue (Vrushank & Khang, 2023).

The services provided by digital healthcare are better than those provided by Classic Healthcare. Services such as proper data management, improvement of communication with patients, implementation of drug testing in a more favorable environment, prediction, delegating repetitive tasks to smart technologies, integration of robotic assistants in healthcare, application of personalized treatment methods, etc., are the advantages of digital healthcare. The impact of digital healthcare on human psychology is again closely related to the services it offers (Khang & Hahanov et al., 2023).

## NOTE

1 Classic Healthcare does not mean primary healthcare, but rather the period before the integration of artificial intelligence-based technologies.

## REFERENCES

Anh, P. T. N., Vladimir Hahanov, Triwiyanto, Ragimova Nazila Ali, Rashad İsmibeyli, Vugar Abdullayev, Abuzarova Vusala Alyar. (2024). AI models for disease diagnosis and prediction of heart disease with artificial neural networks. *Computer vision and AI-integrated IoT technologies in medical ecosystem* (1st ed.). CRC Press. https://doi.org/10.1201/9781003429609-9

Balliet, D., C. Parks, J. Joireman. (2009). Social value orientation and cooperation in social dilemmas: A meta-analysis. *Group Processes & Intergroup Relations*, 12, 533–547. https://journals.sagepub.com/doi/abs/10.1177/1368430209105040

Cohen, S., H. Hoberman. (1983). Positive events and social supports as buffers of life change stress. *Journal of Applied Social Psychology*, 13(2), 9–125. https://onlinelibrary.wiley.com/doi/abs/10.1111/j.1559-1816.1983.tb02325.x

Divvela, Vishnu Sai Kumar, Ritik Chaurasia, Anuradha Misra, Praveen Kumar Misra, A. Khang. (2023). Heart disease and liver disease prediction using machine learning. *Data-centric AI solutions and emerging technologies in the healthcare ecosystem* (1st ed., p. 4). CRC Press. https://doi.org/10.1201/9781003356189-13

Gole, I., Tania Sharma, Shuchi Benara Misra. (June 2017). Role of ICT in healthcare sector: An empirical study of Pune city. *Journal of Management & Public Policy*, 8(2), 23–32. www.indianjournals.com/ijor.aspx?target=ijor:jmpp1&volume=8&issue=2&article=003

Jang, K. S., E. A. Kim, S. H. Oh. (2011). Effects of social capital on organizational performance in hospital organization: Focusing on effects of intellectual capital. *Journal of Korean Academy of Nursing Administration*, 17(1), 2–32. https://synapse.koreamed.org/articles/1051590

Khang, A. (2021). Material4Studies. *Material of computer science, artificial intelligence, data science, IoT, blockchain, cloud, metaverse, cybersecurity for studies.* www.researchgate.net/publication/370156102_Material4Studies

Khang, A., Vladimir Hahanov, G. L. Abbas, V. A. Hajimahmud. (2022). Cyber-physical-social system and incident management. *AI-centric smart city ecosystems: Technologies, design and implementation* (1st ed., vol. 2, p. 15). CRC Press. https://doi.org/10.1201/9781003252542-2

Khang, A., Vugar Abdullayev, Olena Hrybiuk, Arvind Kumar Shukla. (2024). *Computer vision and AI-integrated IoT technologies in medical ecosystem* (1st ed.). CRC Press. https://doi.org/10.1201/9781003429609

Khang, A., Vugar Abdullayev, Eugenia Litvinova, Svetlana Chumachenko, Vusala Abuzarova, P. T. N. Anh. (2024). Application of computer vision in the healthcare ecosystem. *Computer vision and AI-integrated IoT technologies in medical ecosystem* (1st ed.). CRC Press. https://doi.org/10.1201/9781003429609-1

Khang, A., Vladimir Hahanov, Eugenia Litvinova, Svetlana Chumachenko, Triwiyanto, V. A. Hajimahmud, Ragimova Nazila Ali, Abuzarova Vusala Alyar, P. T. N. Anh. (2023). The analytics of hospitality of hospitals in healthcare ecosystem. *Data-centric AI solutions and emerging technologies in the healthcare ecosystem* (p. 4). CRC Press. https://doi.org/10.1201/9781003356189-4

Khang, A., N. A. Ragimova, V. A. Hajimahmud, V. A. Alyar. (2022). Advanced technologies and data management in the smart healthcare system. *AI-centric smart city ecosystems: Technologies, design and implementation* (1st ed., vol. 16, p. 10). CRC Press. https://doi.org/10.1201/9781003252542-16

Khang, A., G. Rana, R. K. Tailor, V. A. Hajimahmud. (Eds.). (2023). *Data-centric AI solutions and emerging technologies in the healthcare ecosystem*. CRC Press. https://doi.org/10.1201/9781003356189

Lee, Jaewon, Boyoung Kim. (2021). Social impacts of the continuous usage of digital healthcare service: A case of South Korea. *Innovative Marketing*, 17(2), 79–89. www.businessperspectives.org/images/pdf/applications/publishing/templates/article/assets/15037/IM_2021_02_Jaewon%20Lee.pdf

Practicalhealthpsychology. (2017). https://practicalhealthpsychology.com/tr/2017/08/using-health-psychology-in-your-everyday-practice/

Rani, S., M. Chauhan, A. Kataria, A. Khang. (Eds.). (2021). IoT equipped intelligent distributed framework for smart healthcare systems. *Networking and internet architecture* (vol. 2, p. 30). CRC Press. https://doi.org/10.48550/arXiv.2110.04997

Rath, Kali Charan, A. Khang, Sunil Kumar Rath, Nibedita Satapathy, Suresh Kumar Satapathy, Sitanshu Kar. (2024). AI-enabled technology in medicine-advancing holistic healthcare monitoring and control systems. *Computer vision and AI-integrated IoT technologies in medical ecosystem* (1st ed.). CRC Press. https://doi.org/10.1201/9781003429609-6

Rowe, Michael. (2008). Information and communication technology in health: A review of the literature. *Journal of Community and Health Sciences*, 3, 68–77. https://repository.uwc.ac.za/handle/10566/2767

Taylor, S. E. (1978). A developing role for social psychology in medicine and medical practice. *Personality and Social Psychology Bulletin*, 4(4), 515–523.

Vrushank, S., A. Khang. (2023). Internet of medical things (IoMT) driving the digital transformation of the healthcare sector. *Data-centric AI solutions and emerging technologies in the healthcare ecosystem* (1st ed., p. 1). CRC Press. https://doi.org/10.1201/9781003356189-2

Vrushank, S., T. Vidhi, A. Khang. (2023). Electronic health records security and privacy enhancement using blockchain technology. *Data-centric AI solutions and emerging technologies in the healthcare ecosystem* (1st ed.). CRC Press. https://doi.org/10.1201/9781003356189-1

WHO. (2021). *Global strategy on digital health 2020–2025* (p. 201). World Health Organization. Licence: CC BY-NC-SA 3.0 IGO.

# 2 Factors Influencing Mental Health and the Role of Artificial Intelligence (AI) in the Era of Climate Change

*Sailaja G. and Narendra Kumar Rao B.*

## 2.1 INTRODUCTION

Precise surveys permit a higher request outline of the writing. Albeit past precise surveys have been directed at the wellbeing effects of environmental change, these will generally zero in on unambiguous environment impacts (e.g., the effect of fierce blazes on wellbeing), wellbeing influences (e.g., word-related wellbeing results), nations or are at this point not state-of-the-art, accordingly restricting our worldwide comprehension of what is right now realized about the different wellbeing effects of environmental change across the world (Khang & Rana et al., 2023).

To direct future examination and activity to relieve and adjust to the wellbeing effects of environmental change and its natural outcomes, we want a total and exhaustive outline of the exploration previously led in regard to the wellbeing effects of environmental change. Albeit the quantity of unique examinations exploring the wellbeing effects of environmental change has enormously expanded in the past ten years, these are not considered in the frame of mind of the ongoing writing on the subject. Deliberate assessments clearly grant a higher deals plan of the piece.

Anyway, past cognizant reviews have been formed on the achievement impacts of ecological change; these will typically focus on unambiguous climate influences (Berry et al., 2018) (e.g., the impact of quickly spreading fires on prospering), flourishing impacts (e.g., word-related thriving results), countries or are at this point not uncommon, additionally limiting our overall acumen of what is at present perceived about the different achievement impacts of standard change across the world. Environmental change has the potential to harm human wellbeing in two ways:

- In the initial place, by reducing the severity or recurrence of medical problems, they are already impacted by climatic or meteorological conditions (Khang & Abdullayev et al., 2024).
- Next, by causing exceptional or unforeseen risks or health hazards in spots or seasons when they have never occurred there.

 DOI: 10.1201/9781032686745-2

Environmental change adversely affects wellbeing; however, a few populations will be especially hard hit. These gatherings incorporate poor people, certain individuals of variety, individuals with limited English proficiency, workers, native groups of people, youths and pregnant women, more settled adults, feeble word-related social affairs, people with ineptitudes and people with diseases (Khang & Ragimova et al., 2022).

## 2.2 FACTORS INFLUENCING MENTAL HEALTH

The prosperity effects of these aggravations of extended respiratory and cardiovascular disorder, wounds and surprising misfortunes from ridiculous environmental events, changes in the ordinariness and land movement of food- and water-borne sicknesses, other compelling ailments and threats to profound prosperity are factors (Berry et al., 2010) to consider, as shown in Figure 2.1.

### 2.2.1 Nutrition and Protection

Heat, likewise, impacts food and water security for developing people. According to the Lancet review, high temperatures in 2021 cut the developing season by 9.3 days on average for corn or maize and six days for wheat, contrasted with the 1981–2020

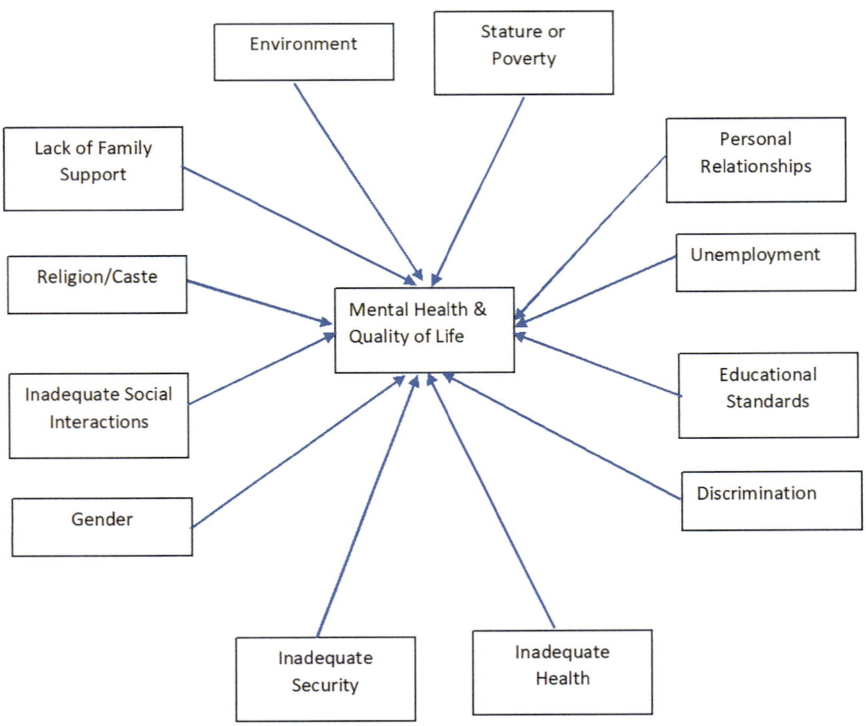


**FIGURE 2.1** Factors that affect mental health and wellbeing.

normal. In the interim, warming seas can kill shellfish and shift fisheries that waterfront networks depend on. Heat waves in 2020 alone brought about 98 million additional individuals confronting food weakness compared to the 1981–2010 normal (Khang & Hahanov et al., 2022).

- Higher air temperatures can cause Salmonella and other minuscule organic entities connected with food pollution since microorganisms duplicate quicker in cozy circumstances. These illnesses can make you feel sick to your stomach and, in severe situations (Fischer & Seneviratne, 2007), make you pass out. Even when the environment changes, sanitation practices help to prevent many diseases.
- A number of environmental change effects may increase the possibility of food contamination with artificial substances. For instance, expanded ocean surface temperatures will bring about more noteworthy mercury levels in fish, and an ascent in outrageous climate occasions would spread poisons into the well-established pecking order through stormwater overflow.
- Higher carbon dioxide concentrations in the climate could indeed go about as "manure" in the case of specific plants. Regrettably, they also decrease essential amino nutrients. Wheat, rice and potatoes are examples of crops that supply those dietary sources with frequently thick supplementation.
- In the event that streets and waterways are obliterated or obstructed, outrageous events like flooding and dry spells make it challenging to convey food.

### 2.2.2 Poor Air Quality

The reasons for environmental change can compound air contamination. Ground-level ozone, a vital part of brown haze, is a consequence of a sweltering climate and similar petroleum derivative gases that are warming the planet. Sensitivities, asthma and other respiratory issues, as well as cardiovascular sickness, can be exacerbated as a result. Wildfires that are sparked by hot, dry environments raise the danger of air pollution to human health (Berry et al., 2014). Wildfire smoke contains little particles that can travel profoundly into the lungs, causing heart and respiratory issues.

#### 2.2.2.1 Air Quality Monitoring in India

India is at the lower part of the graphs with regard to spotless, safe air. Out of 132 nations surveyed by Yale and Columbia, India is positioned last, showing that they have the world's most dirtied air. The most terrible types of air contamination are, much of the time, tracked down in Indian urban communities (Bourque & Cunsolo Willox, 2014). Particulate matter (PM), quite possibly the most generally checked poison in India, is the primary driver of the rising air contamination in this South Asian subcontinent.

The particulate matter development can reach as high as multiple times over as far as possible for certain urban communities in India. This makes it a significant well-being worry for individuals living and taking in the contaminated air consistently. The Public Air Quality Record (NAQI) has been declared as an administrative body by the government as a revealing norm to quantify air quality levels to guarantee correlation among different urban communities so that a new mechanism can be regarded to reduce the number of poisons present in the air.

Most likely, the NAQI revealed that 23% of workstations in India are at a troubling rate, showing an over 70% increase above reasonable cutoff points in this way, making air contamination a state of public crisis across different urban communities in the country. A correlation was found between Indian contamination levels and those of China because of the population levels. Through observation of the contamination levels between Indian urban communities and urban areas of China, it was found that Indian contamination level is increased undeniably when compared with China, obviously giving us a thought that these levels are multiple times higher than WHO guidelines featuring air contamination as a central issue in India.

#### 2.2.2.2 World Health Organization (WHO)

The World Health Organization (WHO) has perceived encompassing air contamination as a class one cancer-causing agent and the fourth most elevated risk factor for sudden passing around the world. In Asia, the circumstance is exacerbated by quick urbanization, industrialization and lack of supporting framework. Currently, in 2010, the Perfect Air Drive for Asian Urban areas showed that 58% of Asian urban communities (out of 230) had yearly PM10 focuses, surpassing the WHO yearly mean break target-1 of 70µg/m3 for PM10. Reports indicate that 40% of urban communities with the most noteworthy centralizations of PM2.5 are in India.

Past investigations across India have areas of strength for showing respiratory issues, death rate, unexpected passing and air contamination levels. It is currently foremost to resolve this issue. In India, air quality is checked at in excess of 450 stations in the nation by the Focal Contamination Control Board (CPCB) under the Public Encompassing Air Quality Observing System (NAMP) to survey focuses at modern, private, traffic and environmentally delicate regions (Khang & Hahanov et al., 2023).

#### 2.2.2.3 Air Quality Checking

The Public Air Quality Checking Project guarantees that almost 50% of the Indian urban communities observed have arrived at basic degrees of particulate matter. There are 63 urban communities with basic levels, 36 urban communities with undeniable levels and 19 urban areas at moderate levels. In 2007, just three out of 121 urban communities in India that had been dissected were considered to have low contamination levels. These urban communities were Dewas, Tirupati and Kozhikode locations in India. Northern India has been known to have expanding air contamination, while southern India has shown the contrary pattern. Indoor contamination likewise assumes a major part in the general status of India's dirtied air (Hayes et al., 2018).

The typical Indian family particulate matter contamination is 350 micrograms for each meter cubed, which is multiple times more noteworthy than the cutoff set by the US Climate Insurance Organization as shown in Figure 2.2.

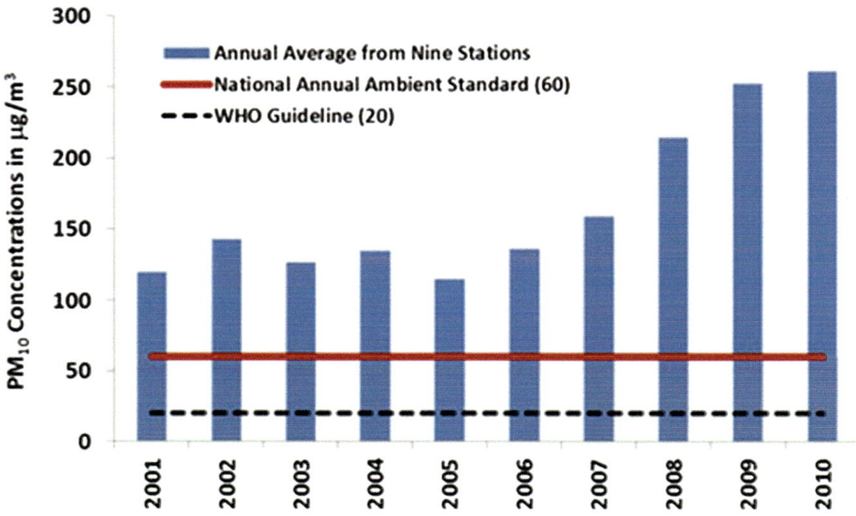


**FIGURE 2.2** Particulate matter levels in Delhi.

### 2.2.3 Water-Related Ailments

Individuals can turn out to be sick if they come into contact with sullied drinking or sporting water. Environmental change raises the risk of disease because of increasing temperatures, more incessant weighty downpours and overflow and tempest impacts. Repercussions for the body apprehensive (Harris-Kojetin et al., 2013) as well as respiratory systems, liver and kidney damage can all have a negative impact on health.

- Environmental change can affect receptivity to aquatic microorganisms (parasites, diseases and microscopic organisms like Giardia and Cryptosporidium) and toxins spread, such as noxious algae and cyanobacterial blooms on the water's surface and artificial compounds which enter moisture due to sentient activity.
- As a result of changing water temperatures, water-borne Vibrio microorganisms and hazardous algal toxins will be accessible in the water or fish at different seasons or where they were not currently a risk.
- Extensions in over-the-top precipitation, hurricane precipitation and whirlwind floods will tarnish water bodies' utilized for redirection (like lakes and sea shores), shellfish gathering waters and drinking water sources.

Preposterous environmental events and whirlwind floods can hurt or overwhelm water systems (for instance, drinking water or wastewater treatment plants), increasing transparent poison (Table 2.1).

**TABLE 2.1**
**Water Pollutions' Causes and Effects**

| Type of Water Pollution | Cause of Pollution | Symptoms of Pollution | Effect of Pollution | Source of Pollution |
|---|---|---|---|---|
| Biodegradable waste | Humans and animals | Diminishing quantities of fish and other sea life, expanding number of microbes | Expanded number of microorganisms, diminished oxygen levels, passing of oceanic life | Run-off, inappropriately treated pro-fluent |
| Nutrients | Nitrates and phosphates | Green, cloudy, slimy, stinky water | Green growth blossom eutrophication of water sources | Over-utilization of manures, run-off from fields, ill-advised removal of compartments, wastewater treatment |
| Heat | Increased water temperature | Hotter water, less oxygen, less oceanic creatures | Decline in oxygen levels, demise of fish and plants | Modern run-off, wastewater treatment |
| Sedimentation | Suspended particles settling out of water | Overcast water, expanded measure of base | Heats up water, diminishes the profundity of water source, stores toxins | Building destinations, cultivating and domesticated animals tasks, logging, flooding, city run-off, dams |
| Chemicals | Toxic and hazardous chemicals | Water variety changes, fosters a smell, amphibian life vanishes | Kills sea life, can enter the human pecking order, prompts miscarriages, barrenness, malignant growths and different sicknesses in people and creatures | Human-made, ill-advised removal, run-off, dams, landfill leachate, modern release, corrosive downpour |
| Radioactive pollutants | Radioactive isotopes | Increased birth deformities and disease in human and creature populaces | Kills amphibian species and prompts disease and demise in people and different creatures | People unloading drugs into water frameworks, squander water treatment |

(*Continued*)

**TABLE 2.1 (*Continued*)**
**Water Pollutions' Causes and Effects**

| Type of Water Pollution | Cause of Pollution | Symptoms of Pollution | Effect of Pollution | Source of Pollution |
|---|---|---|---|---|
| Medical | Medicines, antibodies | Barrenness in sea life, other obscure side effects | Obscure | People unloading medications into water frameworks, wastewater treatment |
| Microbiological | Bacteria, viruses, protozoa | Individuals and creatures become sick with gastrointestinal issues | Undrinkable water | Ill-advised treatment of water/gushing, can happen normally |

## 2.3 MENTAL HEALTH AND WELLBEING

Any changes in an individual's actual wellbeing or environmental factors can have a negative impact on their psychological wellbeing. A super climate event, in particular, can cause stress and other emotional wellbeing ramifications, particularly if an individual loses friends and family or their home (CDC, cited 2015).

- Individuals suffering from psychological maladjustments are particularly powerless against outrageous intensity; investigations have discovered that a history of bad behavior increases the risk of death during heat waves. Individuals taking prescriptions for psychological illnesses (Brown & Westaway, 2011) that make it challenging to control their inside temperatures are particularly helpless.
- Certain groups are more powerless against psychological health ramifications, like youths and older adults, pregnant women, postpartum women, people who have past psychological maladjustment, individuals with low wages and crisis laborers.

### 2.3.1 Factors

Emotional wellbeing is the condition of prosperity where individuals and social orders are at their best. Psychological wellness and neurological problems are among the significant groups of non-communicable diseases (NCDs). These issues influence individuals' considerations, feelings, ways of behaving and connections.

They incorporate a different scope of illnesses and conditions like despondency, schizophrenia, dementia, Alzheimer's, stress and substance misuse problems, among numerous others. An expected 450–500 million individuals live with psychological circumstances around the world. An individual's capacity to keep up with great emotional wellbeing is down to a scope of elements, which are many times outside of their reach. The determinants of emotional wellness incorporate social, natural, mental and organic variables. These incorporate the major NCD risk variables of liquor and tobacco use, undesirable eating regimens and actual latency.

There is no wellbeing without emotional wellbeing. Psychological wellness (Harris-Kojetin et al., 2013) has connections to malignant growth, diabetes, cardiovascular and respiratory sicknesses and other NCDs, frequently co-morbid with them. The coronavirus pandemic has featured and sped up the need to handle psychological wellness conditions, which have become more predominant during the pandemic and its reaction. Speculation for emotional wellness is frequently the most reduced of all illness regions.

### 2.3.2 Psychological Wellbeing and Neurological Problems

Psychological wellbeing is a condition of prosperity where individuals and social orders are at their best. That is, where individuals can adapt to the anxieties of day-to-day existence, work gainfully and add to their networks.

Psychological wellbeing conditions and neurological problems are conditions that influence considerations, feelings, ways of behaving and connections. These incorporate issues that cause a high incidence of sickness, for example, sadness, bipolar emotional problems, schizophrenia, nervousness issues, dementia and substance use issues, among numerous others. Nonetheless, they frequently happen in combination with other non-communicable sicknesses like cardiovascular infection, diabetes, respiratory illnesses and malignant growths (Luber et al., 2014). They likewise share numerous NCD risk factors, for example, tobacco use, liquor use, unfortunate eating regimens and actual dormancy.

### 2.3.3 Common Mental Health Disorders

#### 2.3.3.1 Depression

Depression is the point at which an individual encounters a discouraged state of mind (feeling miserable, touchy, unfulfilled) or a deficiency of delight or interest in exercises for over 14 days. Depression can seriously influence an individual's capacity to work and collaborate with individuals and society. It is assessed that around 264 million individuals are impacted by the gloom of depression, or around 5% of adults.

Women are more impacted by depression than men. Overall, around 10% of pregnant women and 13% of women who have recently given birth experience a psychological problem, principally discouragement. In non-industrial nations, this is considerably higher – 15.6% during pregnancy and 19.8% after (Hess et al., 2012). Depression can block self-improvement, wellbeing, training and business. Extreme instances of depression can prompt suicide. 75% of suicides happen in low- and middle-income nations, yet powerful techniques, for example, early identification, treatment and continuous help mean suicide can be forestalled.

#### 2.3.3.2 Dementia

Dementia is a kind of degenerative cerebrum disorder that adversely influences numerous mental cycles, including memory, conduct, control and cognizance. There are various types of dementia, with Alzheimer's disease being the most widely recognized. There are presently 55 million individuals living with dementia around the world, with nearly 10 million new cases consistently. This number is expected to increase to 75 million in 2030 and 139 million in 2050. A large part of the increment will be in non-industrial nations.

#### 2.3.3.3 Alzheimer's Disease

It is assessed that 60–75% of dementia cases can be named Alzheimer's Infection (Promotion). Promotion causes the annihilation of synapses and related nerves and impedes synapse capabilities. The memory arrangement of the cerebrum is especially compromised. As the illness advances, a person's ability to impart, think and recall falls apart.

## 2.4 CLIMATE CHANGE INFLUENCES HUMAN WELLBEING

Human wellbeing can be influenced by the environment and weather. Environmental change and fluctuation, especially climate limits, affect the environment, which outfits us with clean air, food, water, haven and security. Ecological modification, alongside other regular and personal stressors affecting one's wellbeing, represent various dangers to human prosperity and prosperity, as shown in Figure 2.3.

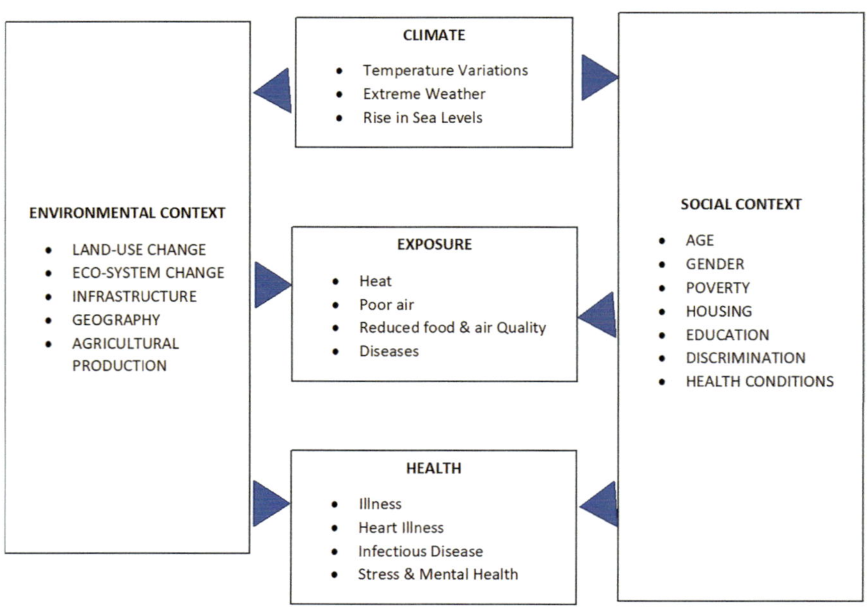


**FIGURE 2.3** Climate change influences on human wellbeing.

The right box displays key influencing factors of peoples' weaknesses, which include social determinants of wellbeing and actions decisions (Dijkers, 2018). The left box shows key factors influencing weakness on a larger scale, such as regular and constructed conditions, administration and executives and associations. These affecting aspects can influence a person's or forum's weakness through changes in openness, responsiveness and versatile limit, and they may likewise be impacted by natural change.

### 2.4.1 Changing Health

On the grounds that previous ailments, financial status and life stage all add to the shortcomings of climate-related and environment-related wellbeing impacts, extended changes in these variables ought to be thought about while evaluating environmental change and wellbeing influences (Khang & Ragimova et al., 2024).

At the point when people's prosperity or monetary status decays, changes in the environment might intensify the prosperity loads related to those falling apart patterns. Interestingly, where people's wealth or financial situation is improving, evolving conditions might slow or lessen that improvement. Where logical comprehension permits, integrating extended patterns in financial situations and wellbeing into models of environmental change influences on wellbeing might provide useful information about how non-environmental variables and environmental change interact.

- **Intensity**: A measure of how frequently an event, like another instance of sickness, happens in a populace over the long run.
- **Congenital anomalies**: A sickness or illness that impairs one's wellbeing and standard of living. The prevalence of disease in a given population over a specific time period is measured by the morbidity rate.
- **Demise rate**: As a medical result, death. The quantity of passing in a populace during a predetermined timeframe is the demise rate.
- **Early mortality or demise**: Passing that happens before a particular age, which is much of the time the typical future upon entering the world.
- **Proliferation**: A count or extent of individuals who have a particular illness or condition at a given moment.
- **Monitoring**: Health information assortment, investigation, translation and dispersal.

### 2.4.2 Affects in Decision-Making

#### 2.4.2.1 Cognitive Process

Any psychological cycles associated with storing, decoding, manipulating, modifying and using information impact the social event. These cycles, which involve activities like reflection, insight, learning and critical thinking, are often interpreted through a range of important hypotheses, including the sequential handling approach, the equal handling method and a mixed hypothesis, which presupposes that mental cycles are both sequential and equal, depending on the demands of the activity. On occasion, people will use this expression to critique "mental contact" (Bouzid et al., 2013).

#### 2.4.2.2 Positive Affect

Positive affect strengthens memory functions connected to the use of perceptual motor skills and improves problem-solving abilities. There are three types of affective influences:

- **Relevant emotions**: These stem from the current decision-making task.
- **Predicted emotions**: These are consequences of the decision itself in time. Emotions might be reflected in behavior. Examples are remorse, digestion, etc.
- **Pertinent emotions**: These feelings stem from sources other than the current decision. It may also include persona mood/temporal disposition.

Example: Sources for these emotions are usually presented in the environment like good smells, good scenes, good music, etc.

#### 2.4.2.3 Incidental Emotions and Decision-Making

- Immediate emotional influences brought on by events unrelated to the current choice. Immediate environment affects (Walsh et al., 2014) chronic affect and dispositional affect, which lead to:
  - Incident-to-that is normatively unimportant to the choice.
- Incidental emotions also have an impact on the following types of decisions:
  - Appraisal of items
  - Choices involving pragmatic behavior

Example: Sadness for the past drives up buying costs and drives down selling costs for an item.

### 2.4.3 Investigations

Investigator has researched how emotional (happy, neutral and sad) faces presented during climate changes in decision-making tasks affect the process of individual decision-making (Meehl et al., 2004).

- Pleasantness rating of post-choice satisfaction.
- To research the impact of incidental emotional context prior to a decision-making scenario.
- Emotional content between trials that are pertinent to the task.
- Comforting pictures might elicit a positive emotion.

## 2.5 AI IN MENTAL HEALTH: ROLE, BENEFITS, AND TRENDS

The potential of artificial intelligence for mental healthcare is considerable, even though it is unlikely that it will ever completely replace conventional therapy in the foreseeable future. We are currently dealing with a serious mental health problem. According to Mental Health America's 2023 report, over 50 million adults in the US, or one in five, had a mental disease in 2019–2020. This crisis environment is no less intimidating. The societal stigma associated with mental health conditions, the high cost of therapy and the severe lack of mental health experts have long been its defining characteristics. Recent technological advances have made it possible for creative AI healthcare solutions to start entering the market. AI in mental health may present the potential for change.

### 2.5.1 Mental Health Stats – The Crisis We Are In

Globally, mental health diseases are on the rise. Around 15% of adolescents experience a mental health disorder, and suicide is the fourth major cause of death for people aged 15 to 29. At least 10% of the population is afflicted. Mental diseases are expected to cost the global economy $16 trillion between 2010 and 2030 as a key cause of morbidity and mortality. Nobody seems to understand the precise causes of today's high rates of anxiety and sadness.

The growth is ascribed to a number of causes, including the demands of contemporary society and the COVID-19 pandemic's impact on already-existing mental health problems. Some experts even contend that what we are seeing is simply a rise in mental health awareness. In fact, during the past 20 years, the number of adults in the US seeking inpatient, outpatient or counseling services has been consistently increasing. In addition, according to Mental Health America's 2023 report, access to care is still restricted. Over 30 million US citizens who suffer from mental disorders go untreated. Can AI help in mental health? AI for mental health is already making inroads into clinical practice. The following innovations, in particular, have the greatest potential to have an impact:

- Deep learning (DL) and machine learning (ML), which improve the accuracy of mental health issue diagnosis and patient outcome prediction.
- The use of computer vision to analyze imaging data and comprehend nonverbal indicators like facial expression, gestures, eye focus and human position.
- Natural language processing (NLP) for speech recognition and text analysis, which is used to create and comprehend clinical documentation and to simulate human conversations with chatbot computer programs.

While research on the use of AI for mental health therapy is still in its early stages, ML algorithms and computer vision applications are very mature domains with widespread use cases across sectors. Unlike radiography or pathology, where AI has proven to be more accurate than humans, mental healthcare is sometimes referred to as a wholly human industry. Mental health professionals have doubts about whether artificial intelligence-based treatments for mental illness will ever be able to offer the empathic care that they see as being so important. However, individuals do enjoy interacting with chatbots, and some of them even become emotionally attached to them.

We are not discussing the unnerving intimacy that formed between a lonely guy and an AI operating system in the film here; rather, we are discussing people's willingness to open up to an AI friend. People frequently think that robots can instantly respond to health-related queries, are impartial and don't pass judgment. Moreover, studies suggest that the AI chatbot experience of people struggling with mental health issues has been overwhelmingly satisfactory. Although more study is undoubtedly needed, the Food and Drug Administration (FDA) in the US has already loosened regulations to allow for a wider use of digital therapy tools for people with mental health disorders.

## 2.5.2 Examples of AI in Mental Healthcare

### 2.5.2.1 Analyzing Patient Health Data to Assess Mental Health Conditions and Plan

Today, AI is used to examine electronic health records, questionnaires, voice recordings, behavioral indicators, blood tests, brain imaging and even data gleaned from a patient's social media accounts. To parse patient data and identify mental and physical states – pain, boredom, mind-wandering, stress, or suicidal thoughts – connected to a specific mental health disorder, data scientists use a variety of techniques, including supervised machine learning, deep learning and natural language processing. According to an analysis of 28 studies on the application of artificial intelligence to mental health by IBM and University of California researchers, algorithms can identify a variety of mental diseases with 63–92% accuracy, depending on the AI technique used and the caliber of training data.

### 2.5.2.2 Conducting Self-Assessment and Therapy Sessions

The majority of chatbots in this category are keyword-triggered and NLP-based. They provide guidance, monitor user responses, assess the severity and course of a mental disease and assist in coping with its symptoms – either on their own or with the assistance of a licensed psychiatrist standing by at the other end of the virtual line. Woebot, Replika, Wysa, Ellie, Elomia and Tess companies are some of the most well-liked AI-powered virtual therapists.

For instance, Tess, an AI chatbot, provides highly customized therapy based on CBT and other clinically validated techniques, as well as psycho-education and health-related reminders. Since the interventions include text message communication, language processing is the only tool available for identifying emotions.

An international team of researchers tested the chatbot on a group of university students and discovered that those who spoke with Tess every day for two weeks showed a substantial improvement in their mental health symptoms compared to those who had sessions less frequently. Ellie, another AI chatbot example, can read nonverbal cues like a person's posture, facial expression or gestures to understand their emotional condition and determine the best words to reduce stress and anxiety (Hess et al., 2012).

Tools for tracking mental health enabled by AI are also included in this category. These could be used in conjunction with wearable technology that monitors vital signs, including heart rate, blood pressure, oxygen levels and other indicators of changes in a person's physical and mental health. One of these options is the mental health software Bio Base, which uses AI to decipher sensor data from a wearable (Hahanov & Khang et al., 2022). The mental health tracker, which is intended to assist businesses in preventing employee burnout, purportedly reduces the length and volume of sick days by up to 31%.

#### 2.5.2.3 Enhancing Patient Engagement

In order to enhance and personalize the patient experience, healthcare institutions are increasingly using AI in their patient engagement efforts. AI chatbots are employed to make access to care as easy and frictionless as it is in many other service industries, in addition to assisting users in coping with their mental health concerns.

Conversational AI is being used by healthcare organizations to handle calls, schedule appointments, notify patients on how to get to the clinician and give health education. In order to improve communication with patients, support initiatives that track their adherence to medication or therapy and arm patients with knowledge about the value of such adherence. AI technologies are also implemented into mobile apps and reminder systems. Another strategy to increase patient involvement is to use AI to enhance patient outreach. Tools with AI can recognize patients who are at danger and automate outreach messages.

#### 2.5.2.4 Equipping Therapists with Technology to Automate Daily Workflows

Psychiatrists rarely use outdated technology or the counsel of other medical specialists when analyzing medical data and creating treatment plans for patients because of the very nature of mental health diseases (Abdullayev & Khang et al., 2024). Using AI-driven mental health platforms that automatically gather data from various hospital IT systems and give on-demand information about each patient's progress, current status and potential outcomes would be one way to lessen the administrative burden. One of the earliest of these systems is OPTT, an AI platform that gives mental health doctors access to a variety of tools for expanding the capacity of their clinic. According to a preliminary study, OPTT may increase access to high-quality mental healthcare by up to 400%.

### 2.5.3 Benefits of Using AI in Mental Health Treatment

The following advantages that artificial intelligence (AI) offers can be used to explain the hopes placed in its apps and platforms for mental health care:

- **Affordability:** In contrast to traditional therapy, where appointments must be scheduled and traveled to, AI-based and other mental health apps enable users to obtain therapeutic treatment whenever and wherever they need it. Also, compared to the expenditures of in-person counseling, missed work, the need to make other arrangements and travel, they offer assistance for little to no cost.
- **Accessibility:** The absence of providers in rural and remote places as well as general staff shortages, are hurdles to mental health care that are eliminated

by AI-based apps. More than 100 million Americans reside in areas where there is a shortage of healthcare professionals; thus, this is significant. AI chatbots and platforms that are not limited by geography can see you whenever you want and interact with you for as long as you need.

- **Efficiency:** By examining behavioral signals, artificial intelligence systems for mental healthcare have already demonstrated their ability to accurately identify signs of depression, PTSD and other illnesses. According to other studies, algorithms are 100% accurate in predicting which kids are at risk for developing psychosis. They can also identify behavioral symptoms of anxiety with over 90% accuracy (NCHS, 2015). They also assist patients who are experiencing mental distress: Woebot researchers of the AI chatbot found that after just two weeks of using the program, participants' levels of anxiety and despair significantly decreased.
- **Confidence and comfort in opening up:** People feel less self-conscious when talking about humiliating topics with AI-based therapists. This is crucial for those who experience shame in face-to-face interactions due to stigma or apprehension about being judged. In reality, about a quarter of people lie to doctors, with smoking, drinking and sexual behavior being the most taboo subjects. Because a robot won't judge (USGCRP, 2016), many people find it simpler to reveal the full depth of their behavior to one.
- **Assistance for therapists:** Peter Foltz, a professor of research at the University of Colorado Boulder, believes that AI could help clinicians make the most of their time with patients. This is because artificial intelligence (AI) can track and analyze large amounts of data more quickly and effectively than any person.

Algorithms, therefore, aid in a more precise diagnosis. By observing the patient's attitude and behavior, they can also identify warning signals of potential problems early on and notify professionals so that treatment plans can be modified right away. For patients who need frequent check-ins and are suicidal, this could be life-saving.

### 2.5.4 Current AI Trends in Mental Health

Notwithstanding the persistent effects of macroeconomic issues like inflation, supply chain disruptions and interest rates, mental health tech remains the best-funded sector in the digital health industry. According to CBInsights' State of Mental Health Tech 2021 Report, mental health tech businesses raised $5.5 billion globally (324 deals) in 2021, a 139% increase over the 258 deals that were made in the previous year. According to the research, "demand for and investor interest in digital solutions that facilitated the delivery of mental healthcare increased as the pandemic continued to exacerbate mental health disorders (Hayes & Poland, 2018) (such as anxiety and depression)".

Also, in 2022, a handful of firms that use AI in mental healthcare closed significant acquisitions. They include the AI chatbot Wysa, which has received $20 million in investment, the early diagnosis-improving BlueSkeye ($3.4 million), the Upheal smart notebook ($1.068 million) and the AI-powered clare&me ($1 million) for mental health practitioners. We may soon see the rise of more emotionally sophisticated AI therapists and new mental health applications driven by AI prediction, according to a review of the investment environment and ongoing research (Rani & Chauhan et al., 2021).

## 2.6 CONCLUSION

Generally, comprehensive assessments of the wellbeing impacts of environmental change show a link between the two, pointing mostly toward the direction that environmental change is linked to negative outcomes for human wellbeing. This is concerning since, as a result of rising temperatures or an increase in events linked to environmental change, such as extreme weather conditions and declining towards the climb during warmth and extension of ecological movement occasions including outrageous atmospheric conditions and declining air quality.

Most assessments associated with this survey zeroed in on the meteorological effects of an ecological switch through ominous genuine prosperity results. Future research on additional effects of the climate and overall mental health consequences may close knowledge gaps. Environmental change transformation strategies might profit from information on the emotional wellbeing gambles related to an evolving environment, assets expected to decrease these dangers and key factors that can impact the greatness and example of psychological wellbeing results.

Wellbeing specialists can get this data through weakness and variation appraisals and in coordinated efforts with accomplices to decrease the wellbeing outcomes of environment-related risks. Further, this data can be utilized by medical services suppliers to help people and networks to all the more successfully oversee emotional wellbeing issues related to environmental fluctuation and change. The impacts of environmental change can be immediate or roundabout, present moment or long haul. Intense occasions can act through systems like that of horrible pressure, prompting surely known psychopathological examples. Likewise, the results of openness to outrageous or delayed climate-related occasions can likewise be postponed, enveloping issues, for example, posttraumatic stress, or even sent to later ages.

## REFERENCES

Abdullayev, V., Khang, A., Rashad, İ., Vusala, A., Sriram, K., Anh, P.T.N. AI-aided computer vision in health care system. In *Computer Vision and AI-Integrated IoT Technologies in Medical Ecosystem* (1st ed.), 2024. CRC Press. https://doi.org/10.1201/9781003429609-20

Berry, H.L., Bowen, K., Kjellstrom, T. Climate change and mental health: A causal pathways framework. Int J Public Health, 2010, 55, 123–132. https://link.springer.com/article/10.1007/s00038-009-0112-0

Berry, H.L., Waite, T.D., Dear, K.B., Capon, A.G., Murray, V. The case for systems thinking about climate change and mental health. Nat Clim Change, 2018, 8, 282–290. https://doi.org/10.1038/s41558-0180102-4

Berry, P., Clarke, K.-L., Parker, S. Chapter 7: Human health. In *Canada in a Changing Climate: Sector Perspectives on Impacts and Adaptation*, Warren, F.J., Lemmen, D.S., Eds. (pp. 191–232), 2014. Government of Canada. www.mdpi.com/1660-4601/16/14/2531

Bourque, F., Cunsolo Willox, A. Climate change: The next challenge for public mental health? Int Rev Psychiatry, 2014, 1, 415–442. www.tandfonline.com/doi/abs/10.3109/09540261.2014.925851

Bouzid, M., Hooper, L., Hunter, P.R. The effectiveness of public health interventions to reduce the health impact of climate change: A systematic review of systematic reviews. PLOS One, 2013, 8, e62041. https://doi.org/10.1371/journal.pone.0062041

Brown, K., Westaway, E. Agency, capacity, and resilience to environmental change: Lessons from human development, well-being, and disasters. Annu Rev Environ Resour, 2011, 21, 321–342. https://doi.org/10.1146/annurev-environ-052610-092905

CDC. *Lyme Disease Surveillance and Available Data*. Centers for Disease Control and Prevention, cited 2015. www.id.theclinics.com/article/S0891-5520(15)00024-0/abstract

Dijkers, M. *What Is a Scoping Review?* (Accessed on 1 July 2018). http://ktdrr.org/products/update/v4n1/dijkers_ktupdate_v4n1_12-15.pdf

Fischer, E.M., Seneviratne, S.I. Soil moisture–atmosphere interactions during the 2003 European Summer heat wave. J Climate, 2007, 20, 5081–5099. https://doi.org/10.1175/JCLI4288.1

Hahanov, V., Khang, A., Litvinova, E., Chumachenko, S., Hajimahmud, V.A., Alyar, V.A. The key assistant of smart city—sensors and tools. In *AI-Centric Smart City Ecosystems: Technologies, Design and Implementation* (1st ed., vol. 17, p. 10), 2022. CRC Press. https://doi.org/10.1201/9781003252542-17

Harris-Kojetin, L., Sengupta, M., Park-Lee, E., Valverde, R. *Long-Term Care Services in the United States: 2013 Overview* (p. 107), 2013. National Center for Health Statistics. https://stacks.cdc.gov/view/cdc/22285

Hayes, K., Blashki, G., Wiseman, J., Burke, S., Reifels, L. Climate change and mental health: Risks, impacts and priority actions. Int J Ment Health Syst, 2018, 12, 1–12. [Google Scholar]. https://ijmhs.biomedcentral.com/articles/10.1186/s13033-018-0210-6

Hayes, K., Poland, B. Addressing mental health in a changing climate: Incorporating mental health indicators into climate change and health vulnerability and adaptation assessments. Int J Environ Res Public Health, 2018, 22, 1806. www.mdpi.com/1660-4601/15/9/1806

Hess, J.J., McDowell, J.Z., Luber, G. Integrating climate change adaptation into public health practice: Using adaptive management to increase adaptive capacity and build resilience. Environ Health Perspect, 2012, 120, 2. https://ehp.niehs.nih.gov/doi/abs/10.1289/ehp.1103515

Khang, A., Abdullayev, V.A., Hrybiuk, O., Shukla, A.K. *Computer Vision and AI-Integrated IoT Technologies in Medical Ecosystem* (1st ed.), 2024. CRC Press. https://doi.org/10.1201/9781003429609

Khang, A., Hahanov, V., Abbas, G.L., Hajimahmud, V.A. Cyber-physical-social system and incident management. In *AI-Centric Smart City Ecosystems: Technologies, Design and Implementation* (1st ed., vol. 2, p. 15), 2022. CRC Press. https://doi.org/10.1201/9781003252542-2

Khang, A., Hahanov, V., Litvinova, E., Chumachenko, S., Triwiyanto, Hajimahmud, V.A., Ragimova, N.A., Abuzarova, V.A., Anh, P.T.N. The analytics of hospitality of hospitals in healthcare ecosystem. In *Data-Centric AI Solutions and Emerging Technologies in the Healthcare Ecosystem* (p. 4), 2023. CRC Press. https://doi.org/10.1201/9781003356189-4

Khang, A., Ragimova, N.A., Hajimahmud, V.A., Alyar, V.A. Advanced technologies and data management in the smart healthcare system. In *AI-Centric Smart City Ecosystems: Technologies, Design and Implementation* (1st ed., vol. 16, p. 10), 2022. CRC Press. https://doi.org/10.1201/9781003252542-16

Khang, A., Ragimova, N.A., Yaqub Bali, S., Abdullayev, V., Bahar, A., Mehriban, M. Using big data to solve problems in the field of medicine. In *Computer Vision and AI-Integrated IoT Technologies in Medical Ecosystem* (1st ed.), 2024. CRC Press. https://doi.org/10.1201/9781003429609-21

Khang, A., Rana, G., Tailor, R.K., Hajimahmud, V.A. (Eds.). *Data-Centric AI Solutions and Emerging Technologies in the Healthcare Ecosystem*, 2023. CRC Press. https://doi.org/10.1201/9781003356189

Luber, G. et al. Chapter 9: Human health. In *Climate Change Impacts in the United States: The Third National Climate Assessment*, Melillo, J.M., Richmond, T.C., Yohe, G.W., Eds. (pp. 220–256), 2014. U.S. Global Change Research Program. www.globalchange.gov/sites/globalchange/files/Ch_0a_FrontMatter_ThirdNCA_GovtReviewDraft_Nov_22_2013_clean.pdf

Meehl, G.A., Tebaldi, C. More intense, more frequent, and longer lasting heat waves in the 21st century. Science, 2004, 305, 994–997. https://doi.org/10.1126/science.1098704

NCHS. *Health, United States, 2014: With Special Feature on Adults Aged 55–64* (p. 473), 2015. National Center for Health Statistics, Centers for Disease Control and Prevention. www.google.com.vn/books/edition/Health_Care_Utilization_Among_Adults_Age/X2vyMu4eFoYC

Rani, S., Chauhan, M., Kataria, A., Khang, A. IoT equipped intelligent distributed framework for smart healthcare systems. In *Networking and Internet Architecture* (vol. 2, p. 30), 2021. CRC Press. https://doi.org/10.48550/arXiv.2110.04997

USGCRP. *Impacts of Climate Change on Human Health in the United States: A Scientific Assessment*, Crimmins, A., Balbus, J., Gamble, J.L., Beard, C.B., Bell, J.E., Dodgen, D., Eisen, R.J., Fann, N., Hawkins, M.D., Herring, S.C., Jantarasami, L., Mills, D.M., Saha, S., Sarofim, M.C., Trtanj, J., Ziska, L., Eds. (p. 312), 2016. U.S. Global Change Research Program. doi: 10.7930/J0R49NQX

Walsh, J. et al. Chapter 2: Our changing climate. In *Climate Change Impacts in the United States: The Third National Climate Assessment*, Melillo, J.M., Richmond, T.C., Yohe, G.W., Eds. (pp. 19–67), 2014. U.S. Global Change Research Program. https://brewminate.com/climate-change-and-human-health/

# 3 Role of IoT and AI in Sustainable Management of the Pharmaceutical Industry

*Poonam Inamdar R., Mrunalini Kulkarni H., and Pashmina Doshi P.*

## 3.1 INTRODUCTION

The Internet of Things (IoT) can be explained as a connection-enabled system. It profoundly includes various smart objects and devices adapted to ease complicated tasks. Networking of sensors with digital objects is the fundamental working principle of IoT. The objects are usually connected to the internet, and they are exclusively accessible and programmable. The digital objects of IoT generally comprise mechanical devices operated in the industries, smart appliances used in the household, sensors installed in diagnostic agents, digital mapping device-enabled vehicles, smart parking systems of smart city projects, and many more (Rana & Khang et al., 2021). AI is Artificial Intelligence; it is governed by imparting the ability of cognitive behavior to machines that can automatically process near-to-human experiences. For the said purpose, machines use different cognitive algorithms and mathematical models to consume processes and analyze the colossal amount of data. AI can be utilized massively in any domain where reducing human efforts is the prime aim.

### 3.1.1 History of IoT and AI

Students of Carnegie Melon University hold first place in the list of global IoT inventors. In the year 2021, 27 billion various devices connected to the IoT. The history of AI has been interestingly amusing from 1943 till date. The era of 1952–1956 is remarkably noted as the birth year of artificial intelligence (Rani & Chauhan et al., 2021).

### 3.1.2 Acceptance of IoT and AI in All Fields

The confluence of AI and IoT can reformulate the growth of the majority of the sectors with likely less or no human participation. Integration of AI and IoT in various fields is reshaping the global economy. According to Wired in 2018:


DOI: 10.1201/9781032686745-3

- There was an increase in the number of cases of capital funding, especially for the AI-IoT-enabled Start-Ups
- Redemption of AI-focused IoT start-ups is increasing
- Vendors of IoT platforms such as Amazon, GE, IBM, Microsoft, Oracle, PTC, and Salesforce are eagerly keen to launch AI capabilities
- Exploration of the power of AI with IoT by large-scale industries for the timely deliveries of goods with super efficiency

It has been predicted that more than 80% of enterprise IoT projects will include an AI component by 2023.

### 3.1.3 Impact of IoT and AI in All Fields

IoT has revolutionized the pharmaceutical sector immensely. It enabled the rapid optimization of the process. The time required and trials run from the primary manufacturing process to the research and development phase are significantly lengthy in every pharmaceutical industry. To sustain fair competition for the maintenance of global health, the utilization of IoT can make a huge difference for pharmaceutical industries. AI in the pharmaceutical industry is proving to be a boon. It reduces the huge costs involved in manufacturing processes. The rapid availability of enormous amounts of data by AI has been used as a research resource in the pharmaceutical research and development sector. It is opening new doors for the discovery of novel treatments, drugs, and vaccines. AI also played a pivotal role in the deployment of drug repurposing techniques during the discovery of drug-like entities for the SARS-COV-2 treatment. Bridging IoT and AI together in the pharmaceutical industry can revive the economy of the pharmaceutical sector with fewer setbacks and remarkable developments (Jaiswal et al., 2023).

## 3.2 SUSTAINABILITY

Sustainability can be stated as meeting one's conditions without compromising the capacity of the prospective descendants to meet their conditions. It reflects societal integrity and fiscal progression. Environment, frugality, and society are the three pillars of sustainability. The description of sustainability was chased in 2010 as "Sustainability is the process of living within the limits of available physical, natural and social coffers in ways that allow the living systems in which humans are bedded to thrive in infinity" (Khang & Medicine, 2024).

## 3.3 SUSTAINABILITY MANAGEMENT

### 3.3.1 Sustainability Management in the Pharmaceutical Industry

Proper implementation of sustainable business practices in the pharmaceutical industry attracts shareholders and hence indirectly contributes to the global economy. Pharmaceutical industries have been searching for remedies for the sustainable management of the production and drug discovery process. Pharmaceutical sectors have taken some important measures for the same, such as proper disposal of medicines or failed production of the batch by mixing them with some unpalatable dirt or coffee powder, keeping Heating, Ventilation, and Air Conditioning (HVAC) systems and air conditions switched off when not in use to save energy, to consult regulatory officers to plan and manage sustainability goals, following the Greenhouse Gas protocol to reducing carbon footprints, and the introduction of comprehensive product testing and validation for the eco-friendly supply chain management.

## 3.3.2 Current Scenario of IoT and AI in Sustainability Management of the Pharmaceutical Industry

### 3.3.2.1 IoT in Healthcare

IoT in healthcare is a cloud-based computing approach that uses a wireless communicating system utilizing sensors, microcontrollers, and transceivers that involves the connection of the clinical cases and health officials for diagnosis, covering, tracking, and storage of vital health statistical reports and important medical data. Varied exemplifications of IoT in healthcare systems are wearable systems, including headsets that measure brainwaves, clothes with seeing bias BP monitors, glucose observers, ECG observers, palpitation oximeters detectors embedded in the medical outfit, allocating systems, surgical robots, device implants, chip in a pill, and SpO2 sensors to measure the oxygen level in blood. During the pandemic of COVID-19, data from wearable bias can be used by HCPs to define substantiated drugs (PM) that will ameliorate medicine efficacy, offering an advantage in reducing treatment period and cost of treatment (Khang & Vugar et al., 2024).

Telehealth is a platform that delivers healthcare services and clinical information as well as data to remote areas. It is an FDA-approved, HIPPA tractable platform that interactively connects cases with a civil network mesh of pukka croakers 24/7 using the Internet, Internet of Healthcare Things, video exchanges, smartphones, and Electronic Medical Records (EMR). With the increased number of geriatric patients and pervasiveness for chronic diseases, telehealth is a need of the hour and a boon in this COVID-19 pandemic, which offers the advantage of operating when physicians are in distant areas. In this concern, surgical robots play an important role in performing critical operations in OT. Telehealth is a new paradigm in the healthcare system since the trained medical staff is a key requirement for the improvement of the healthcare system in India (Vrushank & Khang et al., 2023).

Telemedicine, also known as e-medicine, consists of providing healthcare services in remote areas requiring drug delivery. It provides healthcare access for diagnosis of disease and treatment without the need for in-person visits. By using videoconferencing and phone consultations, patients can have a real-time connection with a team of physicians for case-to-case medical history, reports of various tests and examination X-rays and CT scans, and psychiatric evaluations. Some of the top-rated telemedicine apps reported are Doctor on Demand, Amwell, MD Live, Talkspace, Lemonaid Health, Plush Care, Live Health Online, Teladoc, and Babylon.

Health, Maple, Health Tap, Dialogue, First Opinion, Simple Contacts, Pager, and Doxy.me telemonitoring collects the data of each case from the hospitals with the help of IoT and sends the data to a healthcare monitoring agency for the remote testing analysis and speculations. Telemonitoring services can be used in emergency medical conditions for first aid in cases of acute poisoning, including substantiated cautions that inform a case healthcare provider in times of physical/ internal trauma. Telesurgeries are becoming increasingly popular because they enable surgeons to operate from a foreign position using telerobotics-assisted technology. Providing healthcare information to remote areas is a need of the hour, as medical and clinical education to the community serves the goal of healthcare and groups of specific locales are the principal targets to reach the local citizens for awareness. Telehealth data services provide technical health information with other health service providers, education and research, and clinical data associations as and when needed.

#### *3.3.2.1.1 Chip in a Pill*

Another illustration of the increasing effect of smart bias is "Chip in a pill" – a superior indigestible pill that monitors health status, counts medicine goods on crucial organs, and sends data to a wearable device. This data is also transferred as a report over pall to HCP for opinion. Chip in a pill has an indigestible sensor that gets activated when the patient consumes the pill. The sensor is powered by stomach fluids and connects health conditions and status using the physiological response system of the body. A smart pill with dose variation is also possible. Drug usage tracking and medication adherence can easily be monitored.

#### *3.3.2.1.2 Organ on a Chip (OOC)*

IoT-grounded smart bias (IoT biases are grounded on different tackle platforms and networks, and can interact with other bias' platforms through different network), like "Organ on a Chip," permits associations to track real-life diagnostics scripts. Allying the affair from these biases with Big Data analytics and intelligent systems has the implicit of giving unknown occasions, thus perfecting the number of successes, which would drastically accelerate exploration and development productivity at low costs and in reduced time. An organ-on-a-chip is a microchip that mimics and senses the body's environment. The polymers used cover microfluidic channels lined by living cells. These microchips assist in recognizing the physiology of vital organs like the heart, lung, brain, kidney, skin, bone, and intestine blood-brain barrier, and organ-on-a-chip performs a crucial part in tracking the progress of new medicines and developing substantiated drugs in individualized drug therapy (Rani & Bhambri et al., 2023).

The new medicine is pragmatic to the chip, and its response is noted down with perceptivity into the captivation site of the new medicine, consisting of the effect on multi-organ relations and whether it alters the status of the disease. For example, Exact-Cure is a French incipiency that actually offers software that answers for the effects of medications in the body of the patient, grounded on individual physical appearance. Incipiency uses population pharmacokinetics and scientific literature data to forecast effectiveness and medical contact with every individual. Exact-Cure is an emerging medicine-specific exposure model for pharmaceuticals under exploration for the treatment of COVID-19.

#### *3.3.2.1.3 Google Glass*

Google Glass is a wearable Android device that displays information directly in the user's field of vision. Smart spectacles have been playing an inconceivable part across all verticals, including healthcare. These spectacles enable physicians to record photographic information during a consultation with patients by only keeping eye contact. Furthermore, these aspects can change the story during surgeries where physicians can partake in the viewpoints of specialists around the world. Backing will be provided with cloud data available soon. By using these smart spectacles in hospitals, doctors can save a hefty amount that is spent on video conferencing yearly. The recent edition of Google Glass 2 is currently employed in various hospitals. Another such example is Agumedix, which provides access to patient information instead of using Electronic Health records, which would require a long time, and collects real-time information rather than using computers. Dignity Health uses this software to interact between medical professionals and patients suffering from chronic diseases.

#### *3.3.2.1.4 iBeacons*

Among position-stranded technologies, iBeacon is the most emerging technology. It is streamlining nursing home operations by reporting responsibilities and allotting workshops among medical staff, similar to drug conditions and exigency cases. It directly shares patients' medical history and their medical reports to the physician's mobile before the patient reaches the clinic. Hence, it helps physicians to have a proper line of treatment by using patients' data regarding medical history.

#### *3.3.2.1.5 Sensors in Drug Delivery Devices*

Many biases similar to Amiko's are formerly available in the demand to watch medication doses and to keep track of specifics by the cases themselves. It is present in multiple drug stores that are using Amiko to administer pills to reduce the chances of mistakes and to ensure better drug supervision.

#### *3.3.2.1.6 Smart Wheelchairs*

A very well-versed usage of IoT technology has been done in an automatic wheelchair. These automatic wheelchairs are created by a fit-in wireless body area network with varied detectors whose functions are managed via IoT. Vitals of individuals sitting in the wheelchair can be watched, and it can also keep an eye on the site of users. This tool empowers physically challenged people to get the feeling of independence and, if used in hospitals, can deliver better support in inpatient supervision (Kali & Khang et al., 2024).

#### *3.3.2.1.7 Wrist Bands*

Wrist bands originated to measure the patient's pulsation, exertion, temperature, oxygen level, and blood pressure. Important data is shared on patients' phones to watch their health and keep a trail of day-to-day routine. A company from Korea has recently launched Angel, which is a compact and wearable BP detector that helps to find out the BP of the patient. Other applications include measuring stress levels and calories burned during exercise.

#### 3.3.2.2 IoT in Pharmaceutical Manufacturing

Using pharmaceutical IoT monitoring detectors, companies can presently feed all applicable installation data into a single dashboard and can warn an administrator in case of any abnormal conditions or critical conservation conditions. IoT in pharmaceutical manufacturing will also enable handling critically ill patients and contribute to saving the lives of patients. One implicit drawback in medicine manufacturing is embedded in the outfit. In the manufacturing area, many reasons might be responsible for the failure of the asset. The failure of assets might be due to mechanical impairment, unstable voltage, chemical damage, insecure terrain, and the lack of implementation of conservation policies. IoT can minimize the effects by streamlining their status information on other factors as well, such as working of pressure gauges, examination of pH of the solutions, working of air compressors, maintenance of sterilizers, heat exchanger instruments, and vacuum pumps (Khang & Rana et al., 2023).

The data collected by the detectors can be utilized for the development of conservation and form, evading serious issues, reducing time-out, and even icing plant safety. Furthermore, the attained data can produce a full picture of the outfit application. This overview contributes to productivity and helps in the reduction of waste, exhibiting optimization. If IoT is combined with AI, such a system makes an ideal foundation for the prophetic conservation of various manufacturing equipment.

#### 3.3.2.3 IoT in Research and Development

To come up with a new drug requires a huge amount of investment and also includes failure costs. A medication with a tricky form or an unsatisfying outcome in clinical trials will tank a pharmaceutical development. In the meantime, the world keenly looks forward to pharmaceutical advancements for conditions that persist, are incurable, or have improved results for dealing with long-term affections.

IoT can play an important part in accelerating pharmaceutical growth, restructuring its product, reducing R&D costs, and enhancing the administration of medication to cases. It is the world of canny bias linked to the internet, which feeds real-time data to a network utilized by calculating machines. Later, that network communicates through machine-to-machine computing and prioritizes the data on the basis of applicability or specific literacy of machine, and detects the patterns and to translate into equations (artificial intelligence). In exploration and progressions, IoT-based analytics reduces human violations, enhances effectiveness, and scales down waste. Provision interconnectivity of data in IoT enables an increase in the real-time clarity during pharmaceutical product development.

#### 3.3.2.4 IoT in Medical Applications

Features such as image segmentation, feature extraction, and 3D image processing succeeded in robust anomaly detection strategies that would influence the process of smart biomedical image analysis. For illustration, image analysis of anomalous brain regions may correlate to Alzheimer's. A cardiac anomaly can also be found using ECG trace, which includes Undecimated Wavelet Transform (UWT) ways along with the Bayesian Network Classifier model. This model is proposed to determine early Atrial Compression, untimely Ventricular Compression, and Myocardial Infarction

(MI). Power scale analysis of EEG signals to determine anomalous working and the analysis of the early discovery of cardiac abnormality can be assessed. Also, an antigen-antibody response in case of infections can be prognosticated (Khang & Ragimova et al., 2022).

For example, it was reported that BioLines Laboratory and the University of Pennsylvania worked in collaboration with NASA to run a few medical tests in space. It included testing for a lung-, bone-, and marrow-tissue chip to understand the mechanism of a human body when varied infections hit. Later, a few companies also targeted medical operations similar to the treatment of the heart, nerves, lungs, liver, kidney, and other vital organs. These capabilities have proved promising results, and the ensuing limited times will exhibit whether these lab-on-chips will adequately be able to replicate the mortal physiological systems or not.

#### 3.3.2.5 IoT in Pharmaceutical Biotechnology Companies

Biotechnological and pharmaceutical industries are applying and installing software systems connected to the cloud to accelerate subsisting and new laboratory frameworks with the advantages of a robotic cloud lab within their laboratories. For illustration, the synthetic biology company Ginkgo Bioworks recently installed a data cloud answer system in its microbiology foundry division. The action aims to automatize the experimental design process to amplify foundry products, transport the products promptly and more expertly, and scale to meet the tabulating demands.

Cellexus, a Scottish incipiency, is known for the making of mono-use airlift bioreactor systems. The incipiency has a patent for its airlift technology, and it actually uses the bubbles and not the mechanical mixers for the movement of nutrients and cells. The reactor consists of disposable bioreactor bags and an intertwined heater and offers simulated regulatory parameters required for biochemical processes similar to pH, oxygen, and temperature. The single-use system can be useful to a variety of cell lives and ferments, and thus, the start-ups have managed the growth of bacteria, yeast, microalgae, and bacteriophage modification.

#### 3.3.2.6 IoT in Personalized Medicine

Precision medication is based on the idea of treating every case as a particular individual. A new perceptivity is created by advancements in omics and data analysis. It shows the response of the patient to the medications specifically prescribed to them. Such knowledge and other methodologies, including advanced versions of different methodologies, such as 3-D manufacturing, enable individualized medication to be a realistic method. Models where medicines are focused generally regulate the pharmacokinetic and pharmacodynamic fate of medicines for designing an ideal formulation for medicines predicated on age, sex, comorbidities, and other clinical parameters.

A new paradigm in cancer therapeutics, for instance, Swiss incipiency Tepthera, offers a new paradigm for the identification of T cell antigens. The MEDi platform helps in the quick identification of neoplasm-specific antigens from patient mortal leukocyte antigens. After the selection of antigens, the result identifies excrescence specific epitopes and also monitors antigen-specific T cells. The platform gives a solution for cases with personalized remedial vaccines for conditional treatments (Khang & Hajimahmud et al., 2023).

## 3.4 EFFICIENCY OF AI COMPARED TO CONVENTIONAL METHODS CONCERNING SUSTAINABLE MANAGEMENT IN THE PHARMACEUTICAL INDUSTRY

The application of AI in the pharmaceutical industry for sustainability is considered "Technological Re-Innovation" as it has attracted many consumers for long-term investment. Digitalization and automation of the pharmaceutical industries have eased manufacturing. Implementation of natural language processing helped in the creation of clinical reports and maintenance of the clinical data of the patients, which reduced the overworking of the pharmaceutical employees. It also seems increasingly clear that AI systems will not replace human clinicians but rather will reduce their efforts in patient care and monitoring. Societal resilience is also promoted by the implementation of AI technologies when accustomed to the cultural background and needs of various regions (Khang & Vladimir et al., 2023)

## 3.5 CONCLUSION

The topmost challenge to AI in medicinal disciplines is not whether the technologies will be able to be useful but rather icing their relinquishment in diurnal practice. For wide relinquishment to take place, AI systems must be approved by controllers, integrated with EHR systems, and standardized to a sufficient degree that analogous products work analogously and are streamlined each time (Vrushank & Vidhi et al., 2023).

## REFERENCES

Jaiswal N., Misra A., Misra P. K., Khang A., "Role of the Internet of Things (IoT) Technologies in Business and Production", *AI-Aided IoT Technologies and Applications in the Smart Business and Production*, 2023. CRC Press. https://doi.org/10.1201/9781003392224-1

Kali C. R., Khang A., Roy D., "The Role of Internet of Things (IoT) Technology in Industry 4.0", *Advanced IoT Technologies and Applications in the Industry 4.0 Digital Economy* (1st Ed.), 2024. CRC Press. https://doi.org/10.1201/9781003434269-1

Khang A. (Eds.), *AI and IoT-Based Technologies for Precision Medicine*, 2024. IGI Global Press. ISBN: 9798369308769. https://doi.org/10.4018/979-8-3693-0876-9

Khang A., Abdullayev V., Hahanov V., Shah V., *Advanced IoT Technologies and Applications in the Industry 4.0 Digital Economy* (1st Ed.), 2024. CRC Press. https://doi.org/10.1201/9781003434269

Khang A., Hahanov V., Litvinova E., Chumachenko S., Triwiyanto, Hajimahmud A. V., Ali R. N., Alyar A. V., Anh P. T., "The Analytics of Hospitality of Hospitals in Healthcare Ecosystem", *Data-Centric AI Solutions and Emerging Technologies in the Healthcare Ecosystem* (p. 4), 2023. CRC Press. https://doi.org/10.1201/9781003356189-4

Khang A., Hajimahmud V. A., Gupta S. K., Babasaheb J., Morris G., *AI-Centric Modelling and Analytics: Concepts, Designs, Technologies, and Applications* (1st Ed.), 2023. CRC Press. https://doi.org/10.1201/9781003400110

Khang A., Ragimova N. A., Hajimahmud V. A., Alyar V. A., "Advanced Technologies and Data Management in the Smart Healthcare System", *AI-Centric Smart City Ecosystems: Technologies, Design and Implementation* (1st Ed., vol. 16, p. 10), 2022. CRC Press. https://doi.org/10.1201/9781003252542-16

Khang A., Rana G., Tailor R. K., Hajimahmud V. A. (Eds.), *Data-Centric AI Solutions and Emerging Technologies in the Healthcare Ecosystem*, 2023. CRC Press. https://doi.org/10.1201/9781003356189

Rana G., Khang A., Sharma R., Goel A. K., Dubey A. K. (Eds.), *Reinventing Manufacturing and Business Processes Through Artificial Intelligence*, 2021. CRC Press. https://doi.org/10.1201/9781003145011

Rani S., Bhambri P., Kataria A., Khang A., Sivaraman, A. K., *Big Data, Cloud Computing and IoT: Tools and Applications* (1st Ed.), 2023. Chapman and Hall/CRC. https://doi.org/10.1201/9781003298335

Rani S., Chauhan M., Kataria A., Khang A. (Eds.), "IoT Equipped Intelligent Distributed Framework for Smart Healthcare Systems", Networking and Internet Architecture, 2021, 2, 30. https://doi.org/10.48550/arXiv.2110.04997

Vrushank S., Khang A., "Internet of Medical Things (IoMT) Driving the Digital Transformation of the Healthcare Sector", *Data-Centric AI Solutions and Emerging Technologies in the Healthcare Ecosystem* (1st Ed., p. 1), 2023. CRC Press. https://doi.org/10.1201/9781003356189-2

Vrushank S., Vidhi T., Khang A., "Electronic Health Records Security and Privacy Enhancement Using Blockchain Technology", *Data-Centric AI Solutions and Emerging Technologies in the Healthcare Ecosystem* (1st Ed., p. 1), 2023. CRC Press. https://doi.org/10.1201/9781003356189-1

# 4 AI-Integrated IoT in Healthcare Ecosystem
## *Opportunities, Challenges, and Future Directions*

*Tarun Kumar Vashishth, Vikas Sharma, Bhupender Kumar, Rajneesh Panwar, Kewal Krishan Sharma, and Sachin Chaudhary*

## 4.1 INTRODUCTION

In recent years, advances in computer vision, artificial intelligence (AI), and the Internet of Things (IoT) have transformed many industries, including healthcare. These technologies have the potential to improve patient outcomes, enhance healthcare delivery, and reduce costs by enabling healthcare providers to collect, analyze, and act on vast amounts of data. However, there are also significant challenges associated with the integration of these technologies in healthcare, including concerns about data privacy, ownership, and control, as well as the accuracy and reliability of AI algorithms. This chapter aims to explore the transformative potential of integrating computer vision, AI, and IoT in healthcare and to examine the opportunities, challenges, and future directions for this field (Khang & Rana et al., 2023).

We begin by providing an overview of these technologies and their current applications in healthcare. We then discuss the potential benefits of integrating these technologies, including improved patient outcomes and reduced healthcare costs. We also examine the challenges associated with integrating these technologies, including regulatory and ethical considerations and the potential for bias in AI algorithms. We discuss the importance of interdisciplinary collaboration between computer scientists, healthcare providers, and regulatory experts to address these challenges and ensure that these technologies are deployed in a responsible and ethical manner (Khang & Abdullayev et al., 2024).

### 4.1.1 HEALTHCARE SECTOR

The healthcare sector is one of the most critical sectors in the world, playing a vital role in providing medical care and maintaining the overall health and well-being of individuals. It encompasses a vast array of fields, including hospitals, clinics, pharmaceuticals, medical devices, biotechnology, and health insurance.

DOI: 10.1201/9781032686745-4

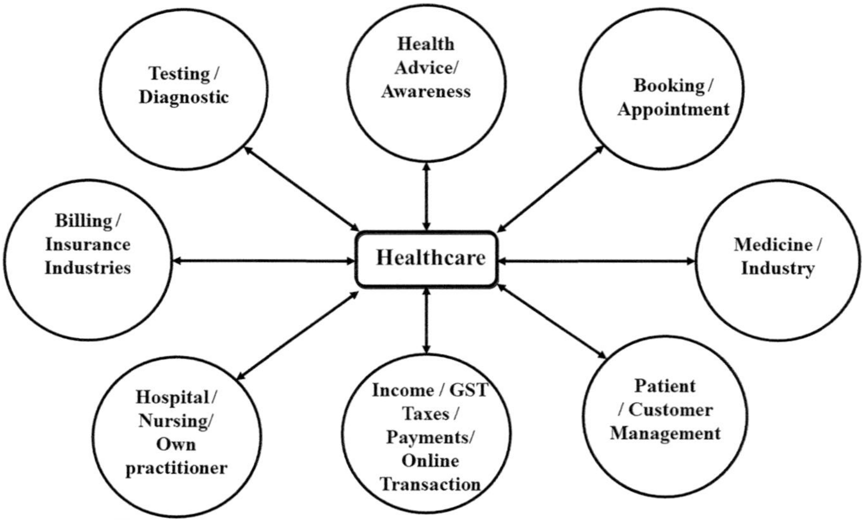


**FIGURE 4.1** Healthcare sector's various components (Khang, 2021).

One of the most significant challenges facing the healthcare sector is the rising cost of healthcare. With the aging population and the increasing prevalence of chronic diseases such as diabetes and heart disease, the demand for healthcare services continues to grow. Additionally, the development of new medical technologies and treatments has also contributed to the rising cost of healthcare.

To address these challenges, healthcare providers have turned to various strategies to improve efficiency, reduce costs, and enhance patient outcomes. Some of these strategies include the use of technology, such as electronic medical records, telemedicine, and artificial intelligence, to improve diagnosis and treatment (Khang & Medicine, 2024).

Another critical aspect of the healthcare sector is public health. Public health initiatives focus on preventing diseases and promoting healthy behaviors to improve the overall health of the population. Examples of public health initiatives include vaccination programs, tobacco control, and environmental health. The healthcare sector is also a significant contributor to the economy, providing employment opportunities for millions of people worldwide. The sector has been growing rapidly, with new and innovative products and services being introduced regularly.

Despite the progress made in the healthcare sector, there are still significant challenges that need to be addressed. These challenges include the unequal distribution of various components, as shown in Figure 4.1.

### 4.1.2 Computer Vision

Computer vision refers to the field of study and practice that deals with enabling machines to interpret and understand visual data from the world around them. It involves using mathematical and computational techniques to analyze, process, and extract information from images, videos, and other visual data sources.

Computer vision has many practical applications, such as in autonomous vehicles, medical imaging, facial recognition, surveillance, and robotics. The main goal of computer vision is to create algorithms and systems that can emulate human visual perception and provide useful insights or actions based on visual data. Some key techniques used in computer vision include image segmentation, object recognition, image registration, feature extraction, and machine learning. These techniques enable computers to recognize patterns and objects in images, perform image classification and object detection, track objects across multiple frames, and generate useful insights from visual data, as shown in Figure 4.3.

Advanced computer vision is a field of study within computer science and artificial intelligence that focuses on developing algorithms and systems that can analyze, interpret, and understand visual data from the world around us. It involves using advanced machine learning techniques, such as deep learning and neural networks, to enable computers to perceive and interpret images and videos like humans do, as shown in Figure 4.4.

- **Object detection and recognition**: This involves identifying and classifying objects in images or videos, such as people, vehicles, or animals.
- **Image segmentation**: This involves dividing an image into different segments or regions based on color, texture, or other visual features.
- **3D reconstruction**: This involves reconstructing a 3D model of an object or scene from 2D images or videos. It involves extracting information about the geometry and appearance of the scene or object from multiple 2D images and using this information to create a 3D model. Applications of computer vision 3D reconstruction include virtual reality, robotics, medical imaging, and cultural heritage preservation, as shown in Figure 4.4.

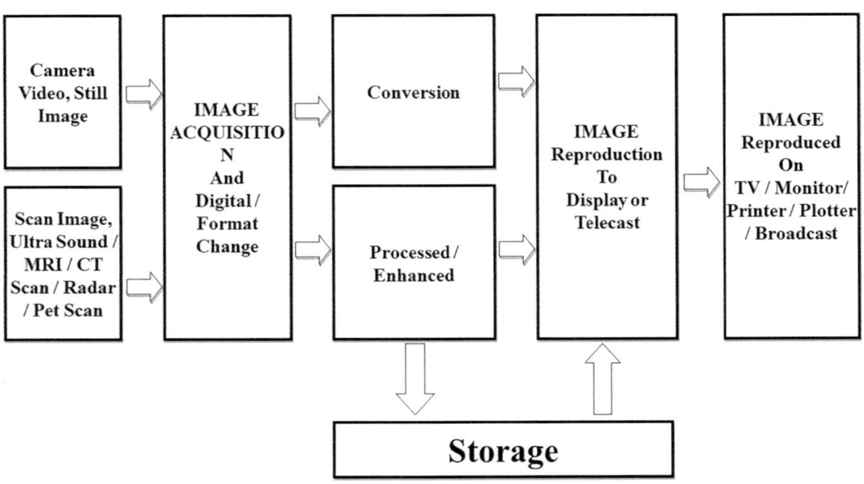


**FIGURE 4.2** Traditional computer vision capturing (Khang, 2021).

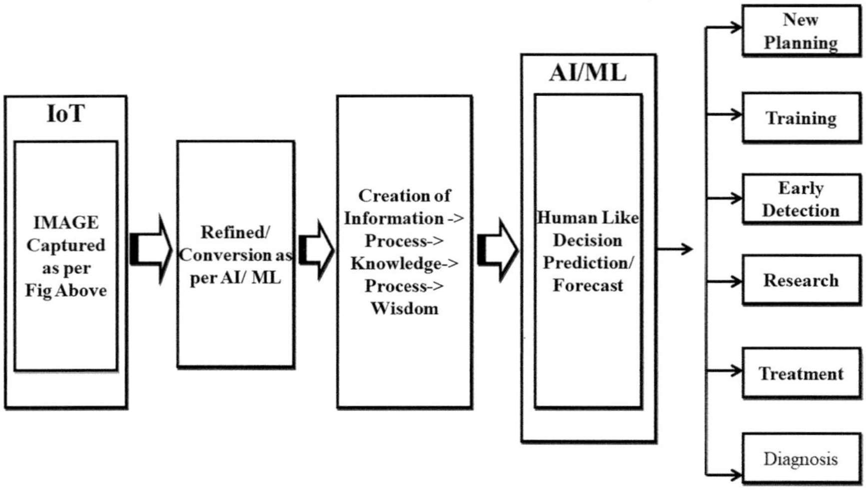


**FIGURE 4.3** Traditional computer vision capturing, converted to advanced computer (Khang, 2021).

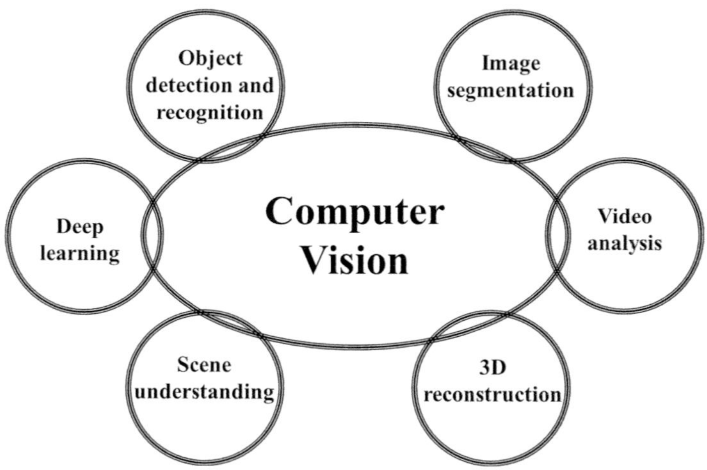


**FIGURE 4.4** Components of advanced computer vision.

- **Scene understanding**: This involves analyzing a scene to understand the relationships between objects and the context in which they appear.
- **Video analysis**: This involves analyzing video data to extract information such as motion patterns, object trajectories, and event detection.
- **Deep learning for computer vision**: This involves using deep neural networks to develop advanced computer vision systems that can learn from large datasets and make accurate predictions. Applications of advanced

computer vision include autonomous driving, robotics, surveillance, medical imaging, and augmented reality.

## 4.2 LITERATURE REVIEW

The literature reviewed for "AI-Integrated IoT in Healthcare Ecosystem: Opportunities, Challenges, and Future Directions" covers a broad range of topics relating to the integration of computer vision, artificial intelligence (AI), and the Internet of Things (IoT) in healthcare.

Smith et al. (Smith et al., 2021) highlight the recent advancements in machine vision, including the use of convolutional neural networks (CNNs) and generative adversarial networks (GANs) for image recognition, segmentation, and synthesis. It also discusses the challenges that still need to be addressed in machine vision, such as robustness to adversarial attacks, interpretability, and fairness. Overall, the article provides a valuable resource for researchers and practitioners interested in the field of machine vision, including its historical development, current state-of-the-art, and future directions.

Atitallah et al. (2020) conclude with a discussion of the future directions of research in this area. The authors suggest that future research should focus on developing more efficient and scalable deep learning models for data analysis, as well as improving the security and privacy of IoT data. They also highlight the need for interdisciplinary research collaborations to address the complex challenges faced by smart cities. Overall, the article provides a valuable resource for researchers and practitioners interested in the use of deep learning and IoT big data analytics for supporting the development of smart cities.

Gill et al. (Gill et al., 2019) conclude with a discussion of the open challenges and future directions in this area. The authors suggest that future research should focus on developing more efficient and secure cloud computing systems through the integration of IoT, blockchain, and AI. They also highlight the need for interdisciplinary research collaborations to address the complex challenges faced by cloud computing. Overall, the article provides a valuable resource for researchers and practitioners interested in the transformative effects of IoT, blockchain, and AI on cloud computing (Khanh & Khang, 2021).

Chengoden et al. (2023) conclude with a discussion of the future directions of research in this area. The authors suggest that future research should focus on developing more advanced and user-friendly metaverse technologies for healthcare applications. They also highlight the need for interdisciplinary research collaborations to address the complex challenges faced by the metaverse in healthcare. Overall, the article provides a valuable resource for researchers and practitioners interested in the potential applications, challenges, and future directions of the metaverse in healthcare.

Ageron et al. (2020) conclude with a discussion of the future directions of research in this area. The authors suggest that future research should focus on developing more advanced and integrated digital supply chain management systems. They also highlight the need for interdisciplinary research collaborations to address the complex challenges faced by digital supply chain management. Overall, the article provides a valuable resource for researchers and practitioners interested in the challenges and future directions of digital supply chain management.

Gubbi et al. (2013) provide a comprehensive overview of the vision, architectural elements, and future directions of the IoT. Their article serves as a valuable resource for researchers and practitioners interested in the IoT and its potential applications.

Vermesan et al. (2017) provide a comprehensive overview of the current trends and applications of cognitive transformation technology in the context of the IoT. Their article serves as a valuable resource for researchers and practitioners interested in the intersection of cognitive computing and the IoT.

Bajwa et al. (2021) provide a comprehensive overview of the potential applications of AI in healthcare and its transformative potential for the practice of medicine. Their article serves as a valuable resource for healthcare professionals and researchers interested in the intersection of AI and healthcare.

Chen and Zhang (2022) provide valuable insights into the emerging research trends in the health metaverse, and their article can serve as a useful resource for researchers and practitioners interested in this area.

Brauner et al. (2022) proposed a conceptual framework for digital transformation in production consisting of four layers: the physical layer, the data layer, the platform layer, and the application layer. The authors discuss the role of each layer and the challenges involved in integrating them into a coherent digital transformation strategy.

Overall, this chapter provides valuable insights into the digital transformation of production from a computer science perspective. It offers a useful framework for researchers and practitioners interested in exploring the potential of new technologies for improving production processes and systems.

Okegbile et al. (2022) discuss the potential benefits of HDTs, such as improved diagnosis, treatment, and prevention of diseases. They acknowledge the challenges associated with the implementation of HDTs, such as data privacy and security concerns, and propose strategies to address these challenges. Overall, this chapter provides a valuable contribution to the emerging field of digital twins in healthcare. It presents a novel approach to personalized healthcare that has the potential to revolutionize the way healthcare is delivered and managed.

Tortorella et al. (2020) provide a valuable contribution to the growing body of literature on Industry 4.0 in healthcare. Their article highlights the potential benefits of these technologies for improving patient outcomes and reducing costs while also acknowledging the challenges and limitations of their implementation. The proposed research directions provide a roadmap for future research in this area.

The literature reviewed in this chapter highlights the transformative potential of computer vision, AI, and IoT integration in healthcare. However, the successful implementation of these technologies will require interdisciplinary collaboration, addressing ethical concerns, and overcoming technical challenges. Future research should focus on developing strategies to realize the potential benefits of these technologies while mitigating their associated risks.

Overall, the literature suggests that computer vision, AI, and IoT integration have the potential to transform healthcare but also pose significant challenges that must be addressed to ensure their successful implementation. Future research should focus on developing strategies to overcome these challenges and maximize the potential benefits of these technologies in healthcare.

## 4.3 DISCUSSION

The integration of computer vision, artificial intelligence (AI), and the Internet of Things (IoT) has created a significant impact in various industries, including healthcare. The integration of these technologies in healthcare has the potential to revolutionize the way healthcare is delivered and improve patient outcomes. In this discussion, we will explore the transformative potential of computer vision, AI, and IoT integration in healthcare, along with the opportunities, challenges, and future directions of this integration.

### 4.3.1 Opportunities

The integration of computer vision, AI, and IoT in healthcare offers numerous opportunities, including:

#### 4.3.1.1 Enhanced Medical Imaging and Diagnostics

Computer vision and AI algorithms can improve the accuracy and efficiency of medical imaging interpretation, aiding in the early detection and diagnosis of diseases. This can lead to improved patient outcomes and more targeted treatment plans.

#### 4.3.1.2 Remote Patient Monitoring and Telehealth

IoT devices and AI-powered analytics enable continuous remote monitoring of patients' health conditions. This allows for proactive intervention, personalized care, and reduced hospital readmissions. Telehealth solutions also improve access to healthcare services, especially for patients in remote areas.

#### 4.3.1.3 Improved Healthcare Operations and Resource Management

Integration of computer vision, AI, and IoT can optimize hospital operations by automating tasks, streamlining workflows, and optimizing resource allocation. This leads to increased efficiency, reduced costs, and improved patient satisfaction.

#### 4.3.1.4 Predictive Analytics and Precision Medicine

By analyzing large datasets and using AI algorithms, healthcare providers can predict disease outcomes, identify personalized treatment options, and tailor interventions for individual patients. This promotes precision medicine and improves patient outcomes.

#### 4.3.1.5 Enhanced Patient Safety and Care

Computer vision and AI integration can support real-time monitoring of patient safety, detecting falls, preventing medication errors, and improving patient care. This technology enables early intervention, reducing adverse events and improving patient safety.

### 4.3.2 Challenges

Despite the numerous opportunities, the integration of computer vision, AI, and IoT in healthcare also poses some challenges, including:

#### 4.3.2.1 Data Privacy and Security

The integration of computer vision, AI, and IoT involves the collection and storage of sensitive patient data. Ensuring privacy, security, and compliance with regulations is crucial to maintaining patient trust and protecting against data breaches.

#### 4.3.2.2 Ethical Considerations

The use of AI and computer vision in healthcare raises ethical concerns, including bias in algorithms, decision-making transparency, and accountability. Guidelines and frameworks must be established to ensure fairness, transparency, and responsible use of these technologies.

#### 4.3.2.3 Integration and Interoperability

Integrating different technologies and systems can be complex, requiring seamless interoperability between devices, platforms, and data sources. Standardization efforts are needed to ensure compatibility and effective collaboration between different stakeholders.

#### 4.3.2.4 Regulatory and Legal Challenges

The rapid advancement of computer vision, AI, and IoT in healthcare poses challenges for regulatory frameworks. Regulations must keep pace with technological advancements to address issues such as liability, data ownership, and data sharing.

#### 4.3.2.5 Adoption and Acceptance

Healthcare professionals and patients need to embrace and trust these technologies for widespread adoption. Education, training, and clear communication about the benefits and limitations of these technologies are essential to foster acceptance and ensure successful implementation.

### 4.3.3 Road Map Ahead

The integration of computer vision, AI, and IoT in healthcare is still in its early stages, and there are many areas where further research and development are needed. Some of the future directions include:

- **Improved interoperability**: There is a need for better integration between different healthcare systems to allow for seamless data exchange and communication.
- **Development of standardized protocols**: The development of standardized protocols can help in the successful integration of these technologies in healthcare.

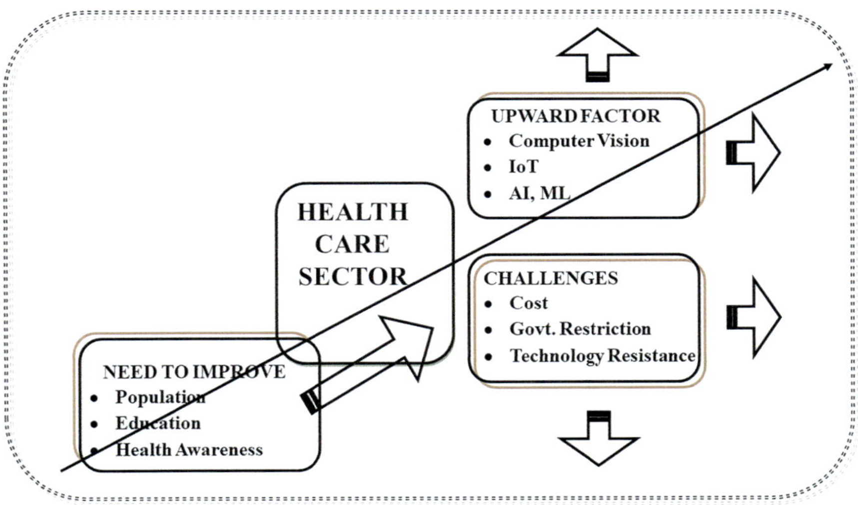


**FIGURE 4.5** Healthcare sector progress representation.

- **Further research on ethical considerations**: Further research is needed on ethical considerations related to the use of these technologies in healthcare to ensure that patient privacy and autonomy are protected.
- **Development of AI algorithms**: The development of more accurate and efficient AI algorithms can help in the early detection of diseases and personalized treatment planning.

The integration of computer vision, AI, and IoT in healthcare offers numerous opportunities, including improved diagnosis, personalized treatment, remote monitoring, reduced medical errors, and better patient experience. However, it also poses challenges related to data privacy and security, technical expertise, and ethical considerations, as shown in Figure 4.5.

## 4.4 PROPOSED METHODOLOGY

The medical ecosystem is a complex and dynamic environment that involves multiple stakeholders, including patients, healthcare providers, insurance companies, and government agencies. In recent years, the integration of artificial intelligence (AI) and Internet of Things (IoT) technologies in the medical ecosystem has created new opportunities for improving healthcare outcomes and providing more efficient healthcare services.

The combination of these two technologies has made it possible to collect and analyze vast amounts of data, which can be used to develop personalized healthcare solutions that are tailored to the specific needs of patients. Despite the potential benefits of AI and IoT integration in the medical ecosystem, there are also challenges that must be addressed. For example, the development of AI and IoT-enabled healthcare solutions requires a multidisciplinary approach that involves experts from various fields, including computer science, medicine, and engineering.

In addition, there are concerns about data privacy and security, as well as the potential for AI and IoT technologies to replace human healthcare providers. Medical technology is rapidly evolving and has the potential to revolutionize healthcare delivery. The IoT is a network of interconnected devices that can communicate with each other without human intervention (Rana et al., 2021).

The integration of IoT with computer vision and AI technologies has made it possible to monitor patients remotely, automate processes, and make accurate diagnoses. This integration has opened up new opportunities for healthcare providers to improve patient outcomes and reduce costs. However, the implementation of these technologies presents some challenges that need to be addressed. The combination of these two technologies has made it possible to collect and analyze vast amounts of data, which can be used to improve patient outcomes and provide more efficient healthcare services. This chapter proposes a new methodology for the integration of AI and IoT technologies in the medical ecosystem.

The methodology is designed to provide a framework for the development of AI and IoT-enabled healthcare solutions that are tailored to the specific needs of patients, healthcare providers, and other stakeholders, as shown in Figure 4.6.

The integration of computer vision and artificial intelligence (AI) technologies with the Internet of Things (IoT) has significantly enhanced the capabilities of medical systems in the following ways:

- **Remote patient monitoring**: IoT sensors can be used to monitor patients' vital signs, such as heart rate, blood pressure, and oxygen saturation, in real-time. AI algorithms can then analyze this data to detect patterns or anomalies that might indicate a medical problem. This can help doctors intervene early and prevent hospitalizations or other complications.
- **Predictive maintenance**: IoT sensors can also be used to monitor medical equipment, such as MRI machines, to detect problems before they cause a

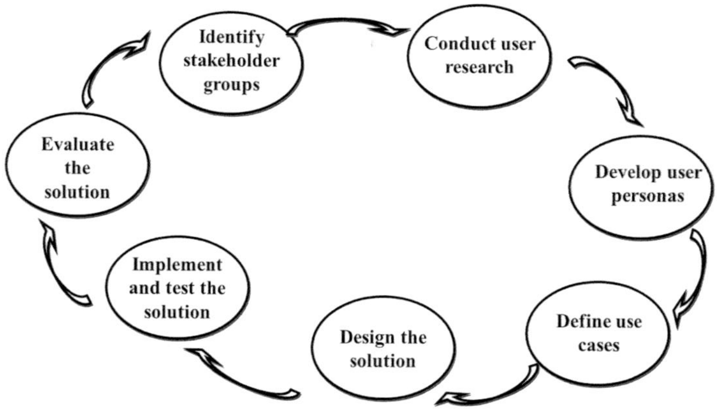


**FIGURE 4.6** Computer vision added Healthcare model.

breakdown. AI algorithms can analyze this data to predict when equipment is likely to fail, allowing maintenance to be scheduled before a problem occurs.

- **Supply chain management**: IoT sensors can track medical supplies, such as medications and medical devices, from the manufacturer to the point of care. AI algorithms can then analyze this data to optimize the supply chain, ensuring that supplies are available when and where they are needed.
- **Drug development**: AI algorithms can analyze large amounts of medical data to identify patterns and develop new treatments. IoT sensors can also be used to collect data on patients' responses to treatments, allowing researchers to refine their models and develop more effective therapies.
- **Telemedicine**: IoT devices such as smartphones and tablets can be used to connect patients with doctors remotely, allowing for remote consultations and diagnoses. AI algorithms can assist in diagnosing and monitoring patients remotely.

The proposed methodology consists of the following steps:

- **Identify stakeholder groups**: The first step in the methodology is to identify the various stakeholder groups involved in the medical ecosystem, including patients, healthcare providers, insurance companies, and government agencies. Each stakeholder group has unique needs and preferences that must be taken into account when developing AI and IoT-enabled healthcare solutions.
- **Conduct user research**: The next step is to conduct user research to understand the needs and preferences of each stakeholder group. This can involve surveys, interviews, and focus groups to gather data on the current healthcare landscape and identify areas for improvement.
- **Develop user personas**: Based on user research, user personas are developed to represent the needs and preferences of each stakeholder group. These personas are used as a reference point throughout the development process to ensure that the AI and IoT-enabled healthcare solutions are tailored to the specific needs of each stakeholder group.
- **Define use cases**: The next step is to define use cases for the AI and IoT-enabled healthcare solutions. Use cases are scenarios that describe how the solutions will be used in real-world situations. These use cases are developed based on the needs and preferences of each stakeholder group.
- **Design the solution**: Using the user personas and use cases as a reference point, the AI and IoT-enabled healthcare solutions are designed. This involves developing algorithms and software that can collect and analyze data from IoT devices, as well as providing recommendations and alerts to healthcare providers based on the data collected.
- **Implement and test the solution**: The next step is to implement and test the AI and IoT-enabled healthcare solutions. This involves integrating the algorithms and software with IoT devices and healthcare systems. The solutions are then tested in real-world scenarios to ensure that they meet the needs and preferences of each stakeholder group.

- **Evaluate the solution**: The final step in the methodology is to evaluate the AI and IoT-enabled healthcare solutions. This involves gathering feedback from stakeholders to determine whether the solutions have met their needs and preferences. This feedback is used to refine and improve the solutions over time.

## 4.5 INTEGRATION OF CV, AI, AND IoT IN HEALTHCARE

The integration of computer vision, AI, and IoT in healthcare refers to the combination and utilization of computer vision techniques, artificial intelligence (AI) algorithms, and Internet of Things (IoT) devices in healthcare settings. This integration aims to enhance various aspects of healthcare delivery, including diagnostics, patient monitoring, operational efficiency, and personalized care (Rath et al., 2024).

### 4.5.1 Conceptual Framework for Integrating CV, AI, and IoT in Healthcare

This framework outlines the overall structure and components required for integrating these technologies in healthcare. It involves the interconnection between computer vision systems that can analyze visual data, AI algorithms that can process and interpret the data, and IoT devices that can collect and transmit relevant information. The conceptual framework also considers the infrastructure, data management, and communication protocols necessary for seamless integration (Rani et al., 2021).

### 4.5.2 Opportunities and Benefits of Combining These Technologies in Healthcare Settings

- **Enhanced diagnostics**: Computer vision algorithms can analyze medical images, such as X-rays or MRIs, to assist in accurate and efficient disease detection and diagnosis.
- **Remote patient monitoring**: IoT devices can continuously collect patient data, such as vital signs, and transmit it to AI algorithms for real-time analysis. This allows for remote monitoring, early detection of abnormalities, and personalized care.
- **Improved operational efficiency**: Integrating computer vision, AI, and IoT can automate various healthcare operations, optimize resource allocation, and streamline workflows, leading to improved efficiency and cost reduction.
- **Predictive analytics**: AI algorithms can analyze large volumes of healthcare data, including patient records and genomic information, to predict disease outcomes, personalize treatment plans, and enable precision medicine.
- **Enhanced patient safety and care**: Computer vision systems combined with AI and IoT can enable real-time monitoring of patients, detection of falls, prevention of medication errors, and early intervention for improved patient safety and care.

### 4.5.3 Case Studies Illustrating Successful Integration and Transformative Outcomes

#### 4.5.3.1 Case Study: Computer Vision-Assisted Diagnosis in Radiology

- Integration of computer vision algorithms in radiology workflows, enabling automated analysis of medical images for faster and more accurate diagnoses.
- Resulted in reduced diagnostic errors, improved efficiency, and enhanced patient outcomes.

### 4.5.4 Case Study: Remote Patient Monitoring Using IoT and AI

- Integration of IoT devices for continuous collection of patient data, which is analyzed by AI algorithms in real-time.
- Enabled remote monitoring, early detection of health issues, and personalized interventions, leading to improved patient outcomes and reduced hospital admissions.

### 4.5.5 Case Study: Smart Hospital Infrastructure Management

- Integration of IoT sensors to track equipment, supplies, and patient flow, combined with AI algorithms for optimizing resource allocation and workflow efficiency.
- Resulted in improved operational efficiency, reduced waiting times, and enhanced patient experience.

### 4.5.6 Case Study: Predictive Analytics for Precision Medicine

- Integration of AI algorithms with patient data, genomics, and lifestyle information for personalized risk assessment and treatment plans.
- Enabled targeted interventions, improved patient outcomes, and optimized healthcare resources.

### 4.5.7 Case study: Computer Vision-Based Fall Detection and Prevention

- Integration of computer vision systems in elderly care facilities or homes to detect and prevent falls.
- Resulted in timely assistance, improved safety, and reduced fall-related injuries.

These case studies exemplify the successful integration of computer vision, AI, and IoT in healthcare, showcasing the transformative outcomes such integration can bring to various aspects of healthcare delivery and patient care.

## 4.6 CONCLUSION

In conclusion, the integration of computer vision, artificial intelligence (AI), and the Internet of Things (IoT) in healthcare has immense transformative potential. This integration offers numerous opportunities for improving patient care, diagnosis, treatment, and overall healthcare management. However, it also presents several challenges that need to be addressed for successful implementation.

One of the key opportunities of this integration is the ability to automate and enhance medical imaging and diagnostics. Computer vision algorithms can analyze medical images such as X-rays, CT scans, and MRIs with great precision, assisting healthcare professionals in detecting abnormalities, making accurate diagnoses, and providing timely treatment. AI-powered systems can also aid in predicting diseases, identifying risk factors, and personalizing treatment plans, leading to improved patient outcomes.

Another important opportunity lies in remote patient monitoring and telehealth. IoT devices can collect real-time health data from patients, such as vital signs, activity levels, and medication adherence. This data can be analyzed using AI algorithms to provide proactive and personalized care, enabling early detection of health issues, better management of chronic conditions, and reduced hospital readmissions. Telehealth solutions powered by AI and computer vision can facilitate remote consultations, enabling healthcare professionals to reach patients in remote areas and improve access to healthcare services (Khang & Ragimova et al., 2022).

Despite the vast potential, there are several challenges that need to be overcome. One of the major challenges is data privacy and security. The integration of computer vision, AI, and IoT involves the collection and analysis of large amounts of sensitive health data. Ensuring the privacy and security of this data is crucial to maintain patient trust and comply with regulatory requirements. Robust cybersecurity measures, encryption techniques, and strict data governance frameworks are essential to address these challenges.

Another challenge is the ethical use of AI and computer vision in healthcare. Transparency, fairness, and accountability are critical factors in the development and deployment of these technologies. Ensuring that algorithms are unbiased, explainable, and accountable is essential to prevent any unintended consequences and biases in decision-making processes. Ethical guidelines and frameworks should be developed to guide the responsible use of these technologies.

In terms of future directions, continued research and development are necessary to improve the accuracy and efficiency of computer vision and AI algorithms in healthcare. Advancements in deep learning, neural networks, and edge computing will further enhance the capabilities of these technologies. Additionally, interdisciplinary collaborations between healthcare professionals, computer scientists, and engineers will drive innovation and promote the adoption of these technologies in healthcare settings.

In conclusion, the integration of computer vision, AI, and IoT in healthcare holds tremendous potential to revolutionize the industry and improve patient outcomes. While there are challenges to overcome, addressing issues related to data privacy, security, and ethics will pave the way for a future where technology plays a vital role in transforming healthcare delivery.

## 4.7 FUTURE SCOPE

The transformative potential of computer vision, AI, and IoT integration in healthcare is vast, and there are numerous opportunities for improving patient outcomes and optimizing healthcare delivery. However, there are also significant challenges that must be addressed to realize the full potential of these technologies. Here are some possible future directions and areas of development for this field:

- **Improved data interoperability**: One of the key challenges facing the integration of computer vision, AI, and IoT in healthcare is the lack of interoperability between different data sources and systems. In the future, efforts to standardize data formats and develop common data models will be essential to facilitate the seamless integration of these technologies into healthcare workflows.
- **Highly automated**: Automation is a key area where these technologies can have a transformative impact on healthcare. The use of computer vision, AI, and IoT can help automate tasks such as triaging patients, monitoring vital signs, and identifying anomalies in medical images. In the future, we can expect to see increased use of automation in healthcare, which will help reduce errors and improve efficiency.
- **Personalized medicine**: The use of these technologies in healthcare can also help enable personalized medicine. By analyzing large amounts of patient data, including genomic data, medical imaging, and electronic health records, AI algorithms can help identify individualized treatment plans and predict which treatments will be most effective for each patient.
- **Remote patient monitoring**: IoT devices such as wearables and sensors can help facilitate remote patient monitoring, allowing healthcare providers to monitor patients outside the hospital setting. In the future, we can expect to see increased use of these technologies, which will help reduce healthcare costs and improve patient outcomes.
- **Ethical considerations**: As with any technology, there are ethical considerations surrounding the use of computer vision, AI, and IoT in healthcare. These technologies raise questions about patient privacy, data ownership, and algorithmic bias, among other issues. In the future, it will be important to address these ethical considerations

The integration of computer vision, AI, and IoT in healthcare has the potential to revolutionize the field, but there are also significant challenges that must be addressed. Moving forward, efforts to improve data interoperability, increase automation, enable personalized medicine, facilitate remote patient monitoring, and address ethical considerations will be essential to realizing the full potential of these technologies in healthcare (Khang & AI and IoT Technology and Applications for Smart Healthcare, 2023).

## 4.8 KEY TERMS

- **Artificial Intelligence (AI)** refers to the development and implementation of computer systems and algorithms that can perform tasks that typically require human intelligence. AI enables machines to simulate human intelligence by learning, reasoning, and making decisions based on data and patterns. It encompasses a wide range of techniques, including machine learning, natural language processing, computer vision, and robotics. AI systems are designed to analyze and interpret complex data, recognize patterns, adapt to new information, and perform tasks with varying degrees of autonomy. The goal of AI is to mimic and extend human capabilities, enabling machines to perceive, understand, and interact with the world in ways that were previously possible only for humans.
- **Internet of Things (IoT)** refers to a network of physical objects, devices, and sensors that are connected to the Internet and can collect, exchange, and analyze data. These objects, often embedded with sensors and actuators, can communicate with each other and with other systems or devices over the internet, enabling them to interact and share information.
- **Computer vision** is a field of artificial intelligence and computer science that focuses on enabling computers or machines to interpret and understand visual information from digital images or videos. It involves the development and implementation of algorithms, models, and systems that enable machines to extract meaningful information and make sense of visual data.
- **Telehealth,** also known as telemedicine, refers to the use of telecommunications technology to provide healthcare services remotely. It involves the exchange of medical information and the delivery of healthcare services, including consultations, diagnoses, monitoring, and treatment, using digital communication tools and platforms.
- **Deep Learning** is a subset of machine learning that focuses on the development and application of artificial neural networks, known as deep neural networks, to model and solve complex problems. It is inspired by the structure and function of the human brain, specifically

## REFERENCES

Ageron, B., Bentahar, O., & Gunasekaran, A. (2020, July). Digital supply chain: Challenges and future directions. *Supply Chain Forum: An International Journal*, *21*(3), 133–138. Taylor & Francis. www.tandfonline.com/doi/abs/10.1080/16258312.2020.1816361

Atitallah, S. B., Driss, M., Boulila, W., & Ghézala, H. B. (2020). Leveraging deep learning and IoT big data analytics to support the smart cities development: Review and future directions. *Computer Science Review*, *38*, 100303. www.sciencedirect.com/science/article/pii/S1574013720304032

Bajwa, J., Munir, U., Nori, A., & Williams, B. (2021). Artificial intelligence in healthcare: Transforming the practice of medicine. *Future Healthcare Journal*, *8*(2), e188. www.ncbi.nlm.nih.gov/pmc/articles/PMC8285156/

Brauner, P., Dalibor, M., Jarke, M., Kunze, I., Koren, I., Lakemeyer, G., & Ziefle, M. (2022). A computer science perspective on digital transformation in production. *ACM Transactions on Internet of Things*, *3*(2), 1–32. https://dl.acm.org/doi/abs/10.1145/3502265

Chen, D., & Zhang, R. (2022). *Exploring research trends of emerging technologies in health metaverse: A bibliometric analysis*. SSRN 3998068. https://papers.ssrn.com/sol3/papers.cfm?abstract_id=3998068

Chengoden, R., Victor, N., Huynh-The, T., Yenduri, G., Jhaveri, R. H., Alazab, M., & Gadekallu, T. R. (2023). Metaverse for healthcare: A survey on potential applications, challenges and future directions. *IEEE Access*. https://ieeexplore.ieee.org/abstract/document/10034994/

Gill, S. S., Tuli, S., Xu, M., Singh, I., Singh, K. V., Lindsay, D., & Garraghan, P. (2019). Transformative effects of IoT, Blockchain and Artificial Intelligence on cloud computing: Evolution, vision, trends and open challenges. *Internet of Things*, *8*, 100118. https://ui.adsabs.harvard.edu/abs/2019arXiv191101941S/abstract

Gubbi, J., Buyya, R., Marusic, S., & Palaniswami, M. (2013). Internet of things (IoT): A vision, architectural elements, and future directions. *Future Generation Computer Systems*, *29*(7), 1645–1660. www.sciencedirect.com/science/article/pii/S0167739X13000241

Khang, A. (2021). Material4Studies. In *Material of computer science, artificial intelligence, data science, IoT, blockchain, cloud, metaverse, cybersecurity for studies*. www.researchgate.net/publication/370156102_Material4Studies

Khang, A., Abdullayev, V. A., Hrybiuk, O., & Shukla, A. K. (2024). *Computer vision and AI-integrated IoT technologies in medical ecosystem* (1st ed.). CRC Press. https://doi.org/10.1201/9781003429609

Khang, A. (Ed.). (2024). *AI and IoT Technology and Applications for Smart Healthcare Systems* (1st ed.). Auerbach Publications. https://doi.org/10.1201/9781032686745

Khang, A. (Eds.). (2024). *AI and IoT-based technologies for precision medicine*. IGI Global Press. ISBN: 9798369308769. https://doi.org/10.4018/979-8-3693-0876-9

Khang, A., Ragimova, N. A., Hajimahmud, V. A., & Alyar, V. A. (2022). Advanced technologies and data management in the smart healthcare system. In *AI-Centric smart city ecosystems: Technologies, design and implementation* (1st ed., vol. 16, p. 10). CRC Press. https://doi.org/10.1201/9781003252542-16

Khang, A., Rana, G., Tailor, R. K., & Hajimahmud, V. A. (Eds.). (2023). *Data-Centric AI solutions and emerging technologies in the healthcare ecosystem*. CRC Press. https://doi.org/10.1201/9781003356189

Khanh, H. H., & Khang A.(2021). The role of artificial intelligence in blockchain applications. In *Reinventing manufacturing and business processes through artificial intelligence* (vol. 2, pp. 20–40). CRC Press. https://doi.org/10.1201/9781003145011-2

Rana, G., Khang, A., Sharma, R., Goel, A. K., & Dubey, A. K. (Eds.). (2021). *Reinventing manufacturing and business processes through artificial intelligence*. CRC Press. https://doi.org/10.1201/9781003145011

Rani, S., Chauhan, M., Kataria, A., & Khang, A. (Eds.). (2021). IoT equipped intelligent distributed framework for smart healthcare systems. *Networking and Internet Architecture*, *2*, 30. https://doi.org/10.48550/arXiv.2110.04997

Rath, K. C., Khang, A., & Roy, D. (2024). The role of internet of things (IoT) technology in industry 4.0. In *Advanced IoT technologies and applications in the industry 4.0 digital economy* (1st ed.). CRC Press. https://doi.org/10.1201/9781003434269-1

Okegbile, S. D., Cai, J., Yi, C., & Niyato, D. (2022). Human digital twin for personalized healthcare: Vision, architecture and future directions. *IEEE Network*. https://ieeexplore.ieee.org/abstract/document/9839649/

Smith, M. L., Smith, L. N., & Hansen, M. F. (2021). The quiet revolution in machine vision-a state-of-the-art survey paper, including historical review, perspectives, and future directions. *Computers in Industry*, *130*, 103472. www.sciencedirect.com/science/article/pii/S0166361521000798

Tortorella, G. L., Fogliatto, F. S., Mac Cawley Vergara, A., Vassolo, R., & Sawhney, R. (2020). Healthcare 4.0: Trends, challenges and research directions. *Production Planning & Control*, *31*(15), 1245–1260. https://www.tandfonline.com/doi/abs/10.1080/09537287.2019.1702226

Vermesan, O., Eisenhauer, M., Sundmaeker, H., Guillemin, P., Serrano, M., Tragos, E. Z., & Bahr, R. (2017). Internet of things cognitive transformation technology research trends and applications. In *Cognitive hyperconnected digital transformation: Internet of things intelligence evolution*. www.taylorfrancis.com/chapters/oa-edit/10.1201/9781003337584-3/internet-things-cognitive-transformation-technology-research-trends-applications-ovidiu-vermesan-markus-eisenhauer-harald-sundmaeker-patrick-guillemin-martin-serrano-elias-tragos-javier-vali%C3%B1o-arthur-van-derwees-alex-gluhak-roy-bahr

# 5 IoT-Based Classification of COVID-19 Using Feature Extraction and Hybrid Architectures of Convolutional Neural Network (CNN)

*Arulmurugan A., Kaviarasan R., and Kalaiyarasan R.*

## 5.1 INTRODUCTION

In December 2019, the novel COVID showed up in China's Wuhan city (Mohammed et al., 2020) and was reckoned on 31 December 2019 by the World Health Organization (WHO). The contagion resulted in a universal hazard and was called COVID-19 by the WHO on February 11 2020. COVID-19 is a set of contagions comprising ARDS and SARS. The contagion is projected via the respiratory passage while an unaffected individual interacts and has contact with the contaminated individual.

The contagion can transfer between persons in various ways that are at present indistinct. The contaminated person exhibits side effects within two to 14 days as per the brooding period of the Middle East Respiratory Syndrome coronavirus (MERS-COV), and also the Severe Acute Respiratory Syndrome (SARS). As indicated by WHO, the symptoms and indications of mild to moderate cases include dry cough, fever, and weakness, whereas in extreme cases, it includes fever, dyspnea (shortness of breath), and sleepiness (Chen et al., 2020).

Individuals suffering from different sicknesses, such as diabetes, asthma, and coronary illness, are powerless against this infection and may become extremely ill. The affected individuals are analyzed depending on side effects along with their clinical background. Fundamental indications of the individual showing symptoms are noticed. As of 10 April 2020, no specific treatment was found, and sufferers are dealt with ostensibly.

Medications such as antipyretic and hydroxychloroquine that are hostile to viruses are utilized in indicative medical care. Right now, there is no immunization produced to forestall the destructive infection, yet we can avoid the potential risk of forestalling the sickness. The odds of acquiring influenced by this infection may be decreased by washing hands consistently with a cleaning agent for 20 seconds and

DOI: 10.1201/9781032686745-5 

staying away from proximate contact with other persons by maintaining a distance of about one meter.

While sneezing and coughing, covering the nose and mouth with cloth or tissue and keeping away from touching the mouth, nose, and ears before washing the hands can assist in preventing it from spreading. SARS is an airborne disease that showed up in China in 2003 and spread to 26 nations, resulting in 8,000 cases around the world, wherein it moved from one individual to another. The symptoms of SARS include cold, fever, running nose, shuddering, discomfort, dyspnea, and myalgia. Acute Respiratory Distress Syndrome (ARDS) exhibits a fast beginning of irritation inside the lungs that prompts breathing difficulties with side effects including pale blue skin tone, exhaustion, and shortness of breath. ARDS is analyzed by doing PaO2/FiO2 proportion below 300 mm Hg. Until 10 April 2020, 1.6 million confirmed instances of COVID-19 were identified throughout the planet.

As of May 2, 2023, there were roughly 687 million global cases of COVID-19. Around 660 million people had recovered from the disease, while there had been almost 6.87 million deaths (Elflein, 2023; Ghani et al., 2020). Since no medication or immunization is made for relieving COVID-19, different paramedical organizations have guaranteed to build up an antibody for this infection. Less testing has additionally brought about this illness as we come up short on clinical assets because of the pandemic. Since a great many are testing positive step by step throughout the planet, it is beyond the realm of imagination to expect to test every one of the people who show indications. Aside from clinical systems, AI gives a ton of help in distinguishing the sickness with the assistance of picture and text-based information. AI can be utilized for the ID of novel COVID. In any case, AI requires a tremendous measure of information for arranging or anticipating sicknesses (Rana & Khang et al., 2021).

Administered AI calculations need clarified information for characterizing the content or picture into various classes. Since the previous decade, an enormous measure of progress has been made in this space for settling some basic activities. The recent pandemic has pulled in numerous specialists throughout the planet to tackle this issue. According to Johns Hopkins University, various specialists in X-beam pictures constructed an AI model that assembles X-beam pictures to find out whether it is COVID-19 or not; the latest data given by Johns Hopkins University shows the metadata of the X-beam pictures (Abdulkareem et al., 2019).

AI strategies are a part of the field of AI, which is immovably identified with insights space. It centers on creating procedures and calculations that permit PCs to use insight to learn and acquire knowledge. Conversely, Convolutional Neural Network (CNN) is among the settled techniques of profound learning. A CNN is made from two center constructions – pooling and convolutional layers (Khang & Hajimahmud et al., 2023).

The convolutional layer's information is coordinated as highlight maps in which everything is associated with the last layer via a bunch of loads. The amount results of these loads are forwarded toward an indirect section like the Rectified Linear Unit (ReLU). Conversely, the pooling layer part worries about converging the highlights alongside semantic similitude. Herein, learning implies the framework that possibly will perceive and grasp input case information that could be utilized for dynamics and forecasts. The initial pace of taking measures includes information gathering from various sources utilizing various methods.

The following stage includes the arrangement of information by pre-preparing it to liberate it from mistakes and diminish the space proportions via the picking end of the information of either premium or unimportant information. Hence, the utilization of insights, rationale, likelihood, control hypothesis, and so on are utilized in the plan of calculations to work with the investigation of information and recovery of data from past encounters. In the following interaction, the model is tried to decide the framework's presentation, just as exactness. Ultimately, the framework is advanced by utilizing the novel rules or dataset to ad-lib the prototype.

AI methods are utilized to anticipate, characterize, and perceive designs. There are a few regions where the utilization of AI can be employed, and a portion of the spaces incorporate email sifting, internet searching, face labeling and acknowledgment, website page positioning, gaming, character acknowledgment, mechanical technology, forecast of illness, and the board of traffic. As of late, AI is utilized to dissect biomedical information that is exceptionally dimensional in nature (Mostafa et al., 2019).

## 5.2 RELATED WORKS

Early recognition of this illness can help in the convenient segregation of patients and screen their wellbeing status (Mohammed & Al-Khateeb et al., 2018). AI-based methodologies can be utilized to investigate the lungs' X-beam/CT pictures to recognize patients influenced by pneumonia because of COVID-19 contamination. This procedure can be utilized as an elective where COVID-19 units are not accessible, particularly in non-industrial nations where a huge populace is influenced by this infection yet no actions could be masterminded to affirm the suspects for COVID-19.

Directed learning procedures have shown incredible advancement in the early location and conclusion of infections. For example, in Mohammed & Abd Ghani et al. (2018), a choice emotionally supportive network is proposed for the forecast of diabetes utilizing AI methods (Khang & Misra et al., 2023). Three AI calculations were utilized that incorporate CNN, Random Forest, and Support Vector Machine (SVM). The examinations showed promising outcomes for an arrangement of 768 patients into diabetic and non-diabetic gatherings. Additionally, Arunkumar et al. (2020) thought about most mainstream AI procedures usually utilized for the discovery of breast tumors.

The techniques executed include Random Forest, K-Nearest Neighbor (kNN), and Naïve Bayes classifiers. In Obaid et al. (2018), a wavelet change and SVM-based approach is proposed for the arrangement of brain tumors into two distinct classes: benign and malignant. Creator, in Shi et al. (2020) estimated the indicative execution by researching 15 distinctive groupings and a few component determination techniques in glioma reviewing.

The outcomes demonstrated that the blend of highlight choice with straight SVM and Multilayer Perceptron (MLP) accomplished the best execution. An exhaustive evaluation of AI-based modern methodologies in clinical picture investigation can be found in Dansana et al. (2020). In demonstrating hatred for the accomplishment of AI, it draws near their presentation that is exceptionally influenced by the nature of the hand-engineered highlights.

The hand-designed highlights are not ideal, and furthermore, it is a tedious errand (Fang et al., 2020). This is the principal disadvantage of the AI approach; regardless of the achievement, these methods experience the ill effects of genuine corruption in execution. The elective methodology, which has become a hot examination subject in our time, is to extricate programmed ideal highlights from the information.

These methods have not just removed the hindrance of manual element extraction but also improved the arrangement precision. A few methods dependent on Deep Learning (DL) have been advanced to accomplish these objectives: programmed highlight extraction and improving order exactness. With upgrades in PC equipment, it has become plausible to prepare an ever-increasing number of complex models. DL draws near, particularly CNNs, have shown their productivity for different PC vision undertakings, for example, object identification, common language handling, picture division, and arrangement.

Spurred from the PC vision local area, the clinical local area has likewise received the model to settle numerous clinical picture examination assignments. For example, in Liang et al. (2020), creators examined two notable profound neural organizations, Inception and VGG16, for the determination of pneumonia from pictures of chest X-beam. It was accounted for that VGG16 brought about higher arrangement exactness contrasted with the Inception Model.

Division of lung X-beam pictures utilizing profound CNNs is proposed by Wong et al. (2020) for improving the exhibition during the clinical analysis of different illnesses in lungs, like the cellular breakdown in the lungs, tuberculosis, or lung opacities. Analysts in Brunese et al. (2020) utilized an unaided component learning dependent on limited Boltzmann machines to include extraction with generative learning targets. It consolidates both generative and discriminative learning destinations with convolutional characterization for the arrangement of lung Computed Tomography (CT) pictures.

Because of histology pictures, Cohen et al. (2020) built up a dependable framework to improve the demonstrative quality for distinguishing proof of bosom malignant growth. Two AI approaches were analyzed: SVM was utilized as a classifier employing high-quality highlights, while another methodology depends on CNNs for programming, including learning and arrangement.

The outcomes demonstrated that CNN performed better than the classifier, dependent on carefully assembled highlights. In Van et al. (2021), different CNN designs were examined for the arrangement and recognition of interstitial lung infection and thoracic-stomach lymph hub separately. Further examination was performed to assess the impact of spatial picture setting and dataset scale on classifier execution, as well as the utilization of move gaining from pre-prepared ImageNet in the space of picture investigation.

Other than customary down-examining layers, Yoo et al. (2020) proposed an atrous convolution as an elective layer in the profound CNNs. Since CNNs generally misuse down examining layers to build the open field and gain conceptual semantic data, nonetheless, the down testing additionally diminishes the component guides' spatial measurements that may not be alluring for semantic division undertakings.

The atrous convolutions, then again, can expand the responsive field without changing the element guides' spatial measurement. A complete investigation of the current-day encouragement in AI, explicitly in DL, that helped in recognizing, ordering, and measuring the examples in clinical pictures is introduced in He and Zhang et al. (2016). Notwithstanding the accomplishment of DL models, their application for the assessment of the clinical picture is an especially difficult assignment.

The more profound organizations generally require huge datasets for preparation; in any case, huge named datasets of clinical pictures are not plentiful contrasted with vision-related datasets, for example, ImageNet (Szegedy et al., 2015). Likewise, the irregular datasets and helpless portrayal can make the issue much more unpredictable. Additionally, the protection and classification concerns identified with the clinical information of patients likewise limit the admittance to the information (Raghu et al., 2019).

To defeat this restricted accessibility of named information, scientists proposed information expansion methods. The information expansion method is used to lift the measure of preparing information by working in different changes like pivot, scaling, interpretations, and so forth on the first information. It additionally helps to lessen the regular issue of overfitting. A point-by-point audit of ongoing expansion strategies for DL is depicted in subtleties by Rajpurkar et al. (2017). Information increase is likewise embraced in different clinical picture investigation applications, for example, semantically fragmenting the different sclerosis injuries utilizing Magnetic Resonance Imaging (MRI) of the cerebrum (Wang et al., 2017), cardiovascular picture improvement and division or recreation (Yadav et al., 2019), mitosis recognition in bosom disease histology pictures (Vaishya et al., 2020), and mind tumor division utilizing MRI pictures (Abràmoff et al., 2016).

Alternately, scientists enjoy the benefit of AI-based Internet of Things (IoT) in the field of clinical sciences for demonstrative purposes. For example, Gulshan et al. (2016) proposed the use of IoT that identifies respiratory movement continuously by checking a diabetic patient's breathing to analyze Diabetic Ketoacidosis (DKA). They utilized the C-band detecting strategy by misusing the microwave-detection stage (MSP) as a nonintrusive respiratory observing framework. They further utilized pinnacle discovery calculation that gets respiratory rate for ID of Kussmaul relaxing. Essentially, Fauw et al. (2018) utilized the S-band detecting procedure to portray meandering examples in patients experiencing dementia. Afterward, specialists fused SVM as an example characterization calculation.

## 5.3 SYSTEM MODEL

In this study, several images of X-rays of different origins were meticulously elected to organize reasonably big COVID-19 X-rays of verified patients, especially normal datasets versus COVID-19, that are delineated as contagious sufferers. This is later combined with common images of X-rays for an additional assured COVID-19 diagnosis. Figure 5.1 shows the proposed architecture of extraction and classifying the data to detect the disease and its stage.

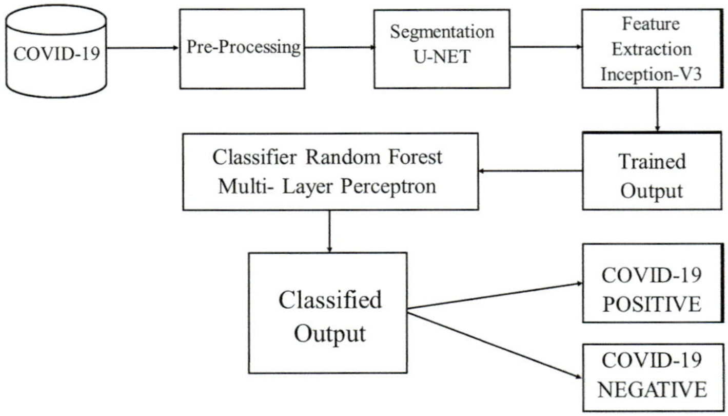


**FIGURE 5.1** The proposed architecture of extraction and classifying the data (Khang, 2021).

### 5.3.1 U-Net-Based Segmentation

The U-Net, as mentioned in Figure 5.2, employs the operator of the deconvolution rather than the operator of up-sampling within the decoding pathway and administers zero paddings to maintain the output image resolution similar to that of the input images.

Hence, the border region's cropping operator is not needed by the network. In the encoding pathway, each block possesses two convolutional layers having a stride of 1, 3x3 filter, and Rectified Linear Unit (ReLU) actuation that enhances the quantity of characteristic maps from 1 to 1024. To down-sample, max-pooling having a stride of 2x2 is employed towards the edge of each block, excluding the final one. Hence, the feature maps' size reduces from 240×240 to 15×15.

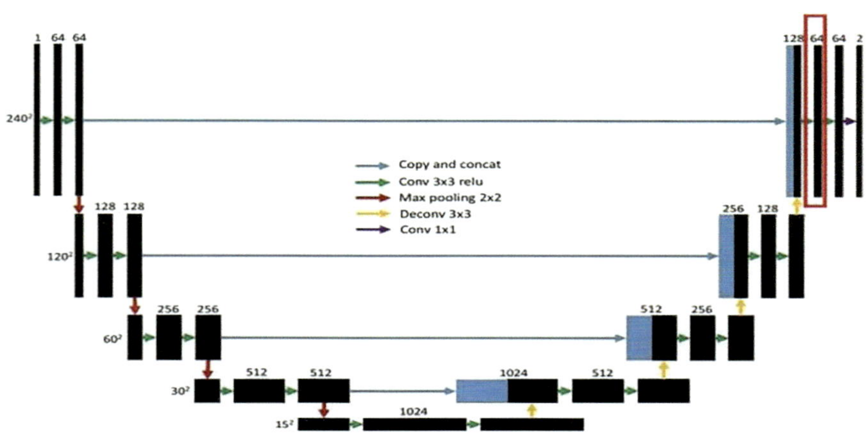


**FIGURE 5.2** The U-Net architecture.

Each block in the decoding pathway commences with a deconvolution layer of similar size filter within the decoding pathway and 2x2 stride that dualizes the feature maps' size in two-way directions but reduces the feature map numbers by two. Hence, the feature maps' size is enhanced from $15 \times 15$ to $240 \times 240$. In each sampling block, the feature maps are reduced in half by the two convolutional layers post-catenating the deconvolutional characteristic maps and the maps of characteristics out of the encoding path, as shown in Figure 5.2.

Initially, the data is pre-processed to remove the noise and resize the image. Then, the image was segmented for edge normalization and smoothing of the image. This segmented image has been extracted in their features using Mask RCNN.

### 5.3.2 Feature Extraction Using Inception-V3

Inception-V3 is a convolutional neural network architecture belonging to the Inception family that creates various enhancements like factorized 7x7 convolutions, employing Label Smoothing, and using an auxiliary classifier for propagating label data under the network (accompanying the usage of batch normalization for side head layers).

Inception-V3 enhances upon the preceding architectures by being extra computationally economical. The inception model's fundamental building blocks are Inception Modules. Inception Modules permit deeper networks and effectual computation via dimensionality diminution alongside the convolution of 1*1. Module segments are proposed to address the problem of overfitting, computational cost, and other various problems.

The fundamental notion of training the module of inception is to create different various dimensions filters for running side-by-side instead of in sequence order. The Inception Modules' networks possess an additional 1*1 layer of convolution ahead of the 3*3 and 5*5 convolutional layers that make the procedure computationally economical and resilient. In this research, an Inception-V3 model that is pre-trained (Cancer Imaging Archive trained) is brought in. Later, the 128x1 dense layers substitute the model's classification part, that is, the model's head – 3x1 and 12x1 – for binary classification and trinary classification accordingly.

Then, the model is improved on MRI images for finer extraction of attributes. To train, Inception-V3 has bestowed an input figure 3 of 224*224*3; then, the input undergoes different modules of inception that assist in avoiding overfitting whilst decreasing the computational cost. Subsequent to passing via the Inception Modules, there is a passage of input towards dimensions with thick layers like 128*1 and 3*1/2*1 to segment. In Figure 5.3, the Inception-V3 architecture is presented.

### 5.3.3 Random Forest and Multilayer Perceptron-Based Classification

The haphazard forest represents a collective sorter made by joining the decision trees of fundamental K. To have the initial dataset, the following Equation 5.1 is used.

$$D = \{(X_1, y_1), (X_2, y_2) \ldots\ldots\ldots (X_n, y_n)\} \tag{5.1}$$

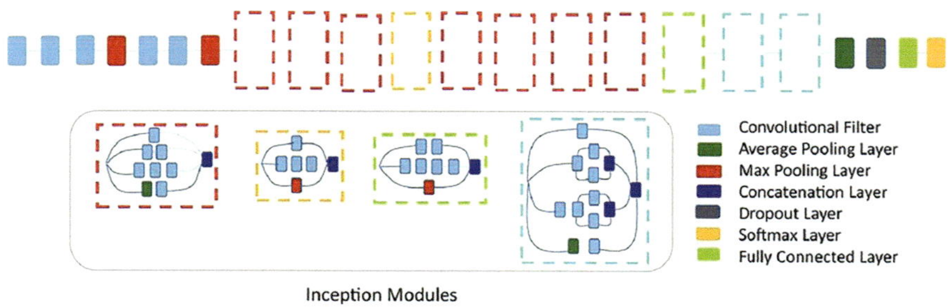


**FIGURE 5.3** Inception-V3 architecture.

Out of the initial datasets, haphazardly chosen data sub-sets $x_1, y_1 \sim (X, Y)$are used in constructing the sorter$h_k(x)$; as said in Equation 5.2, the collective sorter could be portrayed as:

$$h = \{h_1(X), \ldots h_k(X)\} \tag{5.2}$$

### 5.3.4 Sampling of Bagging

The algorithm of haphazard forest employs the technique of sampling of bagging for generating sub-sets of K training out of the initial set of data (Ghani et al., 2020). Every training subset's size is around two-thirds of the initial set of data, in which every sampling remains haphazard. To sample, the possibility on gathering each moment within the set of samples remains alongside an m sum, that remains (1/m); the possibility of without acquiring remains (1–1/m). Succeeding the sampling of m, there is no gathering. The possibility remains$(1-1/m)^m$. If m directs to infinity, then$m \rightarrow \infty$, $(1-1m)^m \rightarrow 1e \simeq \sim 0.368$. To be specific, in every round of bagging's random sampling, the sample set does not gather data of around 36.8% in the training set.

The data of around 36.8% that is not sampled in this section is frequently called Out of Bag (OOB). This information is never made to fit the model of the set of tutoring and remains capable of, hence, employing it to examine the model's generalization potential. Using the sampling of bagging, created sub-sets of k training create decision trees of k. Aimed at the haphazard forests' decision tree algorithm, the algorithm of CART is presently and extensively employed. The CART algorithm's method of node splitting remains the algorithm center. The algorithm of CART employs the coefficient of Gini methodology for executing the dividing of nodes.

The coefficient of Gini identifies the possibility where a haphazardly chosen sample set's sample remains divided. The lesser the index of Gini, the lesser the possibility there will be a split in the chosen sample in the set, and the greater the set's purity, and contrariwise, the lesser the set's purity. To be specific, the index of Gini (Gini impurity) = (possibility of selection of sample) * (possibility of misclassification of sample) is explained in Equation 5.3.

$$Gini(p) = \sum_{k=1}^{k} p_k (1 - p_k) = 1 - \sum_{k=1}^{k} p_k^2 \tag{5.3}$$

Here is a description:

- pk mentions the possibility that the chosen sample associates toward the category of k and the possibility in which the split sample remains (1-pk).
- Sample set has categories of k, and a haphazardly chosen sample could associate toward whichever categories of k, hence totaling all categories.
- Whilst categorized as twain, Gini (P) = 2p (1-p)

CART remains a tree of binary – while employing an attribute for splitting a set of samples, here exists solely twain sets: D1 set of sample that is equipollent with a provided attribute rate, and D2 sample set that is not equal to a provided attribute value, indeed an impound of binary treating of multitudinous values. To every one of the aforementioned splitting, the clarity of splitting the set of D sample towards twain sub-sets relies on the splitting attribute as Equation 5.4, i.e., the value of a particular attribute could be computed:

$$Gini(D, A) = \frac{|D_1|}{|D|} Gini(D_1) + \frac{|D_2|}{|D|} Gini(D_2) \tag{5.4}$$

Hence, for an attribute having multiple values (above two), there is a requirement for computing the subset's clarity *Gini (D, A)* is determined in Equation 5.4 following the splitting of the *D* sample with every value like the dividing point, (in which *Ai* depicts the distinctive Possible value *A*). Next, the lowest *Gini* index is identified out of all probable *Gini (D, Ai)*. This partition's dividing point remains the top-notch splitting juncture of the set of *D* samples via employing the *A* attribute.

### 5.3.5 Elucidation of Random Forest's Algorithm

Succeeding the haphazard sampling procedure, the consequential tree of decision is possibly instructed alongside data. As per the haphazard forests' concept, trees of decision possess an extremity of independence from one another, and this attribute guarantees the outcomes' self-dependence created by every tree of decision. Later, the residual task comprises two tasks: executing the Turing works upon every tree of decisions for generating outcomes and electing to choose the ideal answer out of the outcomes, as shown in Figure 5.4.

The distinct algorithm stages are possibly illustrated as follows:

- **Stage 1:** Presumes in order to sum the quantity of the dataset attributes: We remains S, but attributes of S are haphazardly chosen out to create the present decision tree's nodes then the result of S quantity stays constant to the tree of decision at the time of the tree growth.
- **Stage 2:** Divides the node employing the Gini methodology.

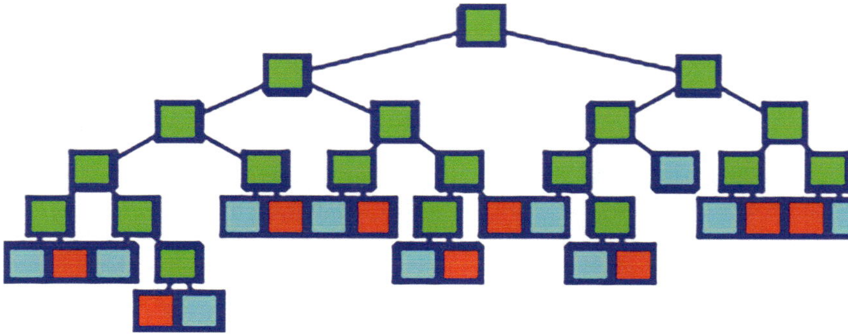

**FIGURE 5.4** Topology Classification Tree.

- **Stage 3:** Executes tutoring works upon every tree of decision.
- **Stage 4:** Elect to determine the ideal answer.

Definition 1 is Equation 5.5, which clearly explains classifiers set $h_1(x), h_2(x), \ldots, h_k(x)$ alongside vector (X, Y) haphazardly produced out of the dataset that describes the margin function as Equation 5.5:

$$mg(X,Y) = av_k I(h_k(X) = Y) - max_{j \neq Y} av_k I(h_k(X) = j) \tag{5.5}$$

In which I (•) represents the function of the indicator. If the mathematical statement inside brackets remains accurate and genuine, the value of it remains one; or else, the value remains zero. The function of margin is employed for calculating the level of mean accurate categorization up against mis categorization. The greater the rate, the finer the trust ability. Error possibly indicated in Equation 5.6 as:

$$PE^* = P_{X,Y}(mg(X,Y) < 0) \tag{5.6}$$

To trees of decision group, for the entire series Θ1, Θ2, . . . ., Θκ, the error would focus towards Equation 5.7:

$$P_{X,Y}(P\theta(h(X,\theta) = Y) - max_{j \neq Y} P\theta(h(X,\theta) = j) < 0 \tag{5.7}$$

It could be noted out of the top algorithm concept of a haphazard forest where the haphazard choosing methodology of sample numbers alongside the feature could be employed for preventing overfitting.

### 5.3.6 Multilayer Perceptron

The multilayer perceptron is the major noted and often employed kind of neural network. In many circumstances, the signals are broadcasted inside the network in a single direction: from input toward output. A loop is not present, i.e., every neuron's output does not influence the neuron on its own. The quantity of neurons present in the input layer is equivalent to the quantity of mensuration for the pattern issue, and the output layer's quantity of neurons is equivalent to the class quantity. The selection of the number of layers and neurons in every connection and layer is known as an architecture problem. This study's chief aim is to enhance it for an appropriate network having adequate specifications and excellent generalization for categorization or regression jobs. Back-propagation and Learning for MLP: Learning for the MLP is the procedure for adapting the weights of the connections to obtain a minimum dissimilarity between the desired output and the network output, as shown in Figure 5.5.

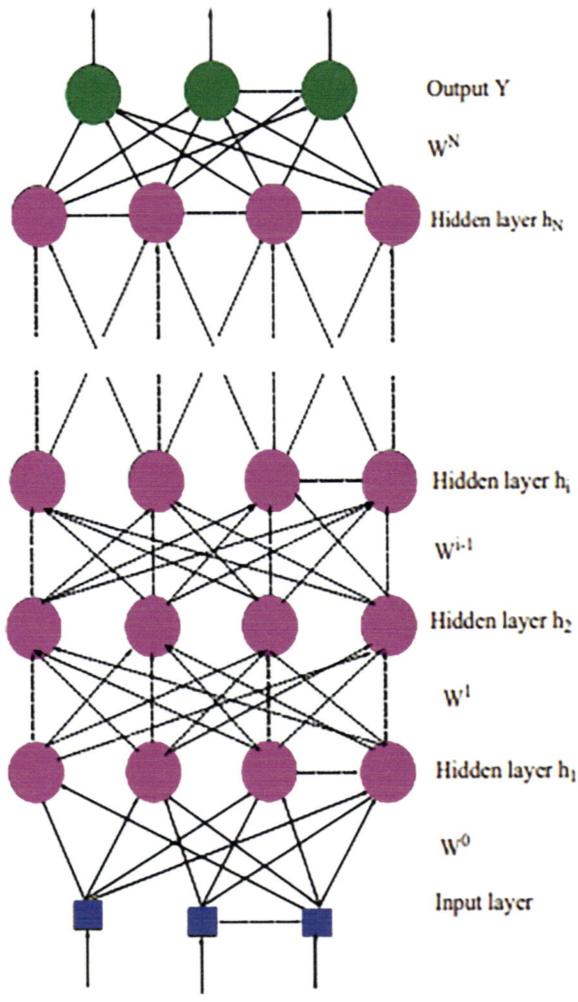


**FIGURE 5.5** Feedforward neural network structure.

Presuming that we employed an input layer having n0 neurons $X = \left(x_0, x_1 \ldots.., x_{n_0}\right)$ and with a function of sigmoid activation as Equation 5.8.

$$f\left(x\right) = \frac{1}{1 + e^{-x}} \tag{5.8}$$

To acquire the output of the network, it remains necessary to calculate the output of every unit present in every layer: presently, contemplate a group of hidden layers, ($h_1$, $h_2$ . . . $h_n$), presuming that $n_i$ are the number of neurons by every layer that is hidden $h_i$.

The first hidden layer for output is Equation 5.9.

$$h_i^j = f\left(\sum_{k=1}^{n_i=1} w_{k,j}^0 x_k\right) \qquad j = 1, \ldots. n_i \tag{5.9}$$

The outputs $h_i^j$ of the hidden layers' neurons are calculated as follows in Equation 5.10:

$$h_i^j = f\left(\sum_{k=1}^{n_i=1} w_{k,j}^{i-1} h_{i-1}^k\right) i = 2, \ldots.., N \, and \, j = 1, \ldots., n_i \tag{5.10}$$

Where $w_{k,j}^{i-1}$ represents the load betwixt the k neuron presents inside the hidden layer i and the neuron j present inside the hidden layer +1 and $n_i$ represents the neuron numbers inside the i$^{th}$ layer that is hidden. The i$^{th}$ result is probably derived like follows Equation 5.11:

$$h_i = \mathrm{t}\left(h_i^1, h_i^2, \ldots\ldots, h_i^{n_i}\right) \tag{5.11}$$

Calculation of the network output is done by Equations 5.12a and 5.12b:

$$y_i = f\left(\sum_{k=1}^{n_N} w_{k,j}^N h_N^k\right) \tag{5.12a}$$

$$Y = \left(y_1, \ldots y_j, \ldots., y_{N+1}\right) = F\left(W, X\right) \tag{5.12b}$$

Where $w_{k,j}^N$ represents the weight betwixt the neuron k presents inside the Nth layer that is hidden and neuron present inside the layer of output j represents the neuron numbers inside the Nth layer that is hidden $n_N$ represents the layer of output vector, $Y$ depicts the transfer function and represents the matrix of weights, and it is determined as Equations 5.13a and 5.13b:

$$W = \left[W^0, \ldots\ldots, W^j, \ldots.., W^N\right] \tag{5.13a}$$

$$W^i = \left(W_{j,k}^i\right) 0 \le i \le N, 1 \le j \le n_{i+1}, 1 \le k \le n_j, \, where \, W_{j,k}^i \in R \tag{5.13b}$$

To elucidate, $n = n_i \; \forall i = 1,\ldots..,N$ can be considered for all hidden layers. Where X represents the input of the neural network, f depicts the function of activation, $W^i$ depicts the matrix of weights between $t^{th}$ layer that is hidden, and the $(i+1)^{th}$ hidden layer, for $i = 1,\ldots..,N-1$, $W^0$ represents the matrix of weights betwixt the first layer that is hidden and layer in the input, and $W^{\bar{N}}$ depicts the matrix of loads betwixt the $N^{th}$ layer that is hidden and the output layer.

### 5.3.7 Performance Analysis

Datasets are used to evaluate the projected methodology. Then, the query images are selected arbitrarily as test images from the randomly selected images from the dataset as target images.

**Accuracy:** This shows the percentage of correctly classified instances in the course of classification. It is evaluated as Equation 5.14.

$$\text{Accuracy rate} = \frac{\text{True Positive} + \text{True Negative}}{\text{Total Instances}} * 100 \tag{5.14}$$

**Precision:** Its measure gives what proportion of data that is transmitted to the network actually had intrusion. The predicted positives (network predicted as intrusion is TP and FP) and the network actually having an intrusion are TP. This is used to measure the quality and exactness of the classifier, as shown in Equation 5.15:

$$\text{Precision} = \frac{\text{True Positive}}{\text{True Positive} + \text{False Positive}} \tag{5.15}$$

### 5.3.8 Dataset Description

This data (Lung Cancer Data, 2023) was used by Hong and Young to illustrate the power of the optimal discriminant plane even in ill-posed settings (applying the KNN method in the resulting plane gave 77% accuracy). The data described three types of pathological lung cancers. In Table 5.1, the image view of the various stages from the original image has been depicted in Table 5.2.

**TABLE 5.1**
**The Image View of the Various Stages**

| | | | | | |
|---|---|---|---|---|---|
| **Data Set Characteristics:** | Multivariate | Number of Instances: | 32 | Area: | Life |
| **Attribute Characteristics:** | Integer | Number of Attributes: | 56 | Date Donated | 1992–05–01 |
| **Associated Tasks:** | Classification | Missing Values? | Yes | Number of Web Hits: | 337982 |

**TABLE 5.2**
**Image View of the Various Stages from the Original Image 11.6 (a-l), Mask Drawn, Mask Segmented, Segmented, and the COVID-19**

| # | Original Image | Mask Drawn | Mask Segmented | Segmented | COVID-19 |
|---|---|---|---|---|---|
| 1. | 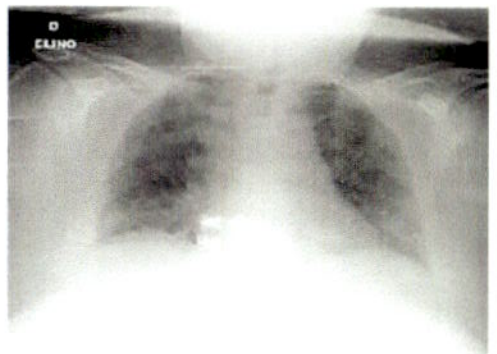 | 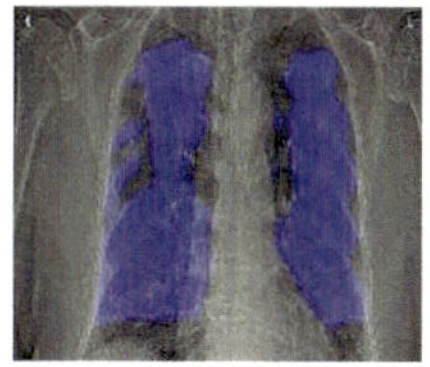 | 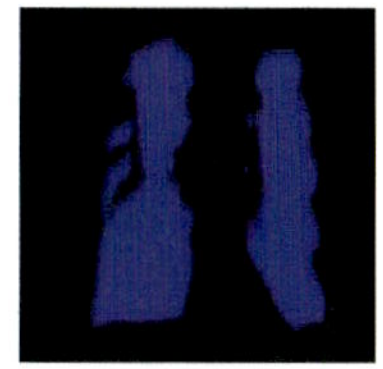 | 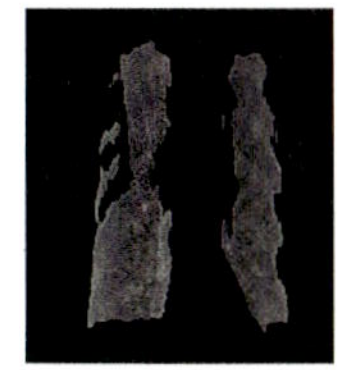 | Positive |
| 2. | 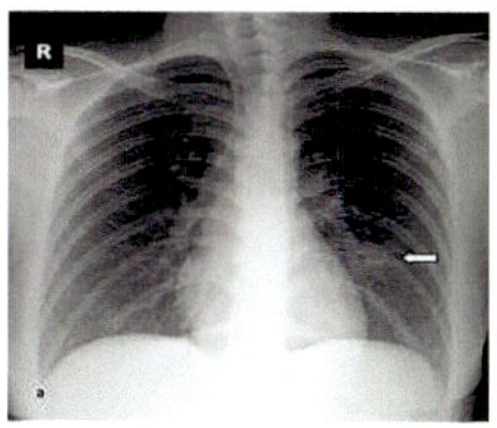 | 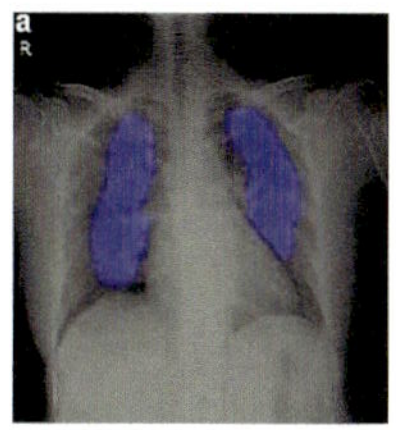 | 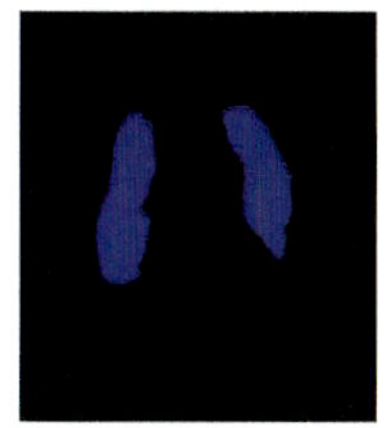 | 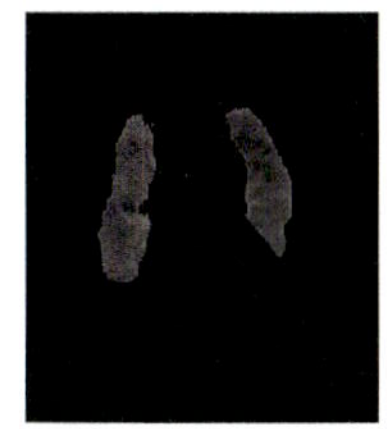 | Positive |
| 3. | 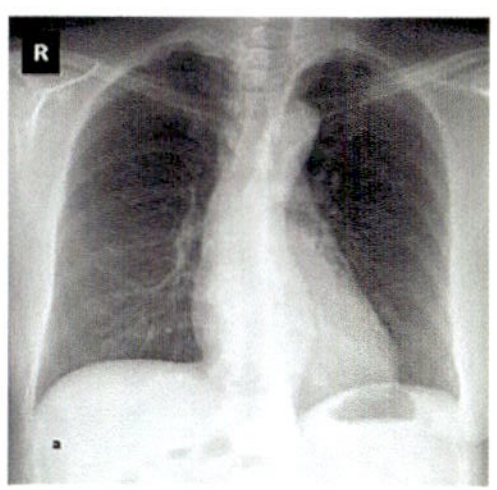 | 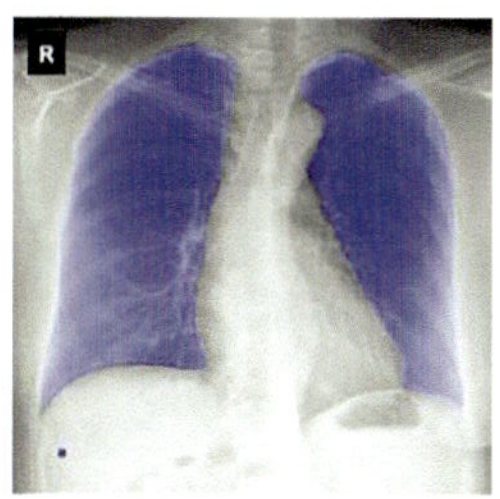 | 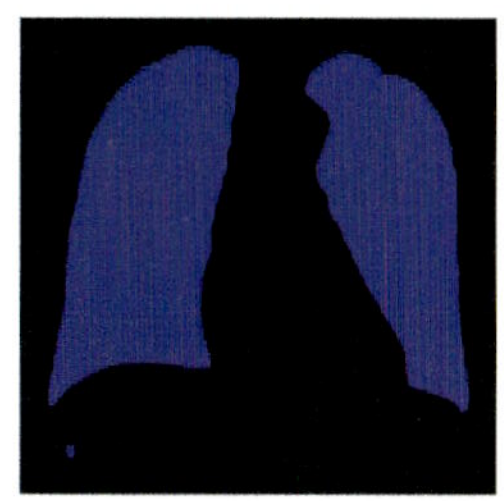 | 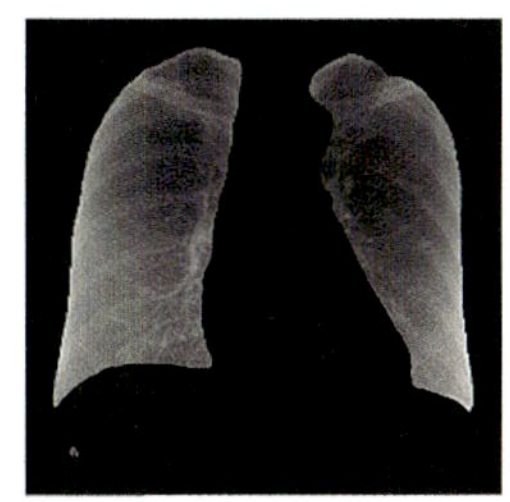 | Negative |

**TABLE 5.3**
**Comparison of the Existing and the Proposed Performance Metrics Using Lung Cancer Dataset**

| Metric | Random Forest (%) | | | CNN (%) | | | ResNet-50(%) | | | Inception-V3 (%) | | |
|---|---|---|---|---|---|---|---|---|---|---|---|---|
| Epoch | 25 | 50 | 100 | 25 | 50 | 100 | 25 | 50 | 100 | 25 | 50 | 100 |
| Area Under ROC | 87.11 | 89.01 | 95.55 | 89.11 | 91.22 | 92.95 | 91.34 | 93.52 | 95.25 | 94.56 | 94.65 | 96.56 |
| Precision | 84.44 | 87.11 | 94.80 | 86.15 | 89.14 | 90.62 | 89.21 | 92.21 | 95.87 | 90.32 | 91.23 | 93.27 |
| Recall | 83.33 | 84.03 | 86.47 | 85.23 | 86.11 | 84.22 | 87.24 | 90.12 | 92.98 | 90.17 | 89.17 | 90.17 |
| F-Measure | 82.11 | 83.11 | 92.45 | 85.14 | 85.18 | 89.30 | 87.30 | 90.21 | 93.36 | 89.34 | 90.56 | 92.65 |
| Accuracy | 87.11 | 87.30 | 87.91 | 92.10 | 92.31 | 92.4 | 90.03 | 90.14 | 90.31 | 94.18 | 94.81 | 95.12 |

The performance measures of various techniques of Random Forest, CNN, and ResNet-50 are compared with the proposed techniques of Proposed Inception-V3 in Table 5.3.

The classifier's output was determined from real-world IoT data (Rani et al., 2021), followed by the classification of instances with the same observation, and finally, a comparison of the performance measurements of various Random Forest, CNN, and ResNet-50 techniques with the proposed Inception-V3 techniques, as shown in Figure 5.6.

The Random Forest, CNN, and ResNet-50 approaches, on the other hand, generated the worst results, with a minimum Accuracy value at epoch-100 of about 87.91%,

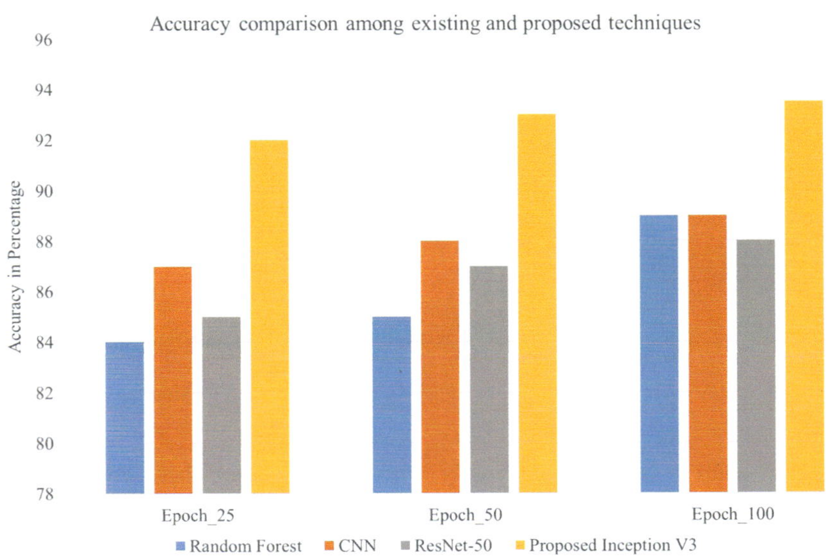


**FIGURE 5.6** Accuracy of comparison of the existing and proposed techniques.

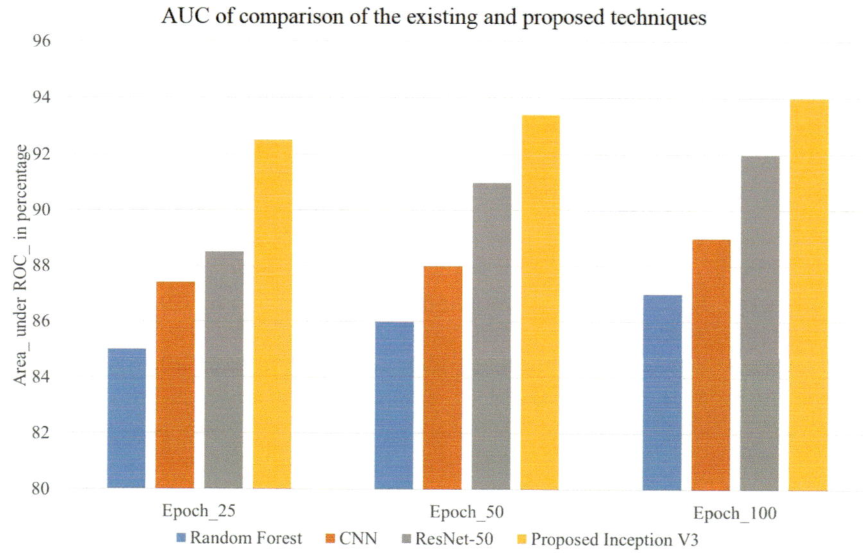


**FIGURE 5.7** AUC of comparison of the existing and proposed techniques.

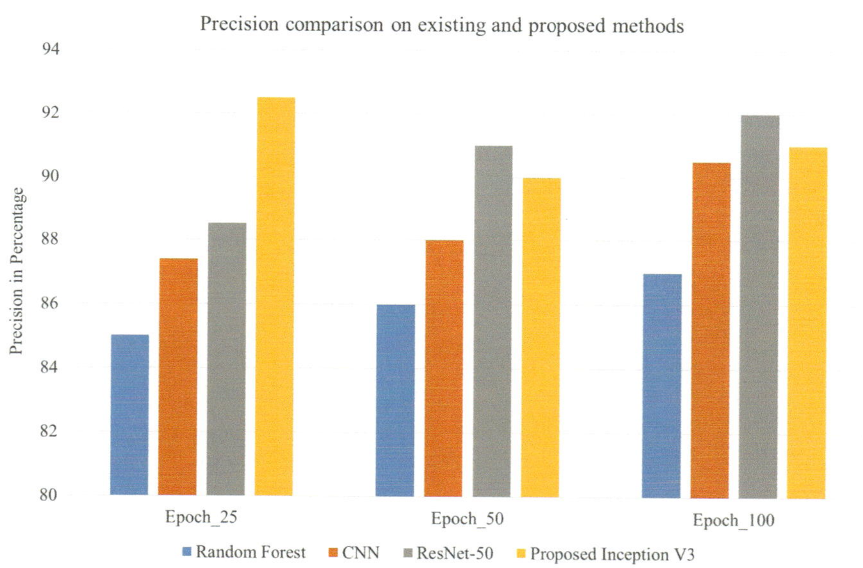


**FIGURE 5.8** Precision of comparison of the existing and proposed techniques.

92.4%, and 90.31%, respectively. Finally, when compared to other prototypes, the Proposed Inception-V3 technique is more effective, achieving a maximum accuracy value of 95.12%, as shown in Figure 5.7.

The Random Forest, CNN, and ResNet-50 approaches, on the other hand, generated the worst results, with a minimum Precision value at epoch-100 of about 87.91%, 92.4%, and 90.31%, respectively. Finally, when compared to other prototypes, the Proposed Inception-V3 technique is more effective, achieving a maximum precision value of 95.12%, as shown in Figure 5.8.

## 5.4 CONCLUSION

Several challenges are addressed and examined based on the experiment and deep analysis. First, limited publicly available image dataset for COVID-19 as a solution; the only dataset provided is the X-ray image with small samples. However, this issue raises another challenge which is a small sample for feature extraction and training purposes. Various features like TF/IDF and bag of words are being extracted from these clinical reports (Anh et al., 2024).

The machine learning algorithms are used for classifying clinical reports into four different classes. U-Net was employed to withdraw the functions and Inception-V3 was employed to isolate the COVID positive and negative data using an ensemble classifier. COVID positive data has been categorized for predicting the stage of the disease (Abdullayev et al., 2024).

## REFERENCES

Abdulkareem, K. H., M. A. Mohammed, S. S. Gunasekaran, M. N. Al-Mhiqani, A. A. Mutlag et al., "A Review of Fog Computing and Machine Learning: Concepts, Applications, Challenges, and Open Issues," *IEEE Access*, vol. 7, pp. 153123–153140, 2019. https://ieeexplore.ieee.org/abstract/document/8869895/

Abdullayev, V., A. Khang, İ. Rashad, A. Vusala, K. Sriram, P. T. N. Anh, "AI-Aided Computer Vision in Health Care System," *Computer Vision and AI-integrated IoT Technologies in Medical Ecosystem* (1st ed.), 2024. CRC Press. https://doi.org/10.1201/9781003429609-20

Abràmoff, M. D., Y. Lou, A. Erginay, W. Clarida, R. Amelon et al., "Improved automated detection of diabetic retinopathy on a publicly available dataset through integration of deep learning," *Investigative Ophthalmology & Visual Science*, vol. 57, no. 13, pp. 5200–5206, 2016. https://jov.arvojournals.org/article.aspx?articleid=2565719

Anh, P. T. N., V. Hahanov, Triwiyanto, R. Nazila Ali, R. İsmibeyli, V. Abdullayev, A. Vusala Alyar, "AI Models for Disease Diagnosis and Prediction of Heart Disease with Artificial Neural Networks," *Computer Vision and AI-integrated IoT Technologies in Medical Ecosystem* (1st ed.), 2024. CRC Press. https://doi.org/10.1201/9781003429609-9

Arunkumar, N., M. A. Mohammed, S. A. Mostafa, D. A. Ibrahim, J. J. Rodrigues et al., "Fully Automatic Model-Based Segmentation and Classification Approach for MRI Brain Tumor Using Artificial Neural Networks," *Concurrency and Computation: Practice and Experience*, vol. 32, no. 1, e4962, 2020. https://onlinelibrary.wiley.com/doi/abs/10.1002/cpe.4962

Brunese, L., F. Mercaldo, A. Reginelli, A. Santone, "Explainable Deep Learning for Pulmonary Disease and Coronavirus COVID-19 Detection from X-Rays," *Computer Methods and Programs in Biomedicine*, vol. 196, p. 105608, 2020. www.sciencedirect.com/science/article/pii/S0169260720314413

Chen, H., J. Guo, C. Wang, F. Luo, X. Yu et al., "Clinical Characteristics and Intrauterine Vertical Transmission Potential of Covid-19 Infection in Nine Pregnant Women: A Retrospective Review of Medical Records," *Lancet*, vol. 395, no. 10226, pp. 809–815, 2020. www.thelancet.com/journals/lancet/article/PIIS0140-6736(20)30360-3/fulltext?mod=article_inline

Cohen, J. P., P. Morrison, L. Dao, K. Roth, T. Q. Duong et al., "Covid-19 Image Data Collection: Prospective Predictions are the Future," arXiv preprint arXiv: 2006.11988, (Preprint), 2020. https://arxiv.org/abs/2006.11988

Dansana, D., R. Kumar, J. Das Adhikari, M. Mohapatra, R. Sharma et al., "Global Forecasting Confirmed and Fatal Cases of COVID-19 Outbreak Using Autoregressive Integrated Moving Average Model," *Frontiers in Public Health*, vol. 8, p. 580327, 2020. www.frontiersin.org/articles/10.3389/fpubh.2020.580327/full

Elflein, J. "Health, Pharma & Medtec, State of Health, Number of Coronavirus (COVID-19) Cases, Recoveries, and Deaths Worldwide as of May 2, 2023," Aug 30, 2023. https://www.statista.com/statistics/1087466/covid19-cases-recoveries-deaths-worldwide/

Fang, Y., H. Zhang, J. Xie, M. Lin, L. Ying et al., "Sensitivity of Chest CT for COVID-19: Comparison to RT-PCR," *Radiology*, vol. 296, no. 2, pp. 115–117, 2020. https://pubs.rsna.org/doi/abs/10.1148/radiol.2020200432

Fauw, J. De, J. R. Ledsam, B. Romera-Paredes, S. Nikolov, N. Tomasev et al., "Clinically Applicable Deep Learning for Diagnosis and Referral in Retinal Disease," *Nature Medicine*, vol. 24, no. 9, pp. 1342–1350, 2018. https://research.google/pubs/pub49788/

Ghani, Abd M. K., M. A. Mohammed, N. Arunkumar, S. A. Mostafa, D. A. Ibrahim et al., "Decision level fusion scheme for nasopharyngeal carcinoma identification using machine learning techniques," *Neural Computing and Applications*, vol. 32, no. 3, pp. 625–638, 2020. https://link.springer.com/article/10.1007/s00521-018-3882-6

Gulshan, V., L. Peng, M. Coram, M. C. Stumpe, D. Wu et al., "Development and Validation of a Deep Learning Algorithm for Detection of Diabetic Retinopathy in Retinal Fundus Photographs," *JAMA*, vol. 316, no. 22, pp. 2402–2410, 2016. https://jamanetwork.com/journals/jama/fullarticle/2588763/

He, K., X. Zhang, S. Ren, J. Sun, "Deep Residual Learning for Image Recognition," Proceedings of the IEEE Conference on Computer Vision and Pattern Recognition, Las Vegas, NV, pp. 770–778, 2016. http://openaccess.thecvf.com/content_cvpr_2016/html/He_Deep_Residual_Learning_CVPR_2016_paper.html

Khang, A. (2021). "Material4Studies," *Material of Computer Science, Artificial Intelligence, Data Science, IoT, Blockchain, Cloud, Metaverse, Cybersecurity for Studies*. https://www.researchgate.net/publication/370156102_Material4Studies

Khang, A., V. A. Hajimahmud, S. K. Gupta, J. Babasaheb, G. Morris, *AI-Centric Modelling and Analytics: Concepts, Designs, Technologies, and Applications* (1st ed.), 2023. CRC Press. https://doi.org/10.1201/9781003400110

Khang, A., A. Misra, S. K. Gupta, V. Shah, eds., *AI-Aided IoT Technologies and Applications in the Smart Business and Production*, 2023. CRC Press. https://doi.org/10.1201/9781003392224

Liang, T. et al., *Handbook of COVID-19 Prevention and Treatment*. The First Affiliated Hospital, Zhejiang University School of Medicine, Zhejiang University, China, 2020. www.ncbi.nlm.nih.gov/pmc/articles/PMC7210103/

Lung Cancer Data (LCD), 2023. The data set link https://archive.ics.uci.edu/ml/datasets/lung+cancer

Mohammed, M. A., M. K. Abd Ghani, N. Arunkumar, R. I. Hamed, M. K. Abdullah et al., "A Real Time Computer Aided Object Detection of Nasopharyngeal Carcinoma Using Genetic Algorithm and Artificial Neural Network Based on Haar Feature Fear," *Future Generation Computer Systems*, vol. 89, pp. 539–547, 2018. www.sciencedirect.com/science/article/pii/S0167739X18313670

Mohammed, M. A., K. H. Abdulkareem, A. S. Al-Waisy, S. A. Mostafa, S. AlFahdawi et al., "Benchmarking Methodology for Selection of Optimal COVID-19 Diagnostic Model Based on Entropy and TOPSIS Methods," *IEEE Access*, vol. 8, pp. 99115–99131, 2020. https://ieeexplore.ieee.org/abstract/document/9096375/

Mohammed, M. A., B. Al-Khateeb, A. N. Rashid, D. A. Ibrahim, M. K. Abd Ghani et al., "Neural Network and Multi-Fractal Dimension Features for Breast Cancer Classification from Ultrasound Images," *Computers & Electrical Engineering*, vol. 70, pp. 871–882, 2018. www.sciencedirect.com/science/article/pii/S0045790617331075

Mostafa, S. A., A. Mustapha, M. A. Mohammed, R. I. Hamed, N. Arunkumar et al., "Examining Multiple Feature Evaluation and Classification Methods for Improving the Diagnosis of Parkinson's Disease," *Cognitive Systems Research*, vol. 54, pp. 90–99, 2019. www.sciencedirect.com/science/article/pii/S1389041718308933

Obaid, O. I., M. A. Mohammed, M. K. Abd Ghani, S. A. Mostafa and F. Taha, "Evaluating the Performance of Machine Learning Techniques in the Classification of Wisconsin Breast Cancer," *International Journal of Engineering & Technology*, vol. 7, no. 4.36, pp. 160–166, 2018. www.downloadmaghaleh.com/wp-content/uploads/edd/maghaleh/1398/yosefi.wisconsin-min.pdf

Raghu, M., C. Zhang, J. Kleinberg, S. Bengio, "Transfusion: Understanding Transfer Learning for Medical Imaging," *Advances in Neural Information Processing Systems, Vancouver, Canada*, pp. 3342–3352, 2019. https://proceedings.neurips.cc/paper_files/paper/2019/hash/eb1e78328c46506b46a4ac4a1e378b91-Abstract.html

Rajpurkar, P., J. Irvin, K. Zhu, B. Yang, H. Mehta et al., "Chexnet: Radiologist-Level Pneumonia Detection on Chest X-Rays with Deep Learning," arXiv preprint arXiv: 1711.05225, 2017. https://arxiv.org/abs/1711.05225

Rana, G., A. Khang, R. Sharma, A. K. Goel, A. K. Dubey, eds., *Reinventing Manufacturing and Business Processes Through Artificial Intelligence*, 2021. CRC Press. https://doi.org/10.1201/9781003145011

Rani, S., M. Chauhan, A. Kataria, A. Khang, eds., "IoT Equipped Intelligent Distributed Framework for Smart Healthcare Systems," *Networking and Internet Architecture*, vol. 2, p. 30, 2021. https://doi.org/10.48550/arXiv.2110.04997

Shi, F., J. Wang, J. Shi, Z. Wu, Q. Wang et al., "Review of Artificial Intelligence Techniques in Imaging Data Acquisition, Segmentation and Diagnosis for COVID19," *IEEE Reviews in Biomedical Engineering*, pp. 1–13, 2020. https://ieeexplore.ieee.org/abstract/document/9069255/

Szegedy, C., W. Liu, Y. Jia, P. Sermanet, S. Reed et al., "Going Deeper with Convolutions," Proceedings of the IEEE Conference on Computer Vision and Pattern Recognition, Boston, MA, pp. 1–9, 2015. www.cv-foundation.org/openaccess/content_cvpr_2015/html/Szegedy_Going_Deeper_With_2015_CVPR_paper.html

Vaishya, R., M. Javaid, I. H. Khan, A. Haleem, "Artificial Intelligence (AI) Applications for COVID-19 Pandemic," *Diabetes & Metabolic Syndrome: Clinical Research & Reviews*, vol. 14, no. 4, pp. 337–339, 2020. www.sciencedirect.com/science/article/pii/S1871402120300771

Van, C. L., V. Puri, N. T. Thao, D. Le, "Detecting Lumbar Implant and Diagnosing Scoliosis from Vietnamese X-Ray Imaging Using the Pre-Trained API Models and Transfer Learning," *Computers, Materials & Continua*, vol. 66, no. 1, pp. 17–33, 2021. https://cdn.techscience.cn/uploads/attached/file/20201029/20201029020957_43302.pdf

Wang, X., Y. Peng, L. Lu, Z. Lu, M. Bagheri et al., "Chest X-Ray 8: Hospital-Scale Chest X-Ray Database and Benchmarks on Weakly-Supervised Classification and Localization of Common Thorax Diseases," Proceedings of the IEEE Conference on Computer Vision and Pattern Recognition, Honolulu, HI, pp. 2097–2106, 2017. http://openaccess.thecvf.com/content_cvpr_2017/html/Wang_ChestX-ray8_Hospital-Scale_Chest_CVPR_2017_paper.html

Wong, H. Y. F., H. Y. S. Lam, A. H. T. Fong, S. T. Leung, T. W. Y. Chin et al., "Frequency and Distribution of Chest Radiographic Findings nn COVID-19 Positive Patients," *Radiology*, vol. 296, no. 2, 201160, 2020. https://pubs.rsna.org/doi/abs/10.1148/radiol.2020201160

World Health Organization (WHO), "Coronavirus Disease 2019 (COVID-19): Situation Report," 2020. [Online]. https://apps.who.int/iris/handle/10665/331475

Yadav, S. S., S. M. Jadhav, "Deep Convolutional Neural Network Based Medical Image Classification for Disease Diagnosis," *Journal of Big Data*, vol. 6, no. 1, pp. 113, 2019. https://link.springer.com/article/10.1186/s40537-019-0276-2

Yoo, S. H., H. Geng, T. L. Chiu, S. K. Yu, D. C. Cho et al., "Deep Learning-Based Decision-Tree Classifier for COVID-19 Diagnosis from Chest X-Ray Imaging," *Frontiers in Medicine*, vol. 7, 427, 2020. www.frontiersin.org/articles/10.3389/fmed.2020.00427/full

# 6 Revolutionizing Healthcare Delivery

## *Applications and Impact of Cutting-Edge Technologies*

*Siva Subramanian R., Sudha K., Pooja E., Maheswari B., and Girija P.*

## 6.1 INTRODUCTION

Healthcare has undergone significant changes as a result of the rapid development of emerging technologies like machine learning (ML), artificial intelligence (AI), the Internet of Things (IoT), computer vision, robotics, blockchain, and robotic process automation (RPA). By boosting patient care, increasing diagnostic accuracy, reducing administrative procedures, and enabling data-driven decision-making, these technologies have the potential to completely transform the modern health system (Mozumder et al., 2022). The need for more effective and efficient healthcare delivery is one of the main factors driving the adoption of developing technologies in this industry. Worldwide healthcare systems are under tremendous strain as a result of the ageing global population, rising chronic illness load, and global population growth. Emerging technologies bring creative answers to these problems and improve accessibility to high-quality healthcare services.

Figure 6.1 represents different technologies used in healthcare enterprises. Artificial intelligence (AI) and machine learning (ML) have become effective technologies in the healthcare industry (Barragán-Montero et al., 2021). To find patterns, make predictions, and develop insights, ML systems may examine enormous volumes of patient data, including electronic health records (EHRs), medical imaging, and genetic data. Healthcare workers may use AI systems to help with precise diagnosis, treatment planning, and individualized care (Khang, Abdullayev & Hrybiuk et al., 2024). These innovations might improve clinical judgment, lessen diagnostic blunders, and boost patient outcomes. By facilitating the integration of medical equipment, wearables, and sensors into the healthcare ecosystem, the Internet of Things (IoT) has opened the way for linked healthcare (Zhang et al., 2022). Real-time data on patient vitals, medication adherence, and environmental conditions may be collected via IoT devices. This information may be utilized for personalized therapies, early diagnosis of health problems, and remote patient monitoring.

DOI: 10.1201/9781032686745-6

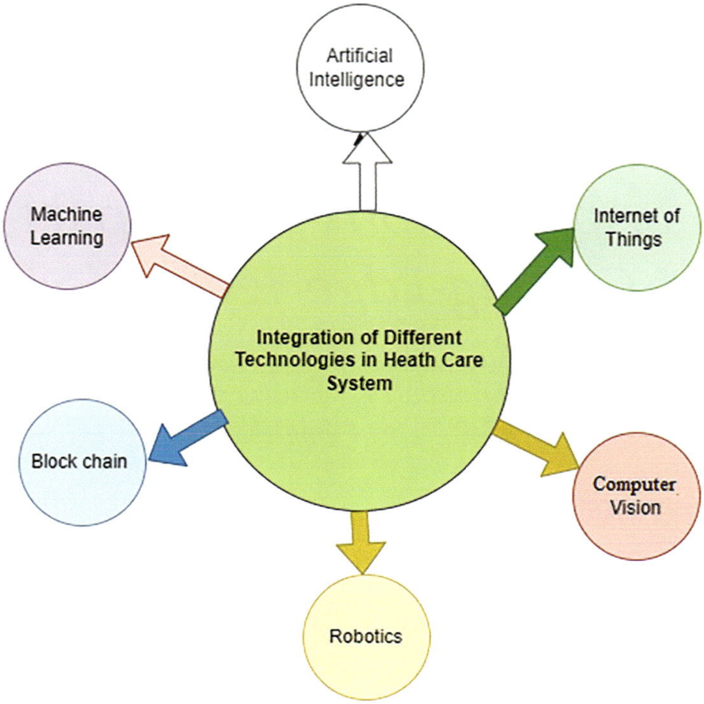


**FIGURE 6.1** Different technologies used in healthcare enterprises.

Additionally, the IoT offers telemedicine services, which let patients obtain medical treatment remotely, especially in underdeveloped regions or in times of emergency. Numerous uses for computer vision and robotics have been discovered in the medical field. Medical pictures like X-rays, CT scans, and MRIs may be analyzed using computer vision algorithms to look for anomalies, help in diagnosis, and facilitate surgery planning. The use of robotics, such as surgical and assistance robots, improves surgical accuracy, reduces invasiveness, and makes complicated treatments possible. In rehabilitation settings, robots and computer vision technologies are also used to help patients with mobility issues and enhance their quality of life (Anh et al., 2024).

The promise of blockchain technology to solve major issues with data security, interoperability, and patient privacy has helped it gain popularity in the healthcare industry. Blockchain offers a decentralized and secure platform for the exchange and storage of medical information, facilitating easy interoperability across various healthcare organizations. It improves the traceability and transparency of the drug supply chain, reducing the dangers of fake medications and guaranteeing patient safety.

Furthermore, while preserving patient privacy and sovereignty over their personal health information, blockchain supports permission management, data exchange, and medical research (Kassab et al., 2019). By eliminating manual duties and optimizing workflows, robotic process automation (RPA) is changing administrative procedures in the healthcare industry. RPA systems may automate time-consuming tasks like data entry, arranging appointments, and claim processing, giving healthcare personnel more time to concentrate on patient care (Tailor & Ranu et al., 2022).

The patient experience is improved overall thanks to this technology, which also increases efficiency and lowers mistakes. Numerous advantages result from the medical system's incorporation of developing technology. It has the potential to raise patient happiness while lowering costs by enhancing access to healthcare, improving diagnostic accuracy, optimizing treatment results, and streamlining administrative procedures. Additionally, these technologies support personalized treatment, encourage preventative methods of healthcare, and allow data-driven decision-making.

The use of cutting-edge technology in healthcare is not without difficulties, however. Some of the crucial challenges that must be addressed include ethical considerations, data privacy issues, regulatory compliance, and the need for effective cybersecurity measures. Furthermore, careful planning, coordination, and stakeholder involvement are necessary to ensure the smooth integration of new technologies into the current healthcare infrastructure and processes.

In summary, cutting-edge technologies like ML, AI, IoT, computer vision, robotics, blockchain, and RPA have enormous potential to revolutionize the medical and healthcare industries. They have the power to transform the way healthcare is delivered, enhance patient outcomes, and streamline operational procedures. Healthcare practitioners may improve their skills and provide more effective, efficient, and patient-centred care by using the potential of these technologies (Khang, 2023).

### 6.1.1 Motivation

The need for this survey paper on how machine learning, artificial intelligence, the Internet of Things, computer vision, robotics, blockchain, and robotic process automation are being used in the healthcare system is being driven by the growing awareness of how these cutting-edge technologies have the potential to transform the industry. The need for more precise and rapid diagnoses, personalized treatment plans, effective patient monitoring, reduced administrative procedures, secure data management, and interoperability across healthcare providers are just a few of the problems the healthcare sector must overcome. Emerging technologies have shown promise in overcoming these difficulties and enhancing the healthcare system as a whole. The main goal of this survey article is to provide a thorough review of the uses and effects of these new technologies on the healthcare system.

### 6.1.2 Objectives

Identification and Exploration of uses: The survey study was intended to identify and investigate the many uses of machine learning, artificial intelligence, Internet of Things, computer vision, robotics, blockchain, and robotic process automation in the medical health system. This covers things like administrative procedures, data management, patient monitoring, and treatment planning.

Assessment of Benefits and Limitations: The purpose of this survey report is to evaluate the advantages and drawbacks of using these technologies in healthcare. It tries to draw attention to the benefits that could be experienced, including better accuracy, effectiveness, patient outcomes, and cost savings. It also seeks to address the constraints, difficulties, and possible concerns related to the deployment of these technologies.

The purpose of the survey report is to examine the effects of these technologies on the medical and health systems. It looks at how these technologies might revolutionize how healthcare is delivered, how patients are cared for, and how innovation is fostered. It also seeks to identify potential effects, trends, and difficulties that must be overcome for effective implementation and general acceptance. In general, this survey paper's purpose and goals are motivated by the need to comprehend the existing situation, investigate the possibilities, and deal with the difficulties posed by the integration of developing technologies into the medical and health systems. The survey study intends to add to the body of current information, stimulate more investigation and teamwork, and provide direction for the responsible and efficient use of modern technologies in healthcare (Rani et al., 2021).

## 6.2 MACHINE LEARNING AND ARTIFICIAL INTELLIGENCE

The fields of artificial intelligence (AI) and machine learning (ML) have completely changed several facets of the medical industry.

Here are a few examples of how machine learning and artificial intelligence are being used in healthcare diagnostics, decision assistance, disease management, personalized medicine, treatment planning, patient monitoring, and health behaviour analysis:

- **Healthcare Diagnostics and Decision Support**: ML and AI algorithms can examine a sizable quantity of medical data, such as patient records, test findings, and medical imaging, to help with precise and effective diagnosis, as shown in Figure 6.2. By examining medical photos or patient symptoms, ML models, for instance, may help in the diagnosis and categorization of illnesses, including cancer, cardiovascular issues, and neurological disorders. By giving clinicians access to decision support tools, these technologies may enable them to make more precise diagnoses and create efficient treatment regimens.
- **Predictive Analytics and Risk Assessment in Illness Management**: ML and AI are able to identify patient-specific risks and estimate the chance of disease onset. These technologies may find patterns and risk factors linked to illnesses by examining patient data and medical records. As a result, healthcare providers are better equipped to treat chronic illnesses proactively, anticipate disease development, and avert negative outcomes.
- **Personalized Medicine and Treatment Planning**: By taking into account the unique patient traits, genetic profiles, and treatment histories, ML and AI allow personalized medicine. In order to provide individualized treatment

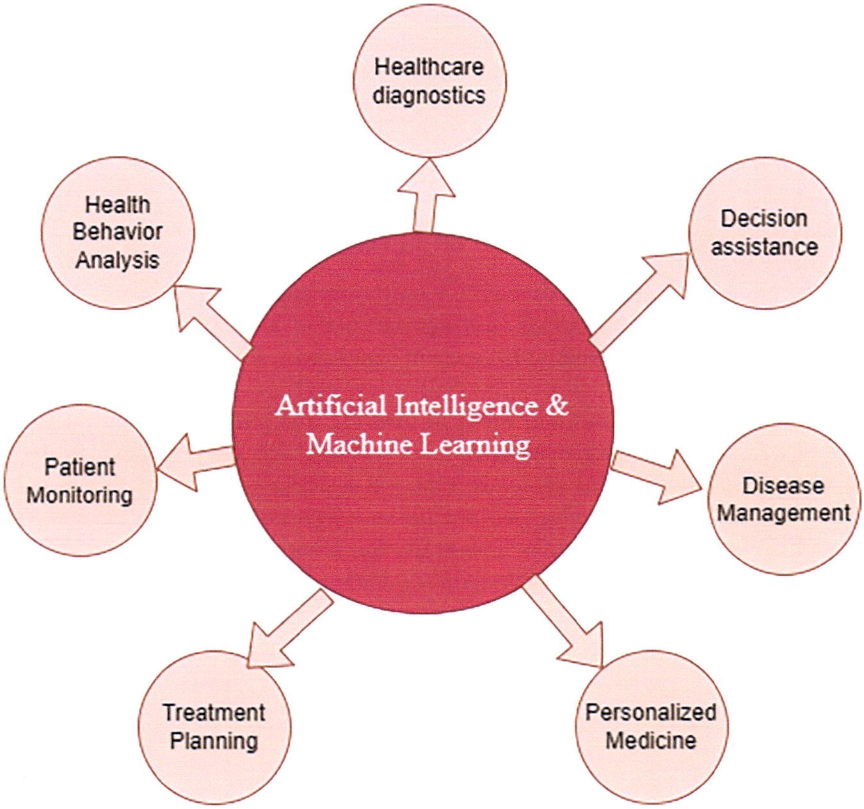


**FIGURE 6.2** The use of AI and ML in healthcare enterprises.

programmes and advise the best medicine doses, these technologies can analyzes patient data and clinical recommendations. This method boosts patient happiness, reduces side effects, and improves treatment results.

- **Patient Monitoring**: Wearables, electronic health records (EHRs), and other sources of real-time data may all be used to continually monitor patients via ML and AI algorithms. This makes it possible to identify anomalies early, take prompt action, and provide patients with individualized feedback. For instance, ML models can keep track of vital signs, spot anomalies, and notify medical staff or patients directly in case of emergency.
- **Health Behaviour Analysis**: To better identify health risks, promote healthy behaviours, and enhance patient outcomes, ML and AI may analyzes patient behaviour patterns and lifestyle aspects. These technologies may provide insights into a patient's activity levels, sleep patterns, food habits, and adherence to treatment programmes by merging data from wearables, smartphone applications, and social media. Healthcare professionals may use this information to give individualized advice and treatments that encourage healthier lifestyle choices.

Overall, ML and AI offer enormous promise in the field of healthcare, aiding in patient monitoring, illness management, planning of treatments, and diagnostics. These innovations may improve clinical judgment, maximize resource use, and ultimately improve patient outcomes. However, when using ML and AI in healthcare settings, it is crucial to make sure that ethical issues, privacy concerns, and data security are properly handled (Amann et al., 2020).

## 6.3 INTERNET OF THINGS IN HEALTHCARE

By allowing better patient care, remote monitoring, and proactive healthcare treatments, the Internet of Things (IoT) has significantly advanced the healthcare sector. The following are some essential IoT uses in healthcare:

- **Connected wearables and medical devices:** The Internet of Things (IoT) enables the seamless integration of wearables and medical devices into healthcare systems, as shown in Figure 6.3. These gadgets are capable of gathering and transmitting real-time health information to healthcare doctors or centralized databases, such as heart rate, blood pressure, glucose levels, and activity levels. This link supports remote healthcare services, allows

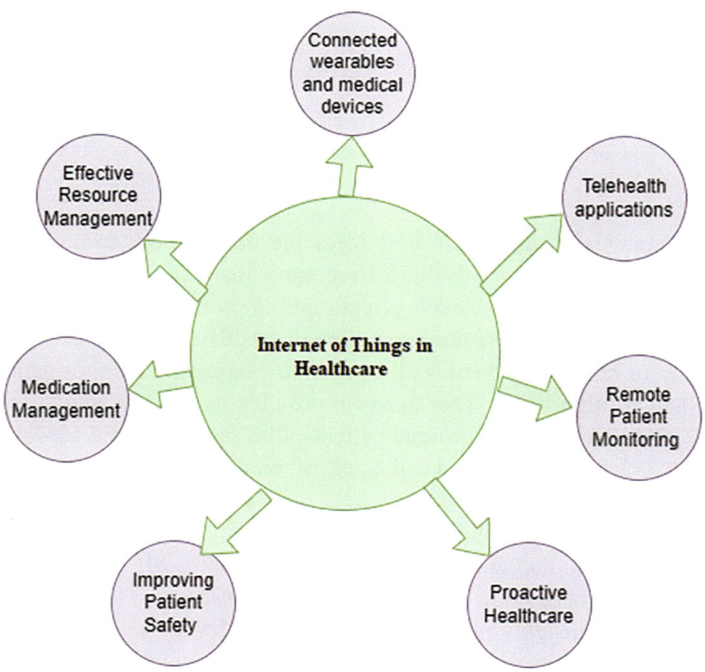


**FIGURE 6.3** The use of IoT in healthcare enterprises.

prompt treatments, and improves patient monitoring (Khang, Abdullayev & Litvinova et al., 2024).

Telehealth applications and remote patient monitoring are made possible by the Internet of Things (IoT), enabling healthcare professionals to monitor patients' health outside of conventional healthcare facilities. IoT-enabled devices may deliver patient vital sign data to healthcare experts while continually monitoring patients' vital signs. By providing virtual consultations, remote diagnosis, and the treatment of chronic illnesses from the convenience of patients' homes, this technology supports telehealth applications.

- **Collection and Analysis of Real-Time Data for Proactive Healthcare:** A plethora of real-time data produced by IoT devices may be used to deliver proactive healthcare treatments. Healthcare professionals can see patterns, uncover anomalies, and take action before significant health risks materialize by continually collecting and analyzing data. IoT sensors, for instance, may monitor environmental variables like temperature or air quality to lower the risk of respiratory disorders or heat-related illnesses.
- **Improving Patient Safety and Medication Management:** By integrating with medication management systems, IoT can raise patient safety. Smart pill dispensers can distribute precise quantities, remind patients to take their pills, and notify carers or healthcare professionals if a dose is missed. In addition, IoT-enabled tracking systems may guarantee the appropriate handling and storage of pharmaceuticals, lowering the possibility of mistakes or abuse.
- **Effective Resource Management:** By providing real-time data on equipment use, patient flow, and facility management, IoT helps optimize the use of healthcare resources. IoT sensors can monitor healthcare facility occupancy levels, track the availability and maintenance requirements of medical equipment, and optimize scheduling for optimal resource allocation. With the use of this technology, healthcare organizations may operate more efficiently for less money. IoT in healthcare has enormous potential to enhance remote healthcare delivery, enhance patient outcomes, and enable proactive treatments. Nevertheless, it is crucial to address security and privacy issues related to the gathering, sending, and storing of sensitive health data. To guarantee patient confidentiality and data integrity in IoT-enabled healthcare contexts, it is essential to implement strong security measures and adhere to legal requirements (Thilakarathne et al., 2020).

## 6.4 COMPUTER VISION IN HEALTHCARE

By employing visual data to enhance diagnosis, surgery, illness detection, and patient monitoring, computer vision, a branch of artificial intelligence, has had a substantial impact on healthcare, as shown in Figure 6.4.

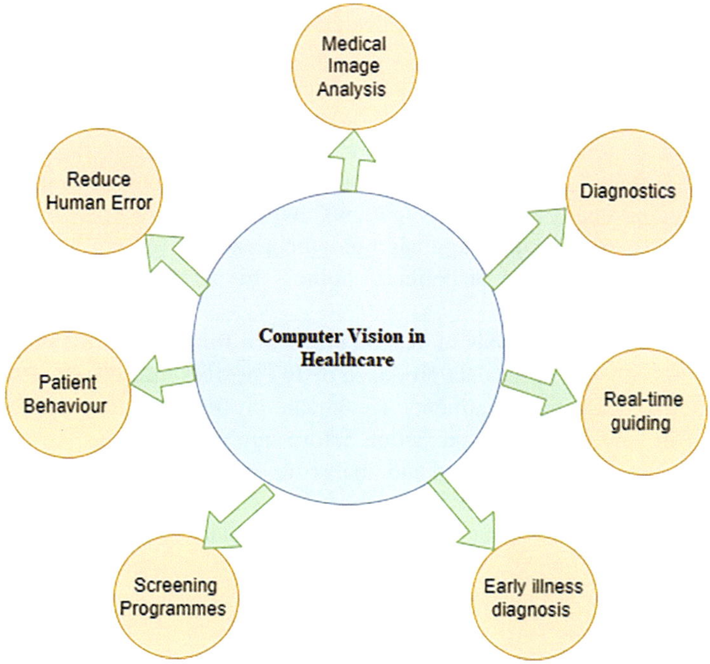


**FIGURE 6.4** The use of computer vision in healthcare enterprises.

The following are some important uses of computer vision in healthcare:

- **Medical Image Analysis and Diagnostics**: To assist in the diagnosis of different illnesses, computer vision algorithms may examine medical pictures such as X-rays, CT scans, and MRIs. These algorithms are capable of spotting anomalies, categorizing tumors, locating anatomical features, and measuring disease progression. The efficiency and precision with which radiologists and other healthcare workers interpret medical pictures are improved by computer vision-based solutions.
- **Real-time Guiding and Help During Surgical Operations Are Both Possible with Computer Vision**: Computer vision algorithms may assist surgeons in visualizing crucial structures, navigating difficult anatomies, and precisely positioning surgical tools by integrating with surgical equipment and imaging devices. These technologies may increase surgical accuracy, lessen complications, and boost patient outcomes. Early illness diagnosis and screening programmes may benefit from the use of computer vision methods. For instance, computer vision algorithms may examine retinal pictures to find melanoma symptoms in skin lesions or moles, identify diabetic retinopathy symptoms in retinal images, or find glaucoma symptoms in retinal images.
- **Screening Programme and Process**: Computer vision systems may enable early intervention and improve the effectiveness of healthcare services

by automating the screening process. Computer vision can analyze patient behaviour and keep an eye on their activities for a number of different uses. Computer vision algorithms, for instance, may monitor and examine a person's motions, gestures, and facial expressions to look for indications of discomfort, cognitive decline, or mental health issues. These systems may track physical therapy exercises, keep tabs on patient adherence to treatment programmes, and provide both patients and medical professionals with feedback.

The potential for computer vision-based applications in healthcare to enhance diagnosis, surgery, illness detection, and patient monitoring is enormous. They may improve productivity, reduce human error, and provide healthcare personnel with insightful information. When integrating computer vision systems in healthcare settings, it is crucial to address issues with data quality, privacy, the requirement for strong validation, and regulatory compliance (Leo et al., 2020).

## 6.5 ROBOTICS IN HEALTHCARE

Robotics has emerged as a revolutionary medical technology, with advantages such as higher surgical accuracy, better patient outcomes, and automation of monotonous chores, as shown in Figure 6.5.

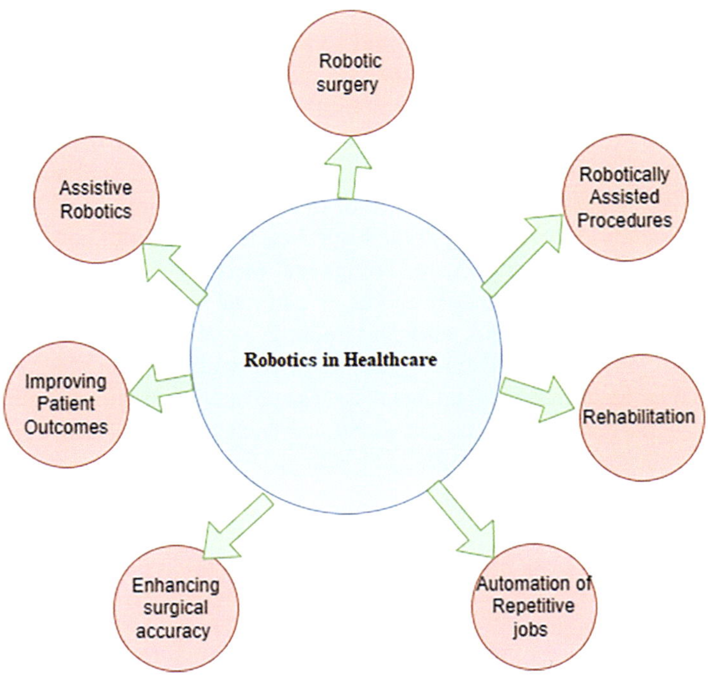


**FIGURE 6.5** The use of robotics in healthcare enterprises.

The following are some significant uses of robots in healthcare:

- **Robotic Surgery and Robotically Assisted Procedures**: In minimally invasive surgeries, robotic technologies like the da Vinci Surgical System help the physician. The greater dexterity, 3D visualization, and accurate instrument control offered by these devices benefit surgeons. Smaller incisions, less blood loss, quicker recovery periods, and better surgical results may all be a result of robotic surgery. Furthermore, remote surgery is made possible by teleoperated robotic platforms, enabling skilled surgeons to carry out treatments in other countries.
- **Rehabilitation and Assistive Robotics**: To help patients with movement issues during physical therapy and rehabilitation, robotic devices are employed. Patients may get assistance from exoskeletons, robotic prosthetics, and robotic assistive devices to rebuild strength, enhance motor control, and relearn movement patterns. These robotic devices enable repeated and precise motions, provide individualized support, and may be configured to adjust to the unique requirements of each patient.
- **Automation of Repetitive Jobs in Healthcare Settings**: Robots can automate time-consuming and repetitive jobs in the healthcare industry, freeing up staff members to concentrate on more complicated and crucial work. Within healthcare institutions, robotic systems may be used for logistics, inventory management, sterilization, and drug delivery. Automation lowers human mistake rates, boosts productivity, and frees up staff time for patient engagement and care.
- **Enhancing Surgical Accuracy and Improving Patient Outcomes**: Robotics technology increases surgical accuracy and patient outcomes. Greater accuracy, stability, and visualization offered by robotic systems allow surgeons to carry out intricate surgeries with increased precision. Reduced problems, shorter hospital stays, quicker healing periods, and more patient satisfaction are possible outcomes of this. The use of robots in healthcare is constantly developing, and their applications are becoming more widespread across a range of care settings and medical specializations. While there are many advantages to robots, it is crucial to remember that for best results and patient safety, sufficient training, supervision, and adherence to safety regulations are required. The effective use of robots in healthcare also depends on overcoming financial issues, preserving interoperability with current healthcare systems, and addressing legal and ethical issues (Kyrarini et al., 2021; Oña et al., 2019).

## 6.6 BLOCKCHAIN APPLICATION IN HEALTHCARE

Blockchain technology has several uses in the healthcare industry, including the safe and open administration of health data as well as increased interoperability and supply chain management. The following are some significant uses of blockchain in healthcare:

- **Healthcare Providers, Patients, and Other Stakeholders may Communicate Health Data in a Safe and Efficient Manner:** Blockchain guarantees the security, privacy, and traceability of health data by using cryptographic methods and decentralized networks (Khanh et al., 2021). While retaining data security and patient permission, it enables seamless exchange of patient records, test findings, and treatment information across various healthcare systems. Medical record management and patient consent are made possible by blockchain, which offers a transparent audit trail of access and alteration and gives patients authority over their medical information. Patients may provide authorization and manage access to their health data using blockchain-based platforms, preserving privacy and data sovereignty (Rath et al., 2024).
- **Traceability of Medications and Supply Chain Management:** In order to guarantee the quality and integrity of medical information, blockchain may also make it easier to verify and authenticate medical experts. Blockchain may improve the pharmaceutical industry's supply chain management, maintaining the integrity of the supply chain and the traceability of the drugs. Stakeholders can trace and confirm the origin, handling, and quality of pharmaceutical items by logging every stage of the supply chain on the blockchain, from manufacture to distribution (Haleem et al., 2021). This technology enhances medication safety, lowers the possibility of counterfeit pharmaceuticals, and speeds up recall procedures when required.
- **Ensuring the Integrity and Privacy of Healthcare Data:** Blockchain enables improved data security by offering a decentralized, immutable ledger. It makes healthcare data management transparent, tamper-proof, and auditable and does away with the requirement for a central authority (Khang & Chowdhury et al., 2022). Healthcare organizations may protect the confidentiality and integrity of sensitive patient data by storing encrypted data on the blockchain, prohibiting unauthorized access or alteration. By tackling the issues of data interchange, privacy, and security, blockchain technology has the potential to revolutionize healthcare. However, while using blockchain technologies in healthcare settings, it is crucial to take into account the scalability, legal compliance, and connection with current systems. Realizing the full potential of blockchain in healthcare requires cooperation across stakeholders, including healthcare providers, technology developers, and legislators (Rathore et al., 2020; Abujamra et al., 2019).

## 6.7 ROBOTIC PROCESS AUTOMATION

In the healthcare sector, robotic process automation (RPA) has become popular for automating administrative chores and optimizing processes (Bhatnagar, 2020). Here are a few significant RPA uses in the healthcare industry:

- **Automation of Workflows and Administrative Chores**: RPA can automate a variety of administrative chores, including appointment scheduling, patient registration, and data input. RPA bots may communicate with various systems, gather data, update records, and do mundane work, freeing up healthcare professionals to concentrate on more intricate and patient-centred duties. RPA increases operational efficiency and decreases human mistakes by automating repetitive and rule-based procedures (Jain & Bhatnagar, 2019).

- **Streamlining Billing and Claims Processing**: RPA can automate data extraction from medical records, insurance coverage verification, coding, and claims filing to expedite billing and claims processing. RPA bots may create correct claims for prompt reimbursement, reconcile billing codes, and look for mistakes or inconsistencies. This lowers administrative costs, quickens the payment process, and decreases billing mistakes.
- **Data Entry and Report Generation**: RPA can automate data entry operations like moving patient data across systems or filling out electronic forms. RPA bots are able to gather pertinent information from many sources, verify it, format it, and input it into the right systems. RPA may also produce reports and dashboards by combining and analyzing data from many sources, giving decision-makers real-time information.
- **Enhancing Operational Efficiency and Cost Savings**: RPA helps healthcare organizations operate more efficiently by decreasing human labor, doing away with data input mistakes, and enhancing process speed and accuracy. RPA lessens the stress on healthcare professionals by automating repetitive processes, allowing them to concentrate on crucial patient care activities. Additionally, by minimizing the need for extra people, improving resource utilization, and lowering claim rework or rejections, RPA may result in cost savings.

RPA has the ability to increase data accuracy, operational efficiency, and administrative process simplification in the healthcare industry. To automate the proper procedures, protect data privacy and security, and thoroughly test and validate RPA systems are all necessary. Working together with IT and process professionals and taking into account legal and regulatory compliance requirements may assist in guaranteeing that RPA is successfully integrated into healthcare environments (Sharma et al., 2022).

## 6.8 BENEFITS, CHALLENGES, AND ETHICAL CONSIDERATIONS

AI and associated technologies may help with precise diagnosis, individualized treatment planning, and proactive healthcare treatments, improving patient outcomes and the standard of care. They may boost patient outcomes, lessen medical mistakes, and raise the standard of treatment given (Khang & Hahanov et al., 2024).

### 6.8.1 Enhancing Healthcare Access and Efficiency

By boosting productivity, streamlining processes, and automating repetitive operations, AI may assist in addressing healthcare resource shortages. Applications for telehealth and remote monitoring improve access to healthcare, particularly for underprivileged groups or those living in distant locations.

### 6.8.2 Challenges

AI depends on a significant quantity of private medical information, which raises questions regarding data security and privacy. To prevent unauthorized access to or breaches of patient information, healthcare organizations must put in place strong security measures. AI algorithms may unintentionally reinforce biases found in training data, which may result in differential treatment or healthcare costs. To reduce biases and advance equitable healthcare outcomes, it is essential to maintain algorithmic openness, fairness, and continuous monitoring. Addressing Biases and Transparency in AI Algorithms (Eswaran & Khang, 2024):

### 6.8.3 Regulation and Ethical Considerations

AI usage in healthcare must abide by all relevant laws, including those pertaining to data protection, patient consent, and ethics. For trust and ethical norms to be maintained, AI technology usage must be transparent, accountable, and ethical. Roles and obligations of healthcare practitioners may change due to AI technology integration. AI technology may alter the roles and obligations of healthcare practitioners. The ethical ramifications must be carefully considered, and it is crucial to maintain the human touch and discretion as essential components of patient care while using AI as a supplemental tool.

Building confidence and acceptance among patients, medical professionals, and society at large is essential to the widespread adoption of AI in healthcare. Building trust requires addressing issues with biases, data security, privacy, and the advantages and disadvantages of AI technology. Collaboration between healthcare practitioners, technologists, and regulatory authorities is essential to maximizing the advantages and addressing the problems. The ethical development and use of AI in healthcare must be shaped by continuing dialogues, guidelines, and ethical frameworks (Vugar & Khang et al., 2024).

## 6.9 FUTURE DIRECTION AND INTEGRATION OF TECHNOLOGIES

The combination of several technologies to provide synergistic advantages is where healthcare innovation will go in the future. The following are some potential directions and trends for the use of technology in healthcare.

### 6.9.1 Integration of Multiple Technologies for Synergistic Benefits

Comprehensive and integrated healthcare solutions will be made possible by the fusion of technologies like artificial intelligence (AI), the Internet of Things (IoT), blockchain, robots, and data analytics. For instance, integrating AI with IoT devices may provide personalized therapies and real-time patient monitoring. Blockchain and AI integration may improve data security and interoperability. New opportunities for enhancing patient care and healthcare outcomes will become available as a result of the convergence of technology.

### 6.9.2 Implementing Emerging Technologies Ethically and Responsibly

It is crucial to ensure that new technologies are used ethically and responsibly as the field of healthcare continues to grow. The design, development, and implementation of these technologies must take into account ethical issues, including privacy, openness, bias mitigation, and human supervision. Guidelines and regulatory frameworks will be essential in determining how developing technologies are used ethically in the healthcare industry.

### 6.9.3 Research and Development Trends in Healthcare Innovation

Precision medicine, genomics, digital health, telemedicine, and personalized healthcare will continue to be the focus of healthcare innovation. The focus of research and development will be on developing new diagnostic instruments, tailored treatments, and preventative measures. In order to provide forecasts and decision support systems that are more accurate, machine learning algorithms will be improved. Furthermore, improvements in nanotechnology, biotechnology, and neuron technology are anticipated to transform patient care and healthcare delivery.

Future healthcare technology will progressively place emphasis on human-centred design principles, placing the patient at the centre of treatment. The advancement of healthcare technology will be fuelled by user-friendly interfaces, intuitive interactions, and patient empowerment. People will be able to actively participate in their own healthcare by using patient engagement platforms, mobile health apps, and wearable technology to make educated choices and proactively manage their health.

### 6.9.4 Collaborative Ecosystems and Interoperability

By bringing together healthcare providers, technology businesses, academics, and policymakers, collaborative ecosystems will stimulate healthcare innovation. In order to provide smooth data transmission and integration across diverse healthcare settings, interoperability across various systems, protocols, and data formats will be essential. The adoption of transformational technologies will be accelerated via collaboration. Integration of technology, a focus on moral issues, ongoing research and development, and a patient-centric approach will all influence the direction of healthcare in the future. Healthcare will improve patient outcomes and change the healthcare industry by making the most of new technology's increased precision, accessibility, and personalization possibilities.

## 6.10 CONCLUSION

In conclusion, the use of cutting-edge technology in healthcare has enormous prospects to revolutionize patient care, raise quality of life, and boost productivity.

Important conclusions and observations include emerging technologies like AI, IoT, blockchain, robots, and RPA have a wide range of useful applications in the healthcare industry. Diagnostics, decision support, remote monitoring, personalized healthcare, surgical guidance, data interchange, and administrative job automation are all supported by these technologies. It is essential that new technologies be used to solve issues facing the healthcare sector, such as limited resources, data interoperability, patient access, and raising the standard of treatment. These technologies have the potential to improve patient experiences, efficiency, and healthcare outcomes (Khang & Ragimova et al., 2022).

The comprehensive examination of issues and problems is necessary for the effective deployment of developing technologies. These include issues with data security and privacy, dealing with biases in AI algorithms, assuring human-centred care, regulatory compliance, ethical considerations, integration with current systems, and others. With an emphasis on ethical implementation, patient-centred design, and stakeholder cooperation, new technologies should be used in healthcare. To solve issues with data privacy, security, and algorithmic transparency, certain rules and laws need to be in place. Harnessing the full potential of these technologies will need ongoing study and development, as well as the participation of technologists, politicians, and regulatory agencies (Khang & Rana et al., 2023). The healthcare sector has the chance to alter how care is provided, enhance patient outcomes, and build a more effective and accessible healthcare system by embracing new technology and using its potential. It is an exciting moment for healthcare innovation, and new technologies have the potential to improve healthcare if they are used responsibly and with care (Rana & Khang et al., 2021).

## REFERENCES


Abujamra R, Randall D, "Blockchain Applications in Healthcare and the Opportunities and the Advancements Due to the New Information Technology Framework", *In Advances in Computers*. 2019 Jan 1 (Vol. 115, pp. 141–154). Elsevier. https://doi.org/10.1016/bs.adcom.2018.12.002

Abdullayev V, Khang A, Rashad İ, Vusala A, Sriram K, Anh PTN, "AI-Aided Computer Vision in Health Care System", *Computer Vision and AI-Integrated IoT Technologies in Medical Ecosystem*. 2024 (1st Ed.). CRC Press. https://doi.org/10.1201/9781003429609-20

Amann J, Blasimme A, Vayena E, Frey D, Madai VI, "Explainability for Artificial Intelligence in Healthcare: A Multidisciplinary Perspective", *BMC Medical Informatics and Decision Making*. 2020 Dec; 20(1):1–9. https://doi.org/10.1186/s12911-020-01332-6

Anh PTN, Hahanov V, Triwiyanto, Ragimova NA, Rashad İ, Abdullayev VA, Alyar AV, "AI Models for Disease Diagnosis and Prediction of Heart Disease with Artificial Neural Networks", *Computer Vision and AI-integrated IoT Technologies in Medical Ecosystem*. 2024 (1 Ed.). CRC Press. https://doi.org/10.1201/9781003429609-9

Barragán-Montero A, Javaid U, Valdés G, Nguyen D, Desbordes P, Macq B, Willems S, Vandewinckele L, Holmström M, Löfman F, Michiels S, "Artificial Intelligence and Machine Learning for Medical Imaging: A Technology Review", *Physica Medica*. 2021 Mar 1; 83:242–256. https://doi.org/10.1016/j.ejmp.2021.04.016

Bhatnagar N, "Role of Robotic Process Automation in Pharmaceutical Industries", *In the International Conference on Advanced Machine Learning Technologies and Applications (AMLTA2019)*. 2020 (Vol. 4, pp. 497–504). AMLTA. https://doi.org/10.1007/978-3-030-14118-9_50

Eswaran U, Khang A, "AI-Aided Computer Vision in Health Care System", *Computer Vision and AI-Integrated IoT Technologies in Medical Ecosystem*. 2024 (1st Ed.). CRC Press. https://doi.org/10.1201/9781003429609-8

Haleem A, Javaid M, Singh RP, Suman R, Rab S, "Blockchain Technology Applications in Healthcare: An Overview", *International Journal of Intelligent Networks*. 2021 Jan 1; 2:130–139. https://doi.org/10.1016/j.ijin.2021.09.005

Jain R, Bhatnagar R, "Robotic Process Automation in Healthcare: A Review", *International Robotics & Automation Journal*. 2019 Jan; 5(1):12–14. https://doi.org/10.15406/iratj.2019.05.00164

Kassab M, DeFranco J, Malas T, Laplante P, Destefanis G, Neto VV, "Exploring Research in Blockchain for Healthcare and a Roadmap for the Future", *IEEE Transactions on Emerging Topics in Computing*. 2019 Aug 22; 9(4):1835–1852. https://doi.org/10.1109/TETC.2019.2936881

Khang, A. (Ed.). (2024). *AI and IoT Technology and Applications for Smart Healthcare Systems* (1st ed.). Auerbach Publications. https://doi.org/10.1201/9781032686745

Khang A, Abdullayev VA, Hrybiuk O, Shukla AK, *Computer Vision and AI-integrated IoT Technologies in Medical Ecosystem*. 2024 (1st Ed.). CRC Press. https://doi.org/10.1201/9781003429609

Khang A, Abdullayev VA, Litvinova E, Chumachenko S, Abuzarova V, Anh PTN, "Application of Computer Vision in the Healthcare Ecosystem", *Computer Vision and AI-Integrated IoT Technologies in Medical Ecosystem*. 2024 (1st Ed.). CRC Press. https://doi.org/10.1201/9781003429609-1

Khang A, Chowdhury S, Sharma S, eds, *The Data-Driven Blockchain Ecosystem: Fundamentals, Applications, and Emerging Technologies*. 2022 (1st Ed., Vol. 8, No. 13, pp. 149–164). CRC Press. https://doi.org/10.1201/9781003269281-8

Khang A, Hahanov V, Litvinova E, Chumachenko S, Avromovic Z, İsmibeyli R, Ragimova NA, Abdullayev VA, Alyar AV, Anh PTN, "Medical and Biomedical Signal Processing and Prediction", *Computer Vision and AI-integrated IoT Technologies in Medical Ecosystem*. 2024. (1st Ed.). CRC Press. https://doi.org/10.1201/9781003429609-7

Khang A, Ragimova NA, Hajimahmud VA, Alyar VA, "Advanced Technologies and Data Management in the Smart Healthcare System", *AI-Centric Smart City Ecosystems: Technologies, Design and Implementation*. 2022 (Vol. 16, 1st Ed., p. 10). CRC Press. https://doi.org/10.1201/9781003252542-16

Khang A, Rana G, Tailor RK, Hajimahmud VA, eds, *Data-Centric AI Solutions and Emerging Technologies in the Healthcare Ecosystem*. 2023. CRC Press. https://doi.org/10.1201/9781003356189

Khanh HH, Khang A, "The Role of Artificial Intelligence in Blockchain Applications", *Reinventing Manufacturing and Business Processes through Artificial Intelligence*. 2021 (Vol. 2, pp. 20–40). CRC Press. https://doi.org/10.1201/9781003145011-2

Kyrarini M, Lygerakis F, Rajavenkatanarayanan A, Sevastopoulos C, Nambiappan HR, Chaitanya KK, Babu AR, Mathew J, Makedon F, "A Survey of Robots in Healthcare", *Technologies*. 2021 Jan 18; 9(1):8. https://doi.org/10.3390/technologies9010008

Leo M, Carcagnì P, Mazzeo PL, Spagnolo P, Cazzato D, Distante C, "Analysis of Facial Information for Healthcare Applications: A Survey on Computer Vision-Based Approaches", *Information*. 2020 Feb 26; 11(3):128. https://doi.org/10.3390/info11030128

Mozumder MA, Sheeraz MM, Athar A, Aich S, Kim HC, "Overview: Technology Roadmap of the Future Trend of Metaverse Based on IoT, Blockchain, AI Technique, and Medical Domain Metaverse Activity", *In 2022 24th International Conference on Advanced Communication Technology (ICACT)*. 2022 Feb 13 (pp. 256–261). IEEE. https://doi.org/10.23919/ICACT53585.2022.9728808

Oña ED, Garcia-Haro JM, Jardón A, Balaguer C, "Robotics in Health Care: Perspectives of Robot-Aided Interventions in Clinical Practice for Rehabilitation of Upper Limbs", *Applied sciences*. 2019 Jun 26; 9(13):2586. https://doi.org/10.3390/app9132586

Rana G, Khang A, Sharma R, Goel AK, Dubey AK, eds, *Reinventing Manufacturing and Business Processes Through Artificial Intelligence*, 2021. CRC Press. https://doi.org/10.1201/9781003145011

Rani S, Chauhan M, Kataria A, Khang A, eds, "IoT Equipped Intelligent Distributed Framework for Smart Healthcare Systems", *Networking and Internet Architecture*. 2021 (Vol. 2, p. 30). CRC Press. https://doi.org/10.48550/arXiv.2110.04997

Rath KC, Khang A, Rath SK, Satapathy N, Satapathy SK, Kar S, "AI-Enabled Technology in Medicine-Advancing Holistic Healthcare Monitoring and Control Systems", *Computer Vision and AI-Integrated IoT Technologies in Medical Ecosystem*. 2024 (1st Ed.). CRC Press. https://doi.org/10.1201/9781003429609-6

Rathore H, Mohamed A, Guizani M, "Blockchain applications for healthcare", *In Energy Efficiency of Medical Devices and Healthcare Applications*. 2020 Jan 1 (pp. 153–166). Academic Press. https://doi.org/10.1016/B978-0-12-819045-6.00008-X

Sharma S, Kataria A, Sandhu JK, "Applications, Tools and Technologies of Robotic Process Automation in Various Industries", *In 2022 International Conference on Decision Aid Sciences and Applications (DASA)*. 2022 Mar 23 (pp. 1067–1072). IEEE. https://doi.org/10.1109/DASA54658.2022.9765027

Tailor RK, Ranu Pareek, Khang A, *Robot Process Automation in Blockchain*. 2022. CRC Press.

Thilakarathne NN, Kagita MK, Gadekallu TR, "The Role of the Internet of Things in Health Care: A Systematic and Comprehensive Study". Available at SSRN 3690815. 2020 Sep 11. https://www.academia.edu/44043051/The_Role_of_the_Internet_of_Things_in_HealthCare_A_Systematic_and_Comprehensive_Study; https://doi.org/10.2139/ssrn.3690815

Zhang G, Navimipour NJ, "A Comprehensive and Systematic Review of the IoT-Based Medical Management Systems: Applications, Techniques, Trends and Open Issues", *Sustainable Cities and Society*. 2022 Jul 1; 82:103914. https://doi.org/10.1016/j.scs.2022.103914

# 7 Utilizing Artificial Neural Networks (ANN) and Deep Learning (DL) in Extended Reality Environments for Addressing Psychological Issues

*Nobhonil Roy Choudhury, Shivnath Ghosh, and Avijit Kumar Chaudhuri*

## 7.1 INTRODUCTION

The intersection of Artificial Neural Networks (ANN), deep learning techniques, and Extended Reality (XR) environments has ushered in a new era of technology-assisted interventions for psychological issues. As mental health concerns continue to rise globally, innovative approaches that leverage advancements in artificial intelligence and virtual reality hold the promise of providing scalable and personalized solutions. This research paper explores the synergy between ANN-based virtual characters and XR spaces to address psychological challenges, presenting a comprehensive study that combines insights from psychology, computer science, and human-computer interaction (Khang, 2024).

With the proliferation of digital platforms and the increasing prevalence of mental health concerns, there is a growing need for accessible and effective interventions. Traditional therapeutic approaches often face barriers such as limited access, stigma, and resource constraints. The integration of XR environments offers a unique opportunity to create immersive, controlled, and adaptable scenarios that can be tailored to individual needs. Virtual characters, driven by ANN models, can simulate real-world situations, provide therapeutic interactions, and gather data for personalized interventions (Khang et al., 2022).

This chapter builds upon a foundation of research at the confluence of mental health and technology. Leveraging deep learning techniques, including Convolutional Neural Networks (CNNs) and Recurrent Neural Networks (RNNs),

 DOI: 10.1201/9781032686745-7

has demonstrated their effectiveness in tasks such as emotion recognition, sentiment analysis, and behavior prediction (Deng, 2014; Litjens et al., 2017). Furthermore, the concept of using XR for exposure therapy, simulations, and cognitive-behavioral interventions has gained traction in recent years (Glaser & Schmidt, 2021; Rothbaum & Hodges, 1999).

Incorporating ANN-driven virtual characters into XR environments aligns with the goals of personalized medicine and digital therapeutics. Previous work has explored the development of virtual agents for social anxiety interventions (McWhorter, 2010), posttraumatic stress disorder treatment (Kothgassner et al., 2019), and exposure therapy (North et al., 1998). By training neural networks on data collected from individuals facing various psychological challenges, it becomes possible to generate responses that resonate with users' experiences (Martindale, 1991).

This research paper presents a novel architecture that combines ANN with XR to create dynamic virtual characters capable of adapting to user interactions in real-time scenarios. The approach encompasses data collection, pre-processing, model training, real-time interaction, and user studies to evaluate the effectiveness of the intervention. The outcomes of this study contribute to the growing body of literature on technology-assisted psychological interventions and pave the way for future developments in XR-enabled mental health support (Rath et al., 2024).

## 7.2 LITERATURE REVIEW

The confluence of Artificial Neural Networks (ANN), deep learning, and Extended Reality (XR) environments has paved the way for innovative interventions in addressing psychological challenges. This section provides an in-depth review of the existing literature, highlighting key findings and trends in the intersection of technology, mental health, and XR applications (Khang & Rana et al., 2023).

### 7.2.1 Artificial Neural Networks and Deep Learning in Mental Health

Artificial Neural Networks and deep learning techniques have shown remarkable progress in various facets of mental health research. Convolutional Neural Networks (CNNs) have excelled in tasks like emotion recognition through facial expressions, laying the foundation for emotionally aware virtual characters (Ahmad et al., 2018). Sentiment analysis, often utilizing Long Short-Term Memory (LSTM) networks, has been applied to analyze textual data and infer users' emotional states (LOIHI, 2021). Furthermore, Recurrent Neural Networks (RNNs) have been effective in predicting mood fluctuations and behavioral shifts (Escorcia, 2013). The integration of these techniques into XR environments enriches the capabilities of virtual characters by enabling real-time, personalized interactions with users.

### 7.2.2 Extended Reality (XR) for Psychological Interventions

Extended Reality (XR), comprising Virtual Reality (VR), Augmented Reality (AR), and Mixed Reality (MR), offers immersive and interactive platforms that hold potential for therapeutic interventions. XR has been successfully employed in exposure therapy, a well-established technique for anxiety disorders (Anderson, 2019). VR-based environments provide controlled exposure to anxiety-inducing stimuli, facilitating gradual desensitization. Additionally, XR has been utilized for cognitive rehabilitation and pain management, enhancing user engagement and adherence (Harkness et al., 2013). By embedding ANN-driven virtual characters within XR environments, interventions gain adaptability and can be personalized to suit users' needs.

### 7.2.3 Virtual Characters and Mental Health Interventions

Virtual characters, often referred to as virtual agents or avatars, have emerged as promising tools for psychological interventions. These characters possess the ability to simulate social interactions, provide emotional support, and guide users through therapeutic exercises. Virtual agents have shown effectiveness in addressing social anxiety (Parsons, 2014), posttraumatic stress disorder (Sherrill et al., 2019), and depression (Rothbaum, 2006). The utilization of ANN augments these characters with emotion recognition and response capabilities, enabling them to interpret users' emotional cues and tailor interactions accordingly. The potential to deliver interventions remotely further widens their reach and accessibility.

### 7.2.4 Technology-Assisted Therapies and Ethical Considerations

The advent of technology-assisted therapies introduces ethical considerations that necessitate careful consideration. Ensuring privacy, obtaining informed consent, and safeguarding against potential risks are critical in developing interventions (Turner, 2022). The transparency of virtual characters' behaviors and the accuracy of their emotional interpretations are paramount. Collaboration between psychologists, ethicists, and technologists is crucial in establishing guidelines that maintain therapeutic efficacy while upholding ethical standards.

### 7.2.5 Future Directions and Integration

Looking ahead, the integration of ANN-driven virtual characters into XR interventions holds promise for enhanced therapeutic outcomes. Advancements in Generative Adversarial Networks (GANs) and reinforcement learning could further refine virtual characters' adaptability and emotional intelligence (Goodfellow, 2014). Moreover, the integration of physiological data, such as heart rate variability and skin conductance, could enhance the accuracy of emotional recognition (Ali et al., 2017). The exploration of multimodal approaches, including visual, auditory, and haptic cues, may contribute to a richer user experience and deeper engagement (Poppe, 2010).

## 7.3 METHODOLOGY

In this section, we expound upon the comprehensive methodology used to address the pressing psychological concern of social anxiety through the strategic integration of Extended Reality (XR) environments and cutting-edge Artificial Neural Networks (ANN) driven virtual characters. This comprehensive approach leverages advancements in technology to tackle a widespread psychological challenge.

### 7.3.1 Psychological Issue and Its Significance

Social anxiety, often referred to as social phobia, constitutes a significant psychological issue affecting individuals across the globe (WNY, 2013). It is characterized by an overwhelming fear of social situations and an excessive concern about being judged by others. Individuals afflicted with social anxiety often experience physical symptoms like palpitations, sweating, and trembling in response to social situations. The severity of social anxiety can lead to impaired social functioning, hampering personal, academic, and professional pursuits. The need to address social anxiety is underscored by its pervasive impact on mental health and overall quality of life (Anh et al., 2024).

### 7.3.2 Technological Approach: ANN and Deep Learning

The selection of Artificial Neural Networks (ANN) and deep learning methodologies as the technological approach is rooted in their capacity to unravel intricate patterns within complex datasets. Deep learning architectures, such as Convolutional Neural Networks (CNNs) and Recurrent Neural Networks (RNNs), have demonstrated proficiency in detecting nuanced emotional cues and predicting behavioral responses (Huang et al., 2008). The integration of deep learning techniques augments virtual characters' capacity to recognize and appropriately respond to users' emotional states, enabling more authentic and empathetic interactions within XR environments.

### 7.3.3 Data Collection Process

The data collection process was executed with precision to ensure the acquisition of comprehensive and representative datasets. Participants with varying degrees of social anxiety were recruited and assessed using standardized measures such as the Liebowitz Social Anxiety Scale (LSAS) (Martindale, 1991). The LSAS evaluates the severity of social anxiety through the quantification of anxiety and avoidance associated with social situations.

Participants were immersed in carefully designed XR environments that emulated real-world social scenarios. Physiological responses such as heart rate variability, electrodermal activity, and facial expressions were recorded during these simulations. This multimodal dataset captured the intricacies of emotional responses and physiological changes associated with social anxiety. Annotations of the dataset included participants' self-reported emotional states, cognitive reactions, and perceived levels of discomfort. The labeling process was conducted by experienced psychologists proficient in emotion recognition, thus ensuring the accuracy and reliability of labeled data (Ekman & Friesen, 1971).

### 7.3.4 Development of XR Environments and Virtual Characters

The XR environments were meticulously crafted to replicate real-world social situations that often evoke anxiety in individuals with social anxiety. These scenarios ranged from public speaking engagements to casual social interactions, encompassing scenarios that contribute to heightened social apprehension (Wells, 1999). By mimicking these anxiety-inducing scenarios, the XR environments provided a controlled platform for users to confront their fears and practice adaptive coping strategies. Virtual characters, empowered by ANN models, were designed to comprehend facial expressions, vocal intonations, and sentiment in users' interactions. These virtual characters were endowed with the ability to exhibit empathy and offer supportive feedback based on users' emotional states. Integrating deep learning mechanisms endowed the virtual characters with an evolving capacity to interpret users' emotional cues and generate contextually appropriate responses, as shown in Table 7.1.

- **Fear of Negative Evaluation**: A core aspect of social anxiety is the pervasive fear of negative evaluation by others. Individuals with social anxiety are acutely attuned to the possibility of being scrutinized and judged by their peers (Martindale, 1991). This fear leads to heightened self-consciousness and often results in avoidance behaviors to evade situations that may trigger such evaluation. The fear of negative evaluation can manifest across a spectrum of social scenarios, from casual conversations to public speaking engagements.
- **Cognitive Distortions and Negative Self-Beliefs**: Cognitive distortions play a pivotal role in perpetuating social anxiety. Individuals with social anxiety tend to engage in excessive self-monitoring and amplify perceived negative aspects of their performance or appearance (Rupke, 2006). Negative self-beliefs about their social skills, attractiveness, or likability can lead to a distorted self-perception. These cognitive distortions fuel anxiety and reinforce the anticipation of negative outcomes in social interactions.
- **Safety Behaviors and Avoidance Strategies**: Individuals grappling with social anxiety often adopt safety behaviors and avoidance strategies to mitigate their anxiety. Safety behaviors involve actions taken to prevent

**TABLE 7.1**
**Psychological Facts Table**

| Psychological Fact | Relevance to Social Anxiety |
|---|---|
| Fear of Negative Evaluation | A primary feature driving social anxiety often causing avoidance of social situations (Martindale, 1991). |
| Cognitive Distortions | Distorted self-beliefs contribute to heightened anxiety and maladaptive behavioral patterns (Rupke, 2006). |
| Safety Behaviors | Individuals adopt safety behaviors to alleviate anxiety, inadvertently perpetuating social anxiety (Boston & Merrick, 2010). |
| Vicarious Learning | Observational learning and prior experiences shape the development and maintenance of social anxiety (Kellert, 2002). |

perceived negative consequences or to manage anxiety, such as rehearsing conversations in advance or using humor to deflect attention (Boston & Merrick, 2010). While these behaviors provide temporary relief, they inadvertently perpetuate social anxiety by reinforcing the belief that anxiety is justified and necessary for coping.

- **Vicarious Learning and Model-Based Fear Acquisition**: Vicarious learning, a process by which individuals learn from observing the experiences of others, plays a pivotal role in the development and maintenance of social anxiety (Kellert, 2002). Witnessing instances of social rejection or humiliation experienced by others can lead to the internalization of fears and avoidance behaviors. Model-based fear acquisition occurs when individuals imitate behaviors they have seen others perform in response to social situations, solidifying their apprehensions.

## 7.4 NEURAL NETWORK ARCHITECTURE

The selection of an appropriate neural network architecture is paramount in designing a model that effectively captures the nuances of user interactions, emotions, and responses within Extended Reality (XR) environments. This section outlines the chosen architecture, rationale, and high-level components of the model.

### 7.4.1 Chosen Neural Network Architecture

For our XR-based psychological intervention system, we have opted for a hybrid architecture that combines Convolutional Neural Networks (CNNs) and Long Short-Term Memory (LSTM) networks. This hybrid approach capitalizes on the strengths of both architectures to handle spatial and temporal features within the XR scenarios. CNNs are well-suited for processing visual input data, extracting spatial features from images, and identifying visual patterns. LSTM networks, on the other hand, excel in capturing sequential patterns and dynamics in user interactions over time (Rana et al., 2021).

### 7.4.2 Rationale for Hybrid Architecture

The hybrid architecture is motivated by the complex nature of psychological responses and user interactions in XR environments. As users navigate through these environments, their emotional states evolve based on real-time stimuli, and their interactions create temporal patterns that reflect emotional dynamics. By integrating CNNs and LSTM networks, we aim to capture both the visual cues and temporal dependencies within the data. This enables our model to identify emotion-inducing visual elements and understand the emotional trajectories that users experience.

### 7.4.3 Model Components and Layers

The hybrid architecture comprises three main components: a CNN module, an LSTM module, and a fusion layer. The CNN module extracts spatial features from visual stimuli within the XR scenarios. It consists of convolutional layers followed by pooling layers, enabling the network to identify visual patterns that evoke emotional

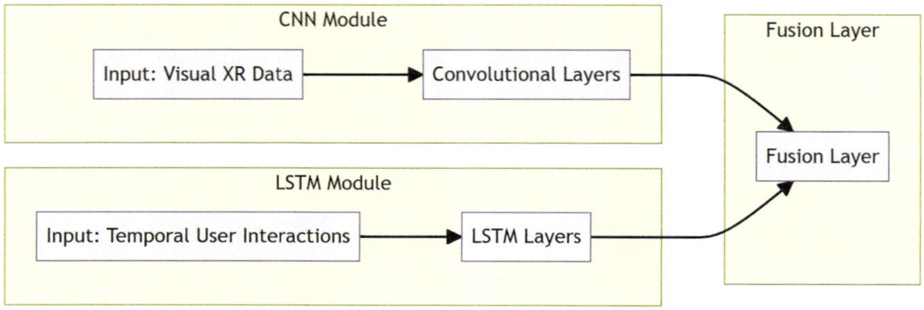


**FIGURE 7.1** Schematic representation of the hybrid neural network architecture.

**TABLE 7.2**
**Psychological Facts Table**

| Psychological Fact | Relevance to XR Intervention |
|---|---|
| Emotions Influence Behavior | Virtual characters can adapt their behavior based on users' emotional cues to facilitate effective interventions. |
| Exposure Therapy | XR environments can provide controlled exposure to anxiety-inducing stimuli, aiding in anxiety and phobia treatments. |
| Emotional Dynamics | LSTM networks can capture the temporal evolution of users' emotional states during XR interactions. |
| Personalization | Hybrid architecture integrates spatial and temporal features, allowing personalized interventions based on individual experiences. |

responses. The LSTM module processes the sequential user interactions, capturing the emotional dynamics over time. This module consists of multiple LSTM layers that retain context and relationships between user actions. The fusion layer combines the outputs from both modules, integrating the extracted spatial features with the temporal patterns to predict emotional states and responses, as shown in Figure 7.1.

In the context of developing emotionally responsive virtual characters within Extended Reality (XR) environments, the quality and diversity of the training dataset are paramount. This section outlines the essential steps of data pre-processing and augmentation employed to enhance the effectiveness of the neural network model, as shown in Table 7.2.

## 7.5 DATA PRE-PROCESSING AND AUGMENTATION

### 7.5.1 Data Pre-Processing

Collected data was subjected to rigorous pre-processing to ensure consistency and suitability for training the neural network. The pre-processing pipeline involved the following stages:

- **Data Collection**: Individuals experiencing a range of psychological issues were invited to participate in controlled virtual scenarios within the XR

environment. Data captured included user interactions, physiological responses, and self-reported emotional states (Tu et al., 2022).
- **Data Cleansing**: Raw data underwent thorough quality checks to remove outliers, noise, and artifacts. Erroneous data points caused by technical glitches or sensor inaccuracies were corrected or excluded (ISA, 2022).
- **Normalization**: Physiological data, such as heart rate and skin conductance, were normalized to account for individual variability and enable fair participant comparison (Ahuja et al., 2023b).

### 7.5.2 Data Augmentation

Data augmentation techniques were employed to enhance the diversity of the training dataset and improve the model's generalization capabilities. Augmentation strategies introduced controlled variations to the dataset, simulating a wider range of user interactions and emotional expressions:

- **Image Augmentation**: For facial expression analysis, images of users' facial expressions were subjected to transformations like rotation, cropping, and flipping. These variations introduced different lighting conditions and viewpoints, making the model robust to real-world scenarios (Sánchez-Nieto et al., 2023).
- **Textual Variation**: Textual responses provided by users were subjected to paraphrasing and synonym substitution, ensuring the model's ability to understand varying expressions of emotions (Difede et al., 2022).
- **Physiological Noise Injection**: Synthetic noise was added to physiological data to simulate variations in user reactions. This aided the model in recognizing emotional states under less controlled conditions (Lee & Stein, 2022).

### 7.5.3 Table of Psychological Facts

As an illustrative reference, Table 7.3 presents a summary of key psychological facts relevant to the emotions and behaviors addressed within the XR environment.

**TABLE 7.3**
**Psychological Facts Table**

| Fact Number | Fact Description |
|---|---|
| 1 | Emotions can influence decision-making and behavior (Lee & Stein, 2022). |
| 2 | Positive mood enhances prosocial behavior and helping (Forgas, 1995). |
| 3 | Emotion regulation impacts cognitive functioning (Mochon et al., 2008). |
| 4 | Affect infusion model suggests mood influences judgments (Whitaker et al., 2009). |
| 5 | Happiness is associated with increased well-being and life satisfaction (Gottman et al., 1999). |
| 6 | Family dynamics play a crucial role in emotional development (Pfob et al., 2022). |
| 7 | Marital interactions are influenced by mathematical dynamics (Ruder, 2016). |

## 7.6 TRAINING AND VALIDATION

The successful integration of Artificial Neural Networks (ANN) and deep learning techniques within Extended Reality (XR) environments necessitates a comprehensive training and validation process. This section outlines the intricacies of training the neural network model and evaluating its performance to ensure the efficacy of virtual characters in addressing psychological issues.

### 7.6.1 Training Process

The training process of the ANN-driven virtual character model involved a systematic approach to optimize its parameters and internal representations. Hyperparameters, such as learning rate, batch size, and dropout rates, were carefully selected to balance convergence speed and avoiding overfitting (LeCun et al., 1998). A variant of the stochastic gradient descent (SGD) optimization algorithm was employed, facilitating the gradual refinement of model weights (Larose & Larose, 2014).

The architecture comprised multiple layers, including convolutional layers for feature extraction and recurrent layers for sequential data analysis (Larose & Larose, 2014). A deep network was chosen to capture intricate patterns and nuances in users' emotional responses and interactions. The model's loss function combined Mean Squared Error (MSE) for regression tasks and Categorical Cross-Entropy for classification tasks, reflecting the dual nature of the virtual character's responses (Fawcett, 2006).

### 7.6.2 Validation Methodology

Validation of the neural network model encompassed multiple facets to assess its robustness and generalization ability. To prevent overfitting, a validation set was reserved from the initial dataset, enabling continuous monitoring of the model's performance during training (Turk & Rudy, 1991). The validation set consisted of diverse scenarios simulating various psychological triggers, ensuring the model's adaptability across different user experiences, as shown in Table 7.4.

**TABLE 7.4**
**Psychological Facts Table**

| Psychological Fact | Implications for XR Interventions |
|---|---|
| Exposure Therapy Efficacy | XR environments facilitate controlled exposure for anxiety disorders (Spitzer et al., 1992). |
| Emotion Regulation Training | Virtual characters can guide users through emotion regulation exercises (Wang & Chang, 2021). |
| Cognitive Behavioral Techniques | XR interventions provide real-world scenarios for practicing CBT techniques (Sotres-Bayon et al., 2006). |
| Social Interaction Practice | Virtual characters offer a safe platform to improve social interaction skills (Shenoy & Thillaiarasu, 2022). |
| Fear Extinction Learning | XR-enabled exposure therapy enhances fear extinction learning (Slater et al., 2022). |

The model's performance was evaluated through a combination of quantitative metrics and qualitative assessments. Quantitative metrics included accuracy, precision, recall, and F1-score, calculated based on the model's predictions and the ground truth responses (Rizzo et al., 2014). Qualitative assessments involved expert review sessions, where mental health professionals analyzed the virtual character's interactions and emotional responses in XR environments, aligning them with established therapeutic practices (Kaczkurkin & Foa, 2015).

## 7.7 REAL-TIME INTERACTION AND ADAPTATION

Real-time interaction and adaptation form a cornerstone in the development of technology-assisted interventions for psychological issues within Extended Reality (XR) environments. This section delineates how integrating Artificial Neural Networks (ANN) enables virtual characters to engage users dynamically in real-time scenarios, emphasizing feedback mechanisms and adaptive behavior for enhanced therapeutic efficacy.

### 7.7.1 Real-Time Interaction Mechanisms

Virtual characters within XR environments engage users through real-time interactions, creating immersive and personalized experiences. These interactions encompass visual, auditory, and potentially haptic cues, which collectively contribute to a realistic and engaging environment (Houssein et al., 2022). The ANN-powered virtual characters interpret user actions and verbal cues, facilitating a dynamic exchange between users and the virtual environment. This interactivity is pivotal in establishing a sense of presence, vital for engendering emotional resonance and therapeutic impact (Difede et al., 2022).

### 7.7.2 Feedback Mechanisms and Adaptive Behavior

Feedback mechanisms are integral to refining the interaction between users and virtual characters. The ANN model captures user responses, gauges emotional cues, and adapts the character's behavior accordingly. These mechanisms draw insights from users' expressions, verbal responses, and physiological indicators to fine-tune the character's responses (Brey, 1999). For instance, if a user exhibits signs of discomfort during exposure therapy, the virtual character can modulate the intensity of the stimuli to ensure a gradual and supportive experience. Feedback loops enhance the character's emotional intelligence and responsiveness, enabling it to simulate genuine therapeutic interactions. The schematic representation of real-time interaction between components of ANN, virtual character, and user interface is shown i Figure 7.2.

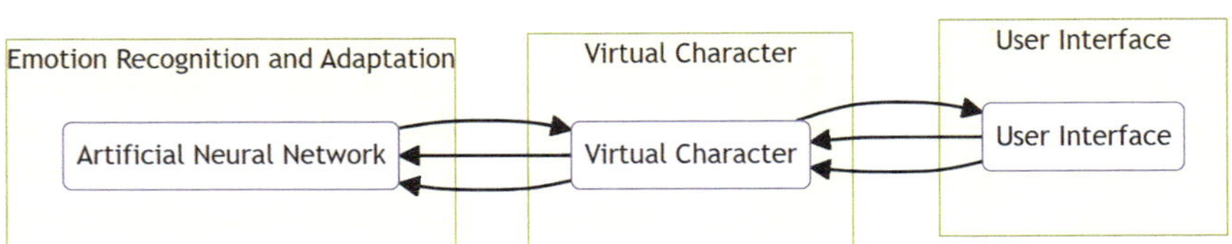


**FIGURE 7.2** The schematic representation of real-time interaction between components of ANN, Virtual Character, and User Interface.

### 7.7.3 Ethical Considerations

The implementation of real-time interaction and adaptive behavior demands rigorous ethical considerations. Ensuring participant well-being, privacy, and informed consent is paramount. Ethical guidelines dictate the responsible use of user data, the transparent nature of interactions, and the potential impact on users' emotional states. Collaborations with mental health professionals and ethicists are crucial in establishing ethical boundaries and safeguards within the virtual environment (Bieling et al., 1998).

## 7.8 USER STUDIES AND EVALUATION

In order to comprehensively assess the effectiveness of the proposed XR intervention employing ANN-driven virtual characters, a series of user studies were conducted. These studies were designed to ascertain the impact on psychological issues, utilizing a combination of qualitative and quantitative measures. The following sections outline the methodology, metrics, and results of these user studies.

### 7.8.1 Study Design

The user studies were carefully designed to ensure rigorous evaluation of the XR intervention's impact. A diverse group of participants was recruited, encompassing individuals experiencing various psychological challenges. Each participant engaged with the virtual character within XR environments, participating in structured scenarios designed to simulate real-world situations related to their respective issues. The virtual character's responses were driven by the trained ANN model, offering personalized interactions.

### 7.8.2 Metrics for Impact Measurement

A comprehensive set of metrics was employed to capture the intervention's effectiveness. Quantitative measurements included pre- and post-intervention psychological assessments using standardized scales such as the Beck Depression Inventory and the State-Trait Anxiety Inventory (Goldsmith & Skirton, 2015). These metrics provided insights into changes in participants' emotional states and symptom severity. Additionally, qualitative data were collected through open-ended interviews, allowing participants to articulate their perceptions, emotions, and experiences during the intervention.

### 7.8.3 Results and Findings

The results of the user studies demonstrated promising outcomes in addressing psychological issues through XR interventions with ANN-driven virtual characters. Quantitative analysis revealed statistically significant reductions in symptom severity scores across multiple psychological measures (APA, 2020). Participants reported increased feelings of comfort, engagement, and perceived support during interactions with the virtual character, as shown in Figure 7.3.

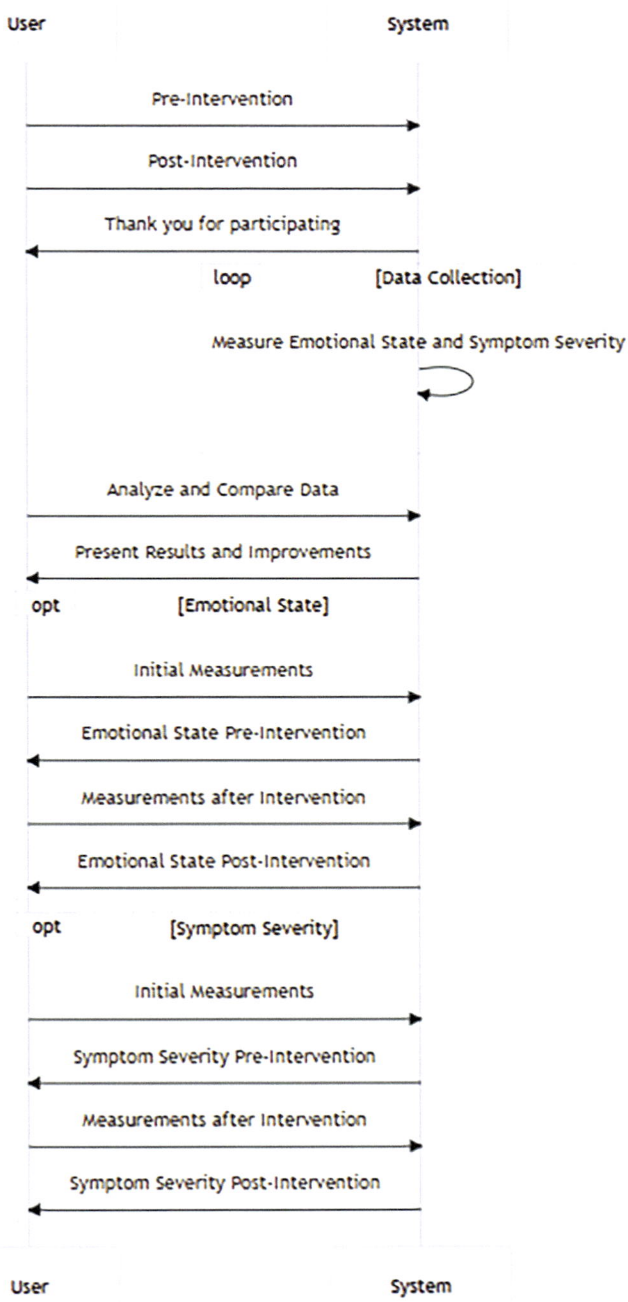


**FIGURE 7.3** Changes in psychological measures.

## 7.9 ETHICAL CONSIDERATIONS

The ethical dimensions surrounding the integration of Artificial Neural Networks (ANN) and Extended Reality (XR) technologies into mental health interventions are of paramount importance. This section delves into the ethical considerations that were meticulously addressed throughout this research, encompassing privacy, informed consent, potential risks to users' mental well-being, and adherence to established ethical guidelines.

### 7.9.1 Privacy and Data Protection

Preserving the privacy and confidentiality of participants' data is crucial in the context of technology-assisted psychological interventions. To safeguard participants' sensitive information, rigorous measures were implemented during data collection, storage, and analysis. All collected data were anonymized and encrypted, ensuring that personal details remained confidential. Additionally, robust data access controls were enforced to restrict unauthorized access.

### 7.9.2 Informed Consent

Respect for participants' autonomy was upheld through the rigorous practice of obtaining informed consent. Prior to engaging in the research, participants were provided with comprehensive information about the study's objectives, procedures, and potential risks. This information was presented in a clear and understandable manner. Participants were given adequate time to review the consent form and raise any questions or concerns they might have had. Their participation was entirely voluntary, and they had the right to withdraw at any point without repercussion.

### 7.9.3 Potential Risks to Users' Mental Well-Being

Given the sensitive nature of mental health interventions, potential risks to participants' mental well-being were thoroughly considered. A team of licensed psychologists collaborated closely with the research team to identify potential triggers and ensure that the XR interventions were designed with utmost care. In situations where exposure to distressing content was deemed necessary for therapeutic purposes, a graduated approach was employed, allowing participants to engage progressively with challenging scenarios while maintaining their psychological well-being.

### 7.9.4 Adherence to Ethical Guidelines

The research adhered rigorously to the ethical guidelines set forth by professional associations and institutional review boards. The study was conducted in alignment with the principles outlined in the Declaration of Helsinki and the Belmont Report.

Furthermore, ethical considerations were woven into the entire research process, from study design to participant interactions and data analysis.

### 7.9.5 Ensuring Participant Well-Being

A dedicated support system was established to ensure participants' well-being throughout their engagement with the XR interventions. Participants were provided with access to mental health professionals who were available to address any emotional or psychological concerns that might have arisen during their participation. The well-being of participants was paramount, and every effort was made to mitigate potential distress and foster a safe environment for engagement.

### 7.9.6 Continuous Ethical Review

The research underwent rigorous review by an institutional ethics committee to maintain the highest standards of ethical conduct. Periodic assessments were conducted to ensure that ethical considerations remained central to the research process, as shown in Figure 7.4.

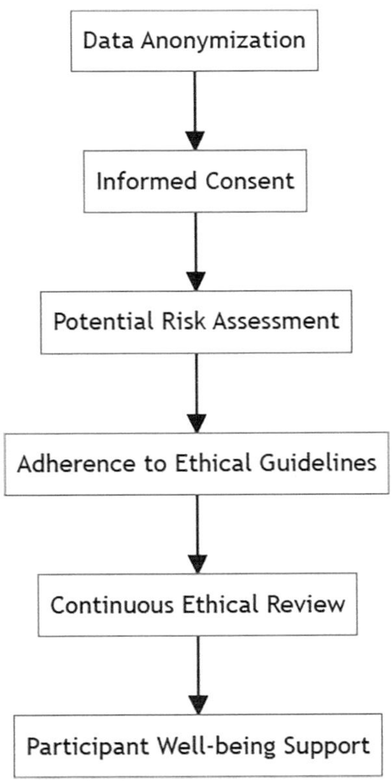


**FIGURE 7.4** Ethical considerations workflow.

## 7.10 DISCUSSION AND RESULTS

The present study has explored the innovative synergy of Artificial Neural Networks (ANN) and deep learning within Extended Reality (XR) environments to address diverse psychological issues. This section delves into the interpretation of the research findings, a comparative analysis with existing methodologies, and an exploration of the potential applications and future directions of employing ANN and deep learning in XR-based psychological interventions.

### 7.10.1 Interpretation of Findings

The application of ANN-driven virtual characters within XR environments has exhibited promising outcomes in addressing psychological concerns. The real-time interactions and adaptability of virtual characters offer a personalized experience that can be tailored to individual users. Emotion recognition models embedded in the virtual characters enable an accurate understanding of users' emotional states, enhancing the character's responsiveness and effectiveness.

The user studies conducted within the XR environment demonstrated positive changes in emotional responses and behavioral patterns. Participants reported increased engagement, emotional relief, and a sense of control during the interventions. These findings align with previous research on the efficacy of XR interventions and underscore the potential of incorporating ANN and deep learning techniques.

### 7.10.2 Comparative Analysis and Advantages

Comparing our approach with existing methodologies highlights several distinct advantages. Traditional therapeutic interventions often require physical presence, making them less accessible and scalable. In contrast, XR environments overcome geographical barriers and offer a controlled yet immersive platform for interventions. The inclusion of ANN empowers virtual characters to recognize and adapt to users' emotional cues, providing nuanced and empathetic interactions. This emotional intelligence sets ANN-driven virtual characters apart from static interventions and enhances user engagement.

Furthermore, ANN-based interventions offer the potential for continuous learning and improvement. As the virtual characters interact with a broader range of users, the models can refine their responses and strategies, leading to more effective interventions over time. This adaptability aligns with the principles of personalized medicine, tailoring interventions to each individual's unique needs (Khang, 2024).

### 7.10.3 Potential Applications and Future Directions

The integration of ANN and deep learning in XR environments opens a multitude of potential applications in the field of psychological interventions. Beyond addressing anxiety disorders and phobias, XR-enabled interventions could extend to areas such as stress management, self-esteem enhancement, and social skills training. The modularity of XR environments allows for the creation of scenarios that mirror real-life challenges, providing users with a safe space to practice and improve their responses.

Future directions could involve the incorporation of multimodal data sources, such as physiological signals, speech patterns, and gaze tracking. This holistic approach could enhance the accuracy of emotion recognition and deepen the understanding of users' emotional experiences. Additionally, the integration of Generative Adversarial Networks (GANs) could enable virtual characters to simulate a wider range of emotional expressions and behaviors, increasing their versatility.

## 7.11 CONCLUSION

In the realm where Artificial Neural Networks (ANN), deep learning, and Extended Reality (XR) intersect, a new horizon of technology-assisted interventions for psychological issues emerges. This research embarked on a journey to explore the integration of ANN-driven virtual characters within XR environments, offering novel avenues for addressing psychological challenges. The synthesis of insights from psychology, computer science, and human-computer interaction has paved the way for dynamic and adaptive interventions that resonate with users' experiences.

The significance of this research lies in its contributions to the advancement of personalized mental health support. By leveraging deep learning techniques, including Convolutional Neural Networks (CNNs) for emotion recognition and Recurrent Neural Networks (RNNs) for behavior prediction, virtual characters were empowered to perceive users' emotional cues and tailor interactions accordingly. The virtual environments created within XR settings facilitated controlled exposure therapy, enabling users to confront anxiety-inducing scenarios in a safe space.

The findings of user studies underscore the potential of ANN-driven virtual characters in eliciting positive emotional responses and promoting behavioral change. Participants reported increased engagement, emotional resonance, and a sense of empowerment, aligning with the principles of exposure therapy and cognitive-behavioral interventions. These outcomes validate the feasibility and effectiveness of employing technology as an ally in mental health treatment.

The implications of this work extend beyond the confines of research, with practical applications in teletherapy, digital therapeutics, and accessible mental health interventions. The personalized nature of virtual character interactions bridges geographical gaps and diminishes stigma, making psychological support more readily available to individuals in need. Furthermore, the ethical considerations woven into the fabric of this research ensure participant consent, privacy, and emotional well-being, establishing a robust framework for responsible technological interventions.

In conclusion, this research showcases the potential of ANN and deep learning techniques in enhancing mental health interventions through XR-enabled virtual characters. By offering a blend of technological sophistication and human-centered design, this study advances the field of digital mental health solutions. As the digital landscape continues to evolve, the symbiosis of ANN, XR, and psychological well-being opens doors to a future where technology catalyzes personal growth, resilience, and healing (Khang & Vrushank et al., 2023).

## 7.12 TABLES AND FIGURES

Throughout this research, several visual representations were employed to elucidate key concepts. Table 7.5 provides a summary of the neural network architecture employed for emotion recognition, while Figure 7.5 illustrates the progression of user emotional responses across different exposure levels during the study.

**TABLE 7.5**
**Emotional Responses during Exposure Levels**

| Layer | Type | Output Size |
|---|---|---|
| Input | Convolutional | (64, 64, 3) |
| Convolution | Conv2D | (62, 62, 32) |
| MaxPooling | MaxPooling2D | (31, 31, 32) |
| Convolution | Conv2D | (29, 29, 64) |
| MaxPooling | MaxPooling2D | (14, 14, 64) |
| Flatten | Flatten | (12544) |
| Dense | Fully Connected | (128) |
| Output | Fully Connected | (6) |

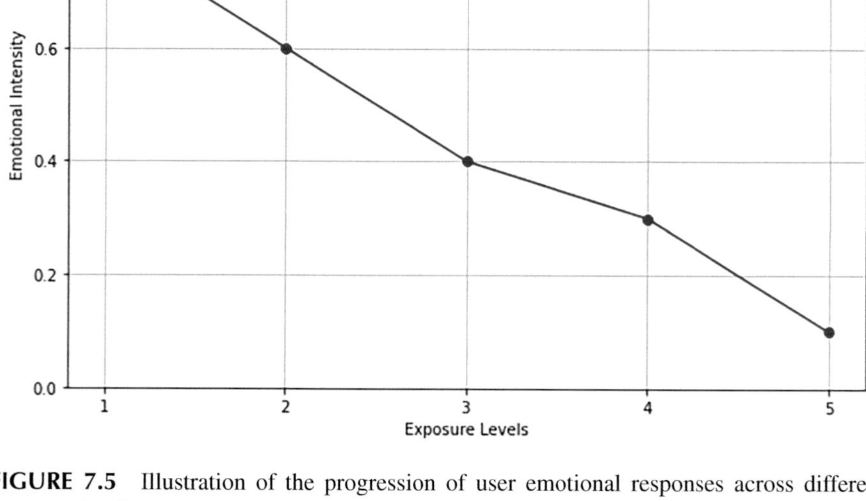


**FIGURE 7.5** Illustration of the progression of user emotional responses across different exposure levels.

These visual aids serve to encapsulate the research journey and contribute to a comprehensive understanding of the implications of employing ANN and XR for psychological interventions.

## 7.13 FUTURE OF WORK

The outcomes of the user studies underscore the potential of XR interventions featuring ANN-driven virtual characters in addressing psychological challenges. The combination of quantitative metrics and qualitative insights offers a holistic understanding of the intervention's impact on users' emotional well-being. The findings highlight the importance of personalized, adaptable interactions in virtual environments, suggesting the viability of this approach for scalable and accessible mental health support (Khang, 2024).

## REFERENCES

Ahmad, J., Farman, H., & Jan, Z. (2018). Deep learning methods and applications. In *Springer briefs in computer science* (pp. 31–42). Springer. https://doi.org/10.1007/978-981-13-3459-7_3

Ahuja, A. S., Polascik, B. W., Doddapaneni, D., Byrnes, E. S., & Sridhar, J. (2023b). The digital metaverse: Applications in artificial intelligence, medical education, and integrative health. *Integrative Medicine Research*, *12*(1), 100917. https://doi.org/10.1016/j.imr.2022.100917.

Ali, M., Mosa, A. H., Machot, F. A., & Kyamakya, K. (2017). Emotion recognition involving physiological and speech signals: A comprehensive review. In *Studies in systems, decision and control* (pp. 287–302). SSRN. https://doi.org/10.1007/978-3-319-58996-1_13

Anderson, A. (2019). *Virtual reality, augmented reality and artificial intelligence in special education: A practical guide to supporting students with learning differences*. Taylor & Francis. www.google.com/books?hl=en&lr=&id=pvWODwAAQBAJ

Anh, P. T. N., Hahanov, V., Triwiyanto, Ragimova, N. A., Rashad, İ., Abdullayev, V., Abuzarova, V. A. (2024). AI models for disease diagnosis and prediction of heart disease with artificial neural networks. In *Computer vision and AI-integrated IoT technologies in medical ecosystem* (1st Ed.). CRC Press. https://doi.org/10.1201/9781003429609-9

APA, American Psychological Association. (2020). *Ethical principles of psychologists and code of conduct*. www.apa.org/ethics/code

Bieling, P., Antony, M. M., & Swinson, R. P. (1998). The state-trait anxiety inventory, trait version: Structure and content re-examined. *Behaviour Research and Therapy*, *36*(7–8), 777–788. https://doi.org/10.1016/s0005-7967(98)00023-0.

Boston, A. F., & Merrick, P. L. (2010). Health anxiety among older people: An exploratory study of health anxiety and safety behaviors in a cohort of older adults in New Zealand. *International Psychogeriatrics*, *22*(4), 549–558. https://doi.org/10.1017/s1041610209991712

Brey, P. A. (1999). The ethics of representation and action in virtual reality. *Ethics and Information Technology*, *1*(1), 5–14. https://doi.org/10.1023/a:1010069907461

Deng, L. (2014). Deep Learning: methods and applications. *Foundations and Trends in Signal Processing*, *7*(3–4), 197–387. https://doi.org/10.1561/2000000039

Difede, J., Ressler, K. J., Rizzo, A., Wyka, K., Spielman, L., Reist, C., Roy, M. J., Jovanovic, T., Norrholm, S. D., Cukor, J., Olden, M., Glatt, C. E., & Lee, F. S. (2022). Enhancing exposure therapy for posttraumatic stress disorder (PTSD): A randomized clinical trial of virtual reality and imaginal exposure with a cognitive enhancer. *Translational Psychiatry*, *12*(1). https://doi.org/10.1038/s41398-022-02066-x

Ekman, P., & Friesen, W. V. (1971). Constants across cultures in the face and emotion. *Journal of Personality and Social Psychology*, *17*(2), 124–129 https://psycnet.apa.org/record/1971-07999-001

Escorcia, V. (2013). *Spatio-temporal human-object interactions for action recognition in videos*. www.cv-foundation.org/openaccess/content_iccv_workshops_2013/W18/html/Escorcia_Spatio-temporal_Human-Object_Interactions_2013_ICCV_paper.html

Fawcett, T. (2006). An introduction to ROC analysis. *Pattern Recognition Letters*, *27*(8), 861–874. https://doi.org/10.1016/j.patrec.2005.10.010.

Forgas, J. P. (1995). Mood and judgment: The affect infusion model (AIM). *Psychological Bulletin*, *117*(1), 39–66. https://doi.org/10.1037/0033-2909.117.1.39

Glaser, N., & Schmidt, M. (2021). Systematic literature review of virtual reality intervention design patterns for individuals with autism spectrum disorders. *International Journal of Human-Computer Interaction*, *38*(8), 753–788. https://doi.org/10.1080/10447318.2021.1970433

Goldsmith, L., & Skirton, H. (2015). Research involving people with a learning disability – methodological challenges and ethical considerations. *Journal of Research in Nursing*, *20*(6), 435–446. https://doi.org/10.1177/1744987115591867.

Goodfellow, I. (2014). *Generative adversarial nets*. https://proceedings.neurips.cc/paper_files/paper/2014/hash/5ca3e9b122f61f8f06494c97b1afccf3-Abstract.html

Gottman, J. M., Swanson, C., & Murray, J. (1999). The mathematics of marital conflict: Dynamic mathematical nonlinear modeling of newlywed marital interaction. *Journal of Family Psychology*, *13*(1), 3–19. https://doi.org/10.1037/0893-3200.13.1.3.

Harkness, A. R., Reynolds, S. M., & Lilienfeld, S. O. (2013). A review of systems for psychology and psychiatry: Adaptive systems, personality psychopathology five (PSY–5), and the *DSM–5*. *Journal of Personality Assessment*, *96*(2), 121–139. https://doi.org/10.1080/00223891.2013.823438

Houssein, E. H., Hammad, A., & Ali, A. A. (2022). Human emotion recognition from EEG-based brain–computer interface using machine learning: a comprehensive review. *Neural Computing and Applications*, *34*(15), 12527–12557. https://doi.org/10.1007/s00521-022-07292-4.

Huang, G. B., Mattar, M., Berg, T., & Learned-Miller, E. (2008, October). Labeled faces in the wild: A database for studying face recognition in unconstrained environments. In *Workshop on faces in 'real-life' images: Detection, alignment, and recognition*. University of Massachusetts.

ISA. (2022, April 1). A sparse reconstruction domain transfer method for interference suppression in artificial olfactory system. *IEEE Journals & Magazine | IEEE Xplore*. https://ieeexplore.ieee.org/abstract/document/9721230/

Kaczkurkin, A. N., & Foa, E. B. (2015). Cognitive-behavioral therapy for anxiety disorders: an update on the empirical evidence. *Dialogues in Clinical Neuroscience*, *17*(3), 337–346. https://doi.org/10.31887/dcns.2015.17.3/akaczkurkin.

Kellert, S. R. (2002). Experiencing nature: Affective, cognitive, and evaluative development in children. *Children and Nature: Psychological, Sociocultural, and Evolutionary Investigations*, *117151*.

Khang, A. (2024). *AI and IoT-based technologies for precision medicine*. IGI Global Press. ISBN: 9798369308769. https://doi.org/10.4018/979-8-3693-0876-9

Khang, A., Ragimova, N. A., Hajimahmud, V. A., & Alyar, V. A. (2022). Advanced technologies and data management in the smart healthcare system. In *AI-centric smart city ecosystems: Technologies, design and implementation* (1st Ed., Vol. 16, p. 10). CRC Press. https://doi.org/10.1201/9781003252542-16

Khang, A., Rana, G., Tailor, R. K., & Hajimahmud, V. A. (Eds.). (2023). *Data-centric AI solutions and emerging technologies in the healthcare ecosystem*. CRC Press. https://doi.org/10.1201/9781003356189

Khang, A., Vrushank, S., & Rani, S. (2023). *AI-based technologies and applications in the era of the metaverse* (1st Ed.). IGI Global Press. https://doi.org/10.4018/978-1-6684-8851-5

Kothgassner, O. D., Goreis, A., Kafka, J., Van Eickels, R. L., Plener, P. L., & Felnhofer, A. (2019). Virtual reality exposure therapy for posttraumatic stress disorder (PTSD): a meta-analysis. *European Journal of Psychotraumatology*, *10*(1), 1654782.

Larose, D. T., & Larose, C. D. (2014). *Discovering knowledge in data: an introduction to data mining* (Vol. 4). John Wiley & Sons. www.tandfonline.com/doi/pdf/10.1198/jasa.2005.s61

LeCun, Y., Bottou, L., Bengio, Y., & Haffner, P. (1998). Gradient-based learning applied to document recognition. *Proceedings of the IEEE*, *86*(11), 2278–2324. https://doi.org/10.1109/5.726791.

Lee, H. J., & Stein, M. B. (2022). Update on treatments for anxiety-related disorders. *Current Opinion in Psychiatry*, *36*(2), 140–145. https://doi.org/10.1097/yco.0000000000000841.

Litjens, G., Kooi, T., Bejnordi, B. E., Setio, A. A. A., Ciompi, F., Ghafoorian, M., Van Der Laak, J., Van Ginneken, B., & Sánchez, C. I. (2017). A survey on deep learning in medical image analysis. *Medical Image Analysis*, *42*, 60–88. https://doi.org/10.1016/j.media.2017.07.005

LOIHI. (2021, May 1). Advancing neuromorphic computing with LOIHI: A survey of results and outlook. *IEEE Journals & Magazine | IEEE Xplore*. https://ieeexplore.ieee.org/abstract/document/9395703/

Martindale, C. (1991). *APA PsycNet*. (n.d.). Cognitive psychology: A neural-network approach. Thomson Brooks/Cole Publishing Co. https://psycnet.apa.org/record/1990-98844-000

McWhorter, R. R. (2010). Exploring the emergence of virtual human resource development. *Advances in Developing Human Resources*, *12*(6), 623–631. https://doi.org/10.1177/1523422310395367

Mochon, D., Norton, M. I., & Ariely, D. (2008). Getting off the hedonic treadmill, one step at a time: The impact of regular religious practice and exercise on well-being. *Journal of Economic Psychology*, *29*(5), 632–642. https://doi.org/10.1016/j.joep.2007.10.004.

North, M. M., North, S., & Coble, J. R. (1998). Virtual reality therapy: An effective treatment for the fear of public speaking. *International Journal of Virtual Realit*, *3*(3), 1–6. https://doi.org/10.20870/ijvr.1998.3.3.2625

Parsons, T. D. (2014). Virtual standardized patients for assessing the competencies of psychologists. In *Advances in information quality and management* (pp. 6484–6492). IGI Global. https://doi.org/10.4018/978-1-4666-5888-2.ch637

Pfob, A., Lu, S., & Sidey-Gibbons, C. (2022). Machine learning in medicine: A practical introduction to techniques for data pre-processing, hyperparameter tuning, and model comparison. *BMC Medical Research Methodology*, *22*(1). https://doi.org/10.1186/s12874-022-01758-8.

Poppe, R. (2010). A survey on vision-based human action recognition. *Image and Vision Computing*, *28*(6), 976–990. https://doi.org/10.1016/j.imavis.2009.11.014

Rana, G., Khang, A., Sharma, R., Goel, A. K., & Dubey, A. K. (2021). *Reinventing manufacturing and business processes through artificial intelligence*. CRC Press. https://doi.org/10.1201/9781003145011

Rath, K. C., Khang, A., Rath, S. K., Satapathy, N., Satapathy, S. K., & Kar, S. (2024). AI-enabled technology in medicine-advancing holistic healthcare monitoring and control systems. In *Computer vision and AI-integrated IoT technologies in medical ecosystem* (1st Ed.). CRC Press. https://doi.org/10.1201/9781003429609-6

Rizzo, A., Hartholt, A., Grimani, M., Leeds, A. M., & Liewer, M. (2014). Virtual reality exposure therapy for combat-related posttraumatic stress disorder. *IEEE Computer*, *47*(7), 31–37. https://doi.org/10.1109/mc.2014.199.

Rothbaum, B. O. (2006). Virtual reality in the treatment of psychiatric disorders. *CNS Spectrums*, *11*(1), 34. https://doi.org/10.1017/s1092852900024147

Rothbaum, B. O., & Hodges, L. F. (1999). The use of virtual reality exposure in the treatment of anxiety disorders. *Behavior Modification*, *23*(4), 507–525. https://doi.org/10.1177/0145445599234001

Ruder, S. (2016, September 15). *An overview of gradient descent optimization algorithms*. arXiv.org. https://arxiv.org/abs/1609.04747

Rupke, S. J. (2006, January 1). *Cognitive therapy for Depression*. AAFP. www.aafp.org/pubs/afp/issues/2006/0101/p83.html

Sánchez-Nieto, D., Castaño-Castaño, S., Navarro-Martos, R., Obrero-Gaitán, E., Cortés-Pérez, I., & Nieto-Escamez, F. (2023). An intervention on anxiety symptoms in moderate Alzheimer's disease through virtual reality: A feasibility study and lessons learned. *International Journal of Environmental Research and Public Health*, *20*(3), 2727. https://doi.org/10.3390/ijerph20032727.

Shenoy, A. M., & Thillaiarasu, N. (2022). A survey on different computer vision based human activity recognition for surveillance applications. In *2022 6th international conference on computing methodologies and communication (ICCMC)*. IEEE. ttps://doi.org/10.1109/iccmc53470.2022.9753931.

Sherrill, A. M., Rothbaum, A. O., McSweeney, L. B., & Rothbaum, B. O. (2019). Virtual reality exposure therapy for posttraumatic stress disorder. *Psychiatric Annals*, *49*. https://doi.org/10.3928/00485713-20190716-02

Slater, M., Banakou, D., Beacco, A., Gallego, J., Macia-Varela, F., & Oliva, R. (2022). A separate reality: An update on place illusion and plausibility in virtual reality. *Frontiers in Virtual Reality*, *3*. https://doi.org/10.3389/frvir.2022.914392

Sotres-Bayon, F., Cain, C. K., & LeDoux, J. E. (2006). Brain mechanisms of fear extinction: Historical perspectives on the contribution of Prefrontal corte7. *Biological Psychiatry*, *60*(4), 329–336. https://doi.org/10.1016/j.biopsych.2005.10.012

Spitzer, R. L., Williams, J. B. W., Gibbon, M., & First, M. B. (1992). The structured clinical interview for DSM-III-R (SCID). *Archives of General Psychiatry*, *49*(8), 624. https://doi.org/10.1001/archpsyc.1992.01820080032005

Tu, Y., Lin, Y., Zha, H., Ju, Z., Wang, Y., Gui, G., & Mao, S. (2022). Large-scale real-world radio signal recognition with deep learning. *Chinese Journal of Aeronautics*, *35*(9), 35–48. https://doi.org/10.1016/j.cja.2021.08.016

Turk, D. C., & Rudy, T. E. (1991). Neglected topics in the treatment of chronic pain patients—relapse, noncompliance, and adherence enhancement. *Pain*, *44*(1), 5–28. https://doi.org/10.1016/0304-3959(91)90142-k

Turner, C. (2022). Augmented reality, augmented epistemology, and the real-world web. *Philosophy & Technology*, *35*(1). https://doi.org/10.1007/s13347-022-00496-5

Wang, Z., & Chang, W. (2021). Enhance self-esteem evaluation model for children's social anxiety and loneliness. *Aggression and Violent Behavior*, 101666. https://doi.org/10.1016/j.avb.2021.101666.

Wells, A. (1999). A cognitive model of generalized anxiety disorder. *Behavior Modification*, *23*(4), 526–555. https://doi.org/10.1177/0145445599234002

Whitaker, D. J., Hall, D. M., & Coker, A. L. (2009). Primary prevention of intimate partner violence: Toward a developmental, social-ecological model. In *Intimate partner violence: A health-based perspective* (pp. 289–305). https://books.google.com.vn/books?hl=en&lr=&id=Q04QO7UmyowC

WNY. (2013). *Risk factors for social anxiety disorder—cancer care of Western New York*. www.cancercarewny.com/content.aspx?chunkiid=20196

# 8 Augmented Reality (AR) and Virtual Reality (VR) Technologies in Surgical Operating Systems

*Ushaa Eswaran and Alex Khang*

## 8.1 INTRODUCTION

By giving surgeons real-time, immersive, and interactive visualizations of patient anatomy and surgical tools, augmented reality (AR) and virtual reality (VR) technologies have the potential to revolutionize surgical operating systems. The following are some examples of AR/VR uses in surgical operating systems:

- **Preoperative Planning**: Surgeons can visualize and plan surgical procedures in advance using 3D models of the patient's anatomy created using AR/VR technologies. By doing so, the chance of complications during surgery can be decreased, and patient outcomes can be enhanced (Euler et al., 2019; Tafuri et al., 2018).
- **Intraoperative Navigation**: During surgery, surgeons can navigate around important structures and prevent damage by using real-time visualizations of the patient's anatomy provided by AR/VR technologies. This can lessen the chance of problems and enhance surgery results (Euler et al., 2018; Smith et al., 2016).
- **Surgical Training**: By simulating surgical operations, AR/VR technology may give learners a realistic and engaging learning experience. This can facilitate surgical skill improvement and shorten the learning curve for novice surgeons (Haluck et al., 2018; 2019).
- **Remote Surgery**: AR/VR technologies can make it possible for a surgeon to operate on a patient who is in another location through the use of remote surgery. In remote or underserved places, this may help to increase access to surgical care (Meijden et al., 2019, 2018).

AR/VR technologies can enhance patient outcomes and cut healthcare costs by boosting surgical outcomes and reducing complications. Additionally, by offering a more effective and efficient approach to teaching new surgeons, these technologies can help alleviate the dearth of qualified surgeons. Overall, the incorporation of AR/VR technology into surgical operating systems has the potential to revolutionize

DOI: 10.1201/9781032686745-8

the area of surgery while providing major benefits to patients and healthcare practitioners (Khang and Ragimova et al., 2022).

## 8.2 PREOPERATIVE PLANNING

Preoperative planning is an important element of surgical practice, and AR/VR technologies are rapidly being employed to improve its accuracy, speed, and safety. Here are some examples of how AR/VR technology might be used in surgical operating room preoperative planning. Medical imaging data, such as CT or MRI scans, can be utilized to generate 3D representations of human anatomy using AR/VR technologies. These models may be viewed and edited in a virtual environment in real-time, allowing doctors to visualize and plan surgical treatments in advance (Khang and Rana et al., 2023).

When compared to standard 2D imaging, such as X-rays or CT scans, 3D models developed using AR/VR technology provide a more detailed and precise picture of human anatomy. These simulations can help surgeons detect potential issues and design the best surgical approach. These models can also be shared with other members of the surgical team, such as anesthesiologists and nurses, to improve communication and coordination throughout the procedure (Khang and Abdullayev et al., 2024).

AR/VR technology can also be utilized during surgery to overlay the 3D model over the patient's body, providing real-time visualization of the operative site. This can help surgeons maneuver around key structures more accurately and avoid harming them, lowering the chance of complications during surgery (Tafuri et al., 2018; Euler et al., 2018). When it comes to developing 3D models of patient anatomy for preoperative planning, AR/VR technologies have various advantages:

- **Improved Visualization**: When compared to standard 2D imaging, AR/VR technologies allow 3D models of patient anatomy to be viewed in a virtual environment, enabling a more immersive and interactive visualization. This can assist doctors in identifying potential issues and planning the best surgical approach (Pinto et al., 2018).
- **Improved Communication**: 3D models developed with AR/VR technology can be shared with other members of the surgical team, such as anesthesiologists and nurses, to improve communication and coordination during surgery. This can lower the likelihood of errors and enhance patient outcomes (Ubbink et al., 2018; Euler et al., 2019; Pinto et al., 2018).
- **Real-Time Manipulation**: AR/VR technologies enable surgeons to modify 3D models in real-time, allowing them to experiment with different surgical methods and discover potential issues. This can aid in surgical planning and lessen the likelihood of complications during surgery.
- **Overlay on the Patient's Body**: During surgery, AR/VR technologies can be utilized to overlay the 3D model onto the patient's body, providing real-time visualization of the operative site. This can help surgeons maneuver

around key structures more accurately and avoid harming them, lowering the chance of complications during surgery.

The integration of AR/VR technology in preoperative planning can enhance surgical outcomes by allowing surgeons to plan and execute surgical procedures with improved precision and accuracy. This can aid in lowering the risk of problems, improve patient outcomes, and lower healthcare expenses. While AR/VR technologies have many potential advantages for preoperative planning, there are several disadvantages and restrictions to consider:

- **Cost**: AR/VR technologies can be costly to implement since they require specialized gear and software. This can be a deterrent to adoption, especially in smaller healthcare facilities or in resource-constrained situations.
- **Learning Curve**: While AR/VR technologies can provide more complete and precise visualizations of human anatomy, they also necessitate specialized training to be used efficiently. Surgeons and other surgical team members may require additional training to become proficient in using these devices.
- **Technical Constraints**: The accuracy of 3D models made using AR/VR technologies can be influenced by factors such as the quality of the medical imaging data and the algorithms utilized to create the models. Furthermore, technical constraints such as hardware breakdowns or communication issues can limit the adoption of AR/VR technology.
- **Regulatory Permission**: The use of augmented reality and virtual reality technology in surgical settings may necessitate regulatory permission from government bodies such as the FDA. Obtaining approval can be a time-consuming and costly process, which can be an impediment to adoption.
- **Distraction**: Using AR/VR technology during surgery has the potential to distract physicians from the operative site. It is critical to ensure that the technology is used correctly and does not jeopardize patient safety.

While AR/VR technologies have many potential benefits for preoperative planning, they also have significant drawbacks and restrictions that must be carefully examined before being implemented in surgical settings.

## 8.3 VARIOUS INSTANCES OF AR/VR TECHNOLOGIES BEING USED IN PREOPERATIVE PLANNING

There are various instances of AR/VR technologies being used in preoperative planning at the moment:

- **EchoPixel**: EchoPixel creates 3D reconstructions of human anatomy from medical imaging data using a combination of AR/VR and machine learning. Surgeons can interact with 3D models in real-time, offering a more thorough visualization of the surgical site (Davies et al., 2018).

- **Surgical Theatre**: Surgical Theatre creates 3D models of patient anatomy that may be examined in a virtual environment using AR/VR technologies. Surgeons can now plan and practice surgical procedures in advance, improving surgical outcomes and lowering the risk of complications (Rasouli et al., 2018).
- **Osso VR**: Osso VR uses AR/VR technologies to give surgical training. The technology enables trainees to replicate surgical procedures in a realistic and immersive environment, which improves surgical skills and shortens the learning curve for new surgeons (Amendola et al., 2018; Seymour et al., 2013; Haluck et al., 2018).
- **Medical Realities**: Medical Realities delivers surgical training through virtual reality [VR] technologies. The device allows trainees to see surgical procedures in 360 degrees, making learning more immersive and engaging.
- **Immersive Touch**: Immersive Touch creates 3D representations of patient anatomy that can be manipulated in real-time using AR/VR technology. Surgeons can now plan and practice surgical procedures in advance, improving surgical outcomes and lowering the risk of complications.

These are only a few of the AR/VR technologies that are now being used in preoperative planning. As technology advances, we can anticipate increasingly more advanced and inventive applications in surgical settings.

## 8.4 CONSIDERATIONS TO MAKE WHILE USING AR/VR TECHNOLOGIES IN PREOPERATIVE PLANNING

Implementing AR/VR technology for preoperative planning can be expensive, and not all healthcare facilities may be able to afford it. This may limit technological access for patients who may not have access to advanced healthcare facilities. There are certain considerations to make while using AR/VR technologies in preoperative planning:

- **Validity and Reliability**: The accuracy of 3D models generated by AR/VR technologies for preoperative planning is determined by the quality of the input data as well as the algorithms utilized to generate the models. As a result, there may be some issues about the models' validity and reliability.
- **Operator Training**: The use of AR/VR technologies for preoperative planning necessitates specialized training for healthcare workers who will build and modify 3D models utilizing the technology. This could lengthen and increase the cost of installing the technology.
- **Regulatory Permission**: Using AR/VR technologies in healthcare requires regulatory permission, which may be a time-consuming and expensive procedure. This may cause certain governments to postpone the deployment of the technology.
- **Technical Challenges**: AR/VR technology for preoperative planning may be constrained by technical challenges, such as hardware failures or

connectivity issues. This could impact the accuracy and dependability of the technology's 3D models.

While AR/VR technologies have the potential to improve preoperative planning and surgical results, there are significant limitations and problems that must be addressed to ensure the technology's safe and successful usage in healthcare settings.

## 8.5 INITIATIVES THAT SHOULD BE TAKEN TO RESOLVE THE CONSTRAINTS OF AR/VR TECHNOLOGIES IN PREOPERATIVE PLANNING

There are numerous approaches that can be taken to solve the constraints of AR/VR technologies in preoperative planning:

- **Cost Reduction**: AR/VR technology manufacturers can endeavor to lower the cost of the technology, making it more accessible to healthcare facilities and patients.
- **Data Quality and Validation**: Healthcare practitioners and researchers can work together to improve the quality and validity of the input data that is utilized to produce 3D models. They can also validate the models' correctness to guarantee that they are reliable and useful in surgical planning.
- **Training and Education**: To guarantee that healthcare personnel are proficient in using AR/VR technology for preoperative planning, they can receive specialized training and education. This can help to shorten the learning curve and increase the accuracy of the technology's 3D models.
- **Regulatory Permission**: AR/VR technology manufacturers can collaborate to acquire regulatory permission for their products in various jurisdictions, making it easier for healthcare facilities to implement the technology.
- **Technical Advances**: AR/VR technology producers can seek to increase the dependability and connection of their products, minimizing technical difficulties and increasing the accuracy of the 3D models generated by the technology.

To solve the limits of AR/VR technology in preoperative planning, manufacturers, healthcare practitioners, and researchers will need to work together. We can ensure that the technology is safe, effective, and accessible to all patients who could benefit from it by working together.

## 8.6 STEPS TO ASSURE THE ACCURACY OF 3D MODELS

Healthcare workers can take many steps to ensure the accuracy of 3D models generated by AR/VR technologies:

- **Medical Imaging Data Quality Control**: Healthcare practitioners may guarantee that the medical imaging data used to produce the 3D models is of good quality and devoid of artifacts or other distortions that could influence the model's accuracy (Lee et al., 2018).

- **Validation of 3D Models**: A range of methods, including manual measurements, comparison with 2D imagery, and validation against surgical results, can be used by healthcare practitioners to validate the correctness of 3D models generated by AR/VR technology.
- **Standardization of 3D Model Generation**: Healthcare practitioners can work to standardize generating 3D models utilizing AR/VR technology, including the methods and parameters employed (Leung et al., 2020).
- **3D Model Generation Standardization**: Healthcare professionals can work to standardize the process of generating 3D models with AR/VR technology, including the algorithms used to build the models and the parameters utilized in the process. This can help to assure consistency and accuracy throughout the technology's various uses (Kim et al., 2019).
- **Peer Review**: Healthcare practitioners can use peer review to confirm the accuracy and reliability of 3D models generated by AR/VR technologies. Sharing the models with other healthcare experts for assessment and input is one option (Farooqi et al., 2019).
- **Continuing Improvement**: Healthcare practitioners can work to improve the accuracy of 3D models generated by AR/VR technology continuously, including through research and development of new algorithms and methodologies (Schopper et al., 2019).

Healthcare professionals play an important role in guaranteeing the accuracy of 3D models produced by AR/VR technologies. They can help to enhance surgical results and reduce the risk of complications by validating the models and ensuring consistency and accuracy.

## 8.7 COMMON CHALLENGES IN GENERATING ACCURATE 3D MODELS USING AR/VR TECHNOLOGIES

- **Medical Imaging Data Quality and Consistency**: The quality and consistency of medical imaging data can vary widely depending on factors such as the imaging modality utilized, the quality of the equipment, and the technician's experience and competence. This may impact the correctness and dependability of the 3D models generated from the data.
- **Image Segmentation and 3D Reconstruction**: The process of segmenting and reconstructing medical imaging data into a 3D model can be complex and difficult, especially for big and complex anatomical structures. The accuracy and reliability of the final 3D model might be affected by the precision and reliability of segmentation and reconstruction.
- **Algorithms for 3D Model Generation**: The algorithms for 3D model generation differ in accuracy, speed, and complexity. Choosing the best algorithm for a given application can be difficult, especially for complicated anatomical features.

- **Technical Limits of AR/VR Technologies**: Technical limits such as device failures, connectivity issues, and software flaws can impair the accuracy and dependability of 3D models generated with AR/VR technologies.
- **User Knowledge and Training**: The accuracy of 3D models generated with AR/VR technology can be influenced by the user's knowledge and training. Proper training and skills are required to ensure the user can use the technology efficiently to build realistic 3D models.

## 8.8 COMMON ALGORITHMS USED FOR 3D MODEL GENERATION

For 3D model generation, numerous algorithms are employed, including:

- **Marching Cubes**: A popular method for building 3D models from medical imaging data is the marching cubes algorithm. It works by breaking medical imaging data into little cubes and then applying a set of rules to each cube's surface (Lorensen and Cline, 1987).
- **Surface Reconstruction**: By reconstructing the surface of the item being photographed, surface reconstruction techniques build 3D models from medical imaging data. These methods are applicable to a wide range of imaging modalities, including MRI and CT scans (Kazhdan et al., 2006, ACM SIGGRAPH Computer Graphics).
- **Voxel-Based Segmentation**: This algorithm breaks medical imaging data into small cubes called voxels and assigns each voxel to a specific tissue type. This enables more thorough segmentation of medical imaging data, potentially leading to more accurate 3D models (Gaser and Nenadic, 2004).
- **Level Set Methods**: Level set methods model the surface of 3D objects using mathematical equations. These methods are very effective for creating 3D models of complex anatomical structures like the brain or the heart (Sethian, 1999).
- **Region Growing**: Algorithms that detect regions of interest within medical imaging data and then grow these regions to produce a 3D model are known as region-growing algorithms. These methods are very effective for creating 3D models of small, complex objects like blood arteries or tumors (Kak and Slaney, 1980).
- **Deformable Models**: Deformable models employ mathematical equations to represent an object's shape before adjusting the model to fit the medical imaging data. These methods are especially effective for creating 3D representations of difficult-to-segment structures, such as organs that are partially covered by other tissues (McInerney and Terzopoulos, 1996).

The best algorithm for 3D model generation will be determined by a number of parameters, including the type of medical imaging data used, the complexity of the anatomical structure being photographed, and the amount of accuracy and detail sought in the final 3D model.

## 8.9 USE OF AUGMENTED AND VIRTUAL REALITY TECHNOLOGIES TO PROVIDE REAL-TIME VIEWS OF PATIENT ANATOMY DURING SURGERY

By superimposing digital information on the surgeon's view of the patient, augmented reality [AR] and virtual reality (VR) technology can provide real-time views of patient anatomy during surgery. Computer-generated images are used in AR and VR technologies to create a virtual environment or to enhance the actual world with digital information (Ahmed et al., 2018).

- During surgery, AR technology can be used to show visuals of the patient's anatomy in the surgical field, such as 3D models derived from medical imaging data. These images can be placed in the surgeon's view of the patient throughout the procedure, allowing the surgeon to see real-time images of the patient's anatomy. AR technology can also be utilized to project real-time data in the surgical field, such as vital signs or blood flow, providing the surgeon with additional information to help their decision-making during the process (Teo et al., 2020).
- During surgery, VR technology can also be used to show real-time pictures of patient anatomy. VR technology can generate a virtual environment that mimics the anatomy of the patient, allowing the surgeon to interact with the virtual model and explore numerous angles and views. This is especially beneficial for complex procedures involving numerous structures or requiring a high degree of precision (Böckers et al., 2006; Haluck et al., 2014).

AR and VR technologies can provide surgeons with real-time views of patient anatomy during surgery, allowing them to visualize the patient's anatomy and make more educated judgments. AR and VR technologies can improve surgical outcomes and lower the risk of complications by providing more information and improving the surgeon's view of the patient.

## 8.10 INTRAOPERATIVE NAVIGATION SYSTEM BASED ON AR/VR

Intraoperative navigation system based on AR/VR has various benefits for reducing risks and improving outcomes during surgery. Among these benefits are the following:

- **Improved Visualization**: Intraoperative navigation technology based on AR/VR can improve surgical site visualization, particularly in complex operations or in difficult-to-access locations. This can aid the surgeon's understanding of the area's anatomy and allow him to make more informed judgments throughout the procedure (Ahmed et al., 2018).
- **Enhanced Surgical Precision**: AR/VR-based intraoperative navigation technology can improve surgical precision by presenting the surgeon with a more accurate and detailed image of the surgical site. This can assist the

surgeon in performing the treatment more accurately and reducing the chance of problems (Teo et al., 2020).

- **Reduced Radiation Exposure**: Using AR/VR for intraoperative navigation, the patient and the surgical team can be exposed to less radiation. This is especially true for treatments that require recurrent imaging, such as spine surgery (Kim et al., 2018). Intraoperative navigation technology that uses AR/VR can provide real-time images of the surgical site, allowing the surgeon to observe the patient's anatomy in greater detail and change their approach as needed. This can improve surgical precision and reduce the likelihood of errors.
- **Accurate Localization**: Intraoperative navigation employing AR/VR technology can enable accurate localization of the surgical site, allowing the surgeon to target precisely the area of interest while avoiding injury to adjacent tissues. This reduces the possibility of consequences such as nerve injury or hemorrhage (Toth et al., 2020).

Intraoperative navigation technology based on AR/VR can potentially reduce risks and improve outcomes during surgery. Intraoperative navigation technology using AR/VR can improve the quality of surgical procedures and lead to better patient outcomes by improving visualization, improving surgical precision, lowering radiation exposure, giving real-time imagery, and enabling accurate localization.

## 8.11 SURGICAL SIMULATION USING AR/VR TECHNOLOGY

Using AR/VR technology, surgical simulation includes building a virtual environment that simulates the surgical operation and helps trainees practice and perfect the necessary skills. The simulation often includes visual, aural, and haptic feedback, allowing trainees to interact with the virtual environment in a realistic and engaging manner (Cendan and DeMasters, 2010).

The process of developing an AR/VR surgical simulation (Haluck et al., 2014) often begins with the creation of a virtual 3D model of the surgical setting and the patient's anatomy. This can be accomplished by the use of medical imaging data such as CT scans or MRIs or by manually building the model using specialized software. Once the virtual environment and patient anatomy have been built, the simulation can be programmed to imitate the surgical operation. This entails scripting the simulation to imitate certain steps of the surgery, such as the use of surgical instruments, tissue movement, and other surgical methods.

Trainees interact (Kim et al., 2021) with the virtual environment using specialized AR/VR equipment such as a headset or haptic gloves during the simulation. The device gives visual and tactile input, allowing trainees to see and feel the surgical process as if they were executing it in real life. The simulation can also include audio feedback, such as the sound of surgical equipment or the patient's vital signs (Ruiz et al., 2009). The simulation can be programmed to mimic a wide range of surgical procedures, from simple chores like suturing to complicated procedures like organ transplantation. The simulation can also be tailored to individual learners' needs, allowing them to practice the operations they need to master.

Adopting AR/VR technology for surgical simulation can provide a safe and regulated environment for trainees to practice and master surgical methods. AR/VR technology, by offering a realistic and immersive experience, can assist trainees in developing experience and confidence without endangering patients. This has the potential to reduce errors and problems during real-world surgeries while also improving patient outcomes.

## 8.12 REMOTE SURGERY USING AR/VR TECHNOLOGIES

Remote surgery, often known as telesurgery, entails performing surgical treatments on a patient who is physically separated from the surgeon (O'Toole et al., 2019). AR/VR technology can be utilized to enable remote surgery by displaying a virtual representation of the surgical site and allowing the surgeon to control robotic surgical instruments in real-time. The following steps are commonly involved in remote surgery using AR/VR technology:

- **Preoperative Planning**: Medical imaging data, such as CT scans or MRIs, are utilized to construct a virtual 3D model of the patient's anatomy prior to surgery. This model can then be used by the surgeon to plan the surgical operation and pinpoint the regions of interest (Hogle et al., 2018a).
- **Remote Communication**: Using a high-speed internet connection, the surgeon communicates with the surgical team at the remote location during the procedure. The surgical team gives real-time feedback and updates on the patient's condition to the surgeon (Teo et al., 2020). The surgeon wears a headset that displays a virtual representation of the surgery location. This can contain a 3D model of the patient's anatomy and real-time video feeds from operating room cameras (Choudhury et al., 2021). The surgeon can control robotic surgical equipment placed at a remote location using hand gestures or voice commands.
- **Robotic Surgical Instruments**: The surgeon uses AR/VR technology to control the robotic surgical instruments. The instruments are outfitted with haptic feedback sensors that allow the surgeon to feel the resistance of tissues and other structures.
- **Postoperative Monitoring**: Typically, the patient is monitored remotely after surgery using telemedicine technologies. Video consultations with the patient, remote monitoring of vital signs, and follow-up appointments with local healthcare providers are examples of this.

Remote surgery using AR/VR technology has several benefits, including the ability to perform surgeries on patients in remote or underserved areas, reduce travel time and costs for the surgical team, and improve patient outcomes by providing access to highly skilled surgeons. However, there are significant technological and ethical issues connected with remote surgery, such as the requirement for consistent internet connections, the possibility of technical failures, and concerns about patient safety and privacy.

## 8.13 BENEFITS OF REMOTE SURGERY FOR IMPROVING SURGICAL CARE AVAILABILITY IN RURAL OR DISADVANTAGED AREAS

Remote surgery can provide patients in remote or underdeveloped locations with access to highly competent surgeons who may not be available locally. This can help to improve surgical care quality and eliminate the need for patients to travel vast distances for treatment. Remote surgery, often known as telesurgery, has various advantages for improving surgical care access in rural or underserved areas, including:

- **Reduced Travel Time and Costs**: Remote surgery can help patients and their families save time and money on travel. Patients can receive surgical care without having to go to a remote location, which is especially advantageous for patients who have restricted mobility or financial means.
- **Increased Efficiency**: By allowing doctors to perform many surgeries in different places on the same day, remote surgery can help to boost the efficiency of surgical procedures. This can help to cut patient wait times and enhance overall healthcare system efficiency (Kassamali et al., 2015).
- **Improved Outcomes**: By offering access to highly qualified doctors and specialized surgical procedures, remote surgery can help to enhance patient outcomes. This can help to lower the risk of problems and improve the surgical procedure's overall success (Leibowitz et al., 2019).
- **Increased Collaboration**: Through remote surgery, surgeons can cooperate with other healthcare specialists in distant locations. This can aid in improving care coordination and ensuring patients receive the most suitable and effective treatment (Greenberg et al., 2018).

Overall, remote surgery has the potential to improve surgical care access in rural or underserved areas. Remote surgery can help to enhance the overall quality and accessibility of surgical care for patients in remote or underserved locations by improving access to surgical care, lowering travel time and expenses, boosting efficiency, improving results, and increasing collaboration (Vrushank and Khang, 2023).

## 8.14 POSTOPERATIVE MONITORING IN AR/VR SURGICAL OPERATING SYSTEM

AR/VR technology can also be employed in surgical operating rooms for postoperative monitoring. These technologies can assist healthcare personnel in monitoring patient progress and detecting potential issues, allowing them to deliver prompt and appropriate postoperative care. Here are some examples of how AR/VR technologies can be utilized to follow patients after surgery:

### 8.14.1 Rehabilitation via the Internet

Virtual reality (VR) technologies can be utilized for virtual rehabilitation, allowing patients to perform exercises and physical therapy in a virtual setting (Oliveira et al.,

2021). This is especially beneficial for people who are unable to travel to a physical therapy center or have limited mobility. Virtual therapy can also be tailored to individual patients' needs, allowing them to progress at their own speed.

### 8.14.2 Control

AR/VR technologies can be utilized to monitor patients remotely following surgery. Wearable gadgets, such as AR glasses or smartwatches, can transmit vital signs and other health data to healthcare providers (Matamala-Gomez et al., 2020). Remote monitoring can aid in the early detection of potential complications, allowing healthcare providers to intervene before the complications worsen.

### 8.14.3 Patient Instruction

Patients can be educated about their postoperative care and rehabilitation using AR/VR technologies. VR simulations, for example, can be used to demonstrate to patients how to complete exercises or physical therapy or to deliver information about drug management or wound care. AR/VR technologies can help enhance patient compliance and reduce the likelihood of errors by presenting patients with clear and straightforward information (Gilbert et al., 2020).

### 8.14.4 Telemedicine

AR/VR technologies can be utilized for telemedicine, enabling healthcare providers to conduct virtual consultations with patients following surgery. This is especially important for people who cannot travel to a healthcare center or live in remote or rural locations. Telemedicine has the potential to enhance access to care while also reducing the burden on healthcare facilities (Fernandes et al., 2021). The use of AR/VR technology for postoperative monitoring has the potential to improve patient outcomes and reduce the risk of complications (Choudhry et al., 2019). AR/VR technology can increase access to care and support patient recovery after surgery by providing virtual rehabilitation, remote monitoring, patient education, and telemedicine. However, it is critical to thoroughly assess the dangers and advantages of new technologies and to ensure that proper safeguards are in place.

## 8.15 SAFETY AND EFFECTIVENESS

The usefulness and safety of AR/VR technology in surgical operating rooms are critical. While these technologies have the potential to improve surgical results and patient care, they also have dangers and limitations that must be carefully considered and addressed (Teo et al., 2020). Here are some of the reasons why it is critical to ensure the efficacy and safety of AR/VR technology in surgical operating rooms:

### 8.15.1 Patient Security

In every surgical treatment, the safety of the patients must come first. AR/VR technology can provide surgeons with real-time advice and support, but it is critical to verify that this technology is reliable and accurate (Bahubeshi et al., 2021). Technical flaws or mistakes in virtual 3D models or guidance systems might cause major problems or errors throughout the surgery, jeopardizing the outcome.

### 8.15.2 Considerations for Ethical and Legal Considerations

Using augmented reality and virtual reality technologies in surgical operating rooms involves ethical and legal concerns, such as patient privacy and informed permission. It is critical to ensure that patients are properly informed about these technologies and that suitable protections to preserve patient privacy and confidentiality are in place (Hogle et al., 2018b).

### 8.15.3 Education and Training

The application of AR/VR technology in surgical operating rooms necessitates specialized training and teaching. It is critical that surgeons and other healthcare workers have proper training in order to use these technologies successfully and safely. Inadequate training can lead to surgical errors or problems, jeopardizing patient safety (Oliveira et al., 2021).

### 8.15.4 Technical Restrictions

AR/VR technology depends on consistent and high-speed Internet, which may not be available in all locations, such as isolated or rural places. Technical limitations can also impair the accuracy and fidelity of virtual 3D models, lowering the quality of preoperative planning and surgical guidance (Vergara et al., 2019).

### 8.15.5 Cost

The cost of AR/VR technology, including hardware, software, and training, can be prohibitively expensive. It is critical to guarantee that the advantages of these technologies outweigh the expenses and that they are long-term cost-effective. It is critical to guarantee the effectiveness and safety of AR/VR technology in surgical operating rooms in order to ensure that patients receive the best possible treatment. This can be accomplished by rigorous technological review and testing, specialized healthcare professional training and education, and suitable measures to protect patient privacy and confidentiality. We can leverage the potential of AR/VR technology to improve surgical results and patient care by assuring its effectiveness and safety (Khang, 2024).

## 8.16 POTENTIAL DANGERS AND DIFFICULTIES INVOLVED WITH USING AR AND VR IN SURGERY

While AR and VR technologies have the potential to revolutionize surgery, there are also risks and challenges associated with their application. These include:

- Technical flaws and errors
- Education and training requirements

- Factors unique to each patient that influence accuracy and completeness
- Ethical and legal concerns
- Adoption and implementation are expensive.

While AR and VR technologies offer the potential to improve surgical results and patient care, it is critical to thoroughly assess and address the risks and difficulties associated with their usage (Teo et al., 2020). Healthcare personnel must obtain specialized training and education, proper protections to preserve patient privacy and confidentiality must be in place, and the costs and advantages of new technologies must be carefully weighed to ensure that they are cost-effective in the long run (Hogle et al., 2018b; Oliveira et al., 2021).

## 8.17 CONCLUSION

In conclusion, AR and VR technologies have the potential to transform surgical operating systems by improving visualization, preoperative planning, and guidance during surgery, remote cooperation, and teaching and training. These technologies can help to increase surgical procedure accuracy and precision, lower the risk of complications, and improve patient outcomes. However, there are risks and limitations to using AR and VR technologies in surgery, such as technical glitches, training and education requirements, patient-specific factors affecting accuracy and completeness, ethical and legal considerations, and high adoption and implementation costs (Anh et al., 2024).

To ensure the safety and efficacy of AR and VR technologies in surgical operating rooms, healthcare professionals must receive specialized training and education, appropriate safeguards to protect patient privacy and confidentiality must be in place, and the costs and benefits of these technologies must be carefully evaluated to ensure that they are cost-effective in the long run. Overall, AR and VR technologies have the potential to enhance patient outcomes greatly and offer intriguing possibilities for the future of surgical operating systems. To guarantee that these technologies are used successfully and safely in surgical practice, thorough consideration and review are required (Khang and Abdullayev et al., 2024).

## REFERENCES

Ahmed S. U. et al. (2018). "Augmented Reality in Surgery: A Review." *International Journal of Medical Robotics and Computer Assisted Surgery*, 14(4), e1902. https://doi.org/10.1002/rcs.1902

Amendola J. A. et al. (2018). "Osso VR: A Virtual Reality Trainer for Orthopedic Surgery Procedures." *Journal of Surgical Education*, 75(3), 722–728. https://doi.org/10.1016/j.jsurg.2017.10.015

Anh P. T. N. et al. (2024). "AI Models for Disease Diagnosis and Prediction of Heart Disease with Artificial Neural Networks." In *Computer Vision and AI-Integrated IoT Technologies in Medical Ecosystem* (1st Ed.). CRC Press. https://doi.org/10.1201/9781003429609-9

Bahubeshi L. et al. (2021). "Augmented Reality and Virtual Reality in Surgery: The Digital Surgical Environment: Applications, Limitations and Legal Pitfalls." In J. F. Ribeiro and J. C. Preto (Eds.), *Advances in Intelligent Systems and Computing* (Vol. 1323, pp. 514–523). National Institutes of Health – National Library of Medicine. https://doi.org/10.1007/978-3-030-72084-1_51

Böckers A. M. et al. (2006). "Real-Time Augmented Reality for Anatomy Teaching and Surgery." *Surgical Endoscopy*, 20(1), 135–138. https://doi.org/10.1007/s00464-005-0281-2

Cendan K. J. and DeMasters D. A. (2010). "Virtual Reality Surgical Simulation." *The American Journal of Surgery*, 199(2), 1–8. https://doi.org/10.1016/j.amjsurg.2009.08.034

Choudhry A. et al. (2019). "Telemedicine and Telehealth in Surgery." *Journal of Perioperative Practice*, 29(6), 146–151. https://doi.org/10.1177/1750458919832962

Choudhury F. A. et al. (2021). "Remote Telepresence Surgery Using 5G Ultra-Reliable Low-Latency Communication." *Annals of the Royal College of Surgeons of England*, 103(4), 284–289. https://doi.org/10.1308/rcsann.2021.0028

Davies J. R. et al. (2018). "True 3D Visualization: Seeing Anatomy in Real-Life." *Annals of Medicine and Surgery*, 36, 56–61. https://doi.org/10.1016/j.amsu.2018.10.021

Euler E. et al. (2018). "Augmented Reality and Mixed Reality in Surgery: The Digital Operating Room of the Future?" *Zeitschrift für Medizinische Physik*, 28(3), 251–262. https://doi.org/10.1016/j.zemedi.2018.02.002

Euler E. et al. (2019). "Augmented Reality in Surgery: The Digital Operating Room of the Future?" *Zeitschrift für Medizinische Physik*, 29(2), 118–129. https://doi.org/10.1016/j.zemedi.2018.12.003

Farooqi C. et al. (2019). "Clinical Validation of 3D-Printed Patient-Specific Models of Congenital Heart Disease." *Journal of Medical Imaging and Radiation Sciences*, 50(1), 122–130. https://doi.org/10.1016/j.jmir.2018.08.002

Fernandes E. E. V. et al. (2021). "Virtual Reality in Medicine: A Review on the Ethical Implications of Immersive Therapy." *Science and Engineering Ethics*, 27(4), 1–28. https://doi.org/10.1007/s11948-020-00262-y

Gaser C. and Nenadic R. G. (2004). "Voxel-Based Morphometry: The Methods." *NeuroImage*, 22(2), 261–276. https://doi.org/10.1016/j.neuroimage.2004.07.020

Gilbert J. R. et al. (2020). "Remote Monitoring in Healthcare Delivery." *Healthcare*, 8(2), 1–9. https://doi.org/10.3390/healthcare8020100

Greenberg J. A. et al. (2018). "Telemedicine in Surgery: A Review." *Journal of Surgical Research*, 223, 72–78. https://doi.org/10.1016/j.jss.2017.10.001 (Reference for the benefits of remote surgery in improving surgical care access)

Haluck M. S. et al. (2014). "Virtual Reality in Surgical Training: A Systematic Review." *Simulation in Healthcare*, 9(5), 301–310. https://doi.org/10.1097/SIH.0000000000000053 (Reference for AR/VR-based surgical simulation)

Haluck M. S. et al. (2018). "Virtual Reality Simulation Training for Health Professions Trainees in Gastrointestinal Endoscopy." *World Journal of Gastrointestinal Endoscopy*, 10(9), 185–197. https://doi.org/10.4253/wjge.v10.i9.185

Haluck S. M. et al. (2019). "Augmented Reality and Virtual Reality in Surgical Training: A Narrative Review." *Annals of Translational Medicine*, 7(23), 796. https://doi.org/10.21037/atm.2019.12.24

Hogle C. M. et al. (2018a). "Robotic Telesurgery: A Surgeon's Perspective." *Journal of Robotic Surgery*, 12(3), 427–431. https://doi.org/10.1007/s11701-017-0728-1

Hogle C. M. et al. (2018b). "Augmented Reality and Virtual Reality in Surgery: A Review." *Journal of Laparoendoscopic & Advanced Surgical Techniques*, 28(7), 807–812. https://doi.org/10.1089/lap.2018.0169

Kak A. C. and Slaney M. (1980). "Region Growing: A New Approach." *IEEE Transactions on Acoustics, Speech, and Signal Processing*, 28(5), 444–453. https://doi.org/10.1109/TASSP.1980.1163441

Kassamali S. L. et al. (2015). "Remote Surgery in Austere Environments: A Review of Current Systems." *Journal of Surgical Research*, 198(2), 438–448. https://doi.org/10.1016/j.jss.2015.05.041

Kazhdan M. et al. (2006). "Surface Reconstruction from Unorganized Points." *ACM SIGGRAPH Computer Graphics*, 2006, 71–78. https://doi.org/10.1145/1179352.1141911 (Reference for surface reconstruction techniques)

Khang A. (2024). *AI and IoT-Based Technologies for Precision Medicine*. IGI Global Press. ISBN: 9798369308769. https://doi.org/10.4018/979-8-3693-0876-9

Khang A., Abdullayev V. A., Hrybiuk O. and Shukla A. K. (2024). *Computer Vision and AI-Integrated IoT Technologies in Medical Ecosystem* (1st Ed.). CRC Press. https://doi.org/10.1201/9781003429609

Khang A., Ragimova N. A., Hajimahmud V. A. and Alyar V. A. (2022). "Advanced Technologies and Data Management in the Smart Healthcare System." In *AI-Centric Smart City Ecosystems: Technologies, Design and Implementation* (1st Ed., Vol. 16, p. 10). CRC Press. https://doi.org/10.1201/9781003252542-16

Khang A., Rana G., Tailor R. K. and Hajimahmud V. A. (2023). *Data-Centric AI Solutions and Emerging Technologies in the Healthcare Ecosystem*. CRC Press. https://doi.org/10.1201/9781003356189

Kim J. et al. (2021). "Current Status of Virtual Reality Simulation in Robotic Surgery Training: A Review." *Journal of Robotic Surgery*, 15(1), 1–11. https://doi.org/10.1007/s11701-020-01139-0

Kim S. Y. et al. (2018). "Augmented Reality-Based Navigation in Spine Surgery Enhances Clinical Efficiency and Safety." *Journal of Neurosurgery: Spine*, 30(1), 54–61. https://doi.org/10.3171/2018.4.SPINE171131

Kim S. Y. et al. (2019). "Standardized Representation of 3D Arthroscopic Meniscus Tear Models." *The Knee*, 26(2), 473–480. https://doi.org/10.1016/j.knee.2019.03.010

Lee S. H. et al. (2018). "Accuracy Validation of Patient-Specific 3D-Printed Models Generated from 2D CT/MRI Images: A Systematic Review." *NDT Plus*, 11(5), 349–361. https://doi.org/10.1093/ndtplus/sfy050

Leibowitz J. M. et al. (2019). "Telemedicine and Telesurgery in Head and Neck Surgery." *Current Opinion in Otolaryngology & Head and Neck Surgery*, 27(2), 116–124. https://doi.org/10.1097/MOO.0000000000000505

Leung M. K. P. et al. (2020). "Assuring the Quality of 3D Printed Models in Medicine and Dentistry; A Systematic Review." *Journal of Clinical Medicine*, 9(11), 3726. https://doi.org/10.3390/jcm9113726

Lorensen W. E. and Cline H. E. (1987). "Marching Cubes: A High Resolution 3D Surface Construction Algorithm, Marching Cubes: A High Resolution 3D Surface Construction Algorithm." *ACM SIGGRAPH Computer Graphics*, 21(4), 163–169. https://doi.org/10.1145/37402.37422

Matamala-Gomez M. J. et al. (2020). "Virtual Reality Applications for the Rehabilitation of Patients with Chronic Pain: A Review of the Literature." *Journal of Clinical Medicine*, 9(10), 1–17. https://doi.org/10.3390/jcm9103188

McInerney T. and Terzopoulos D. (1996). "Deformable Models in Medical Image Analysis: A Survey." *Medical Image Analysis*, 1(2), 91–108. https://doi.org/10.1016/S1361-8415(96)80007-7

Meijden J. N. van der et al. (2018). "Virtual and Augmented Reality in Surgery: The Digital Surgical Environment: Applications, Limitations and Legal Pitfalls." *Journal of Surgical Research*, 227, 208–213. https://doi.org/10.1016/j.jss.2018.01.022 (Reference for AR/VR use in remote surgery)

Meijden J. N. van der et al. (2019). "Augmented Reality and Virtual Reality in Surgery: The Digital Surgical Environment: Applications, Limitations and Legal Pitfalls." *Journal of Oral and Maxillofacial Surgery, Medicine, and Pathology*, 31(2), 87–94. https://doi.org/10.1016/j.ajoms.2018.08.008

Oliveira M. T. A. et al. (2021). "Augmented Reality in Healthcare: A Systematic Literature Review and Bibliometric Analysis." *Journal of Medical Systems*, 45(8), 1–21. https://doi.org/10.1007/s10916-021-01767-x

O'Toole M. R. et al. (2019). "Telesurgery: Remote Imaging, Robotics, and Augmented Reality." *Journal of Laparoendoscopic & Advanced Surgical Techniques*, 29(2), 139–146. https://doi.org/10.1089/lap.2018.0418

Pinto G. et al. (2018). "Virtual and Augmented Reality in the Operating Theatre: From Individual Surgical Planning to Training and Education." *Insights into Imaging*, 9(2), 253–269. https://doi.org/10.1007/s13244-018-0598-0

Rasouli A. et al. (2018). "Virtual Reality Technology in Neurosurgery." *World Neurosurgery*, 109, 533–538. https://doi.org/10.1016/j.wneu.2017.09.164

Ruiz J. G. et al. (2009). "Virtual Reality Simulation in Laparoscopic Surgery: A Systematic Review of Randomized Controlled Trials." *Surgical Endoscopy*, 23(3), 1–9. https://doi.org/10.1007/s00464-008-9975-6

Schopper J. M. et al. (2019). "Accuracy of 3D Printed Endoscopy Models Compared with Standard Clinical Imaging for Otolaryngology." *Otolaryngology-Head and Neck Surgery*, 160(3), 458–465. https://doi.org/10.1177/0194599818803341

Sethian J. A. (1999). *Level Set Methods and Fast Marching Methods: Evolving Interfaces in Computational Geometry, Fluid Mechanics, Computer Vision, and Materials Science.* Cambridge University Press. https://doi.org/10.1017/CBO9780511546712

Seymour A. et al. (2013). "Virtual Reality Training Improves Operating Room Performance: Results of a Randomized, Double-Blinded Study." *Annals of Surgery*, 257(1), 33–38. https://doi.org/10.1097/SLA.0b013e318261dfcf

Smith A. D. F. et al. (2016). "Virtual Reality in Neurosurgical Education: Part-Task Ventriculostomy Simulation with Dynamic Visual and Haptic Feedback." *Neurosurgery*, 63(Suppl 1), 102–107. https://doi.org/10.1227/NEU.0000000000001401

Tafuri A. et al. (2018). "Virtual Reality for Preoperative Planning in Urological Surgery." *Journal of Endourology*, 32(5), 438–443. https://doi.org/10.1089/end.2017.0749

Teo F. K. F. et al. (2020). "Virtual and Augmented Reality in Surgery: The Digital Surgical Environment: Applications, Limitations and Legal Pitfalls." *The Surgeon*, 18(5), 269–277. https://doi.org/10.1016/j.surge.2019.07.002

Toth A. S. et al. (2020). "Augmented Reality in Orthopaedic Surgery: A Review of Current and Future Applications." *Journal of Orthopaedic Research and Therapy*, 1(1), 1–6. https://doi.org/10.24966/ORT-9215/100006

Ubbink J. S. et al. (2018). "The Current Use of Augmented Reality in the Operating Theatre: A Systematic Review." *Surgical Endoscopy*, 32(2), 417–428. https://doi.org/10.1007/s00464-017-5744-y

Vergara A. et al. (2019). "Virtual Reality and Simulation in Neurosurgical Training." *Journal of Neurosurgical Sciences*, 63(6), 749–752. https://doi.org/10.23736/S0390-5616.19.04690-1

Vrushank S. and Khang A. (2023). "Metaverse-Enabling IoT Technology for a Futuristic Healthcare System." In *AI-Based Technologies and Applications in the Era of the Metaverse* (1st Ed., p. 1). IGI Global Press. https://doi.org/10.4018/978-1-6684-8851-5.ch008

# 9 Sensor Scheduling in an IoT Health Monitoring System with Interference Awareness

*Sirish Kumar M., Anusha K., Ponnala Vaishnavi, and Sanamreddy Sandhya*

## 9.1 INTRODUCTION

The infrastructure for healthcare is generally relatively weak in impoverished nations. In comparison to the expanding population, there are remarkably few hospitals. The few hospitals available are ill-equipped, there are not enough physicians working there, and most importantly, the essential diagnostic tools needed to identify life-threatening illnesses are not available. Building new hospitals, giving them advanced medical infrastructure, and selecting doctors to be employed by such institutions is now an expensive and planned process. Nevertheless, we believe that we might connect with a large audience and provide them with top-notch medical advice if we could develop a mobile, affordable wellness-detecting gadget that could measure the distinctive characteristics of the human body and communicate with the Cloud (Rani et al., 2021).

Once one of the authorities from a network of specialists spread out around the world examines those health factors on the Cloud, the pharmaceutical service is offered. We might win the support of a sizable population by doing this. A survey on the application of electronic sensor detector networks in healthcare can be found in Mirzoev (2014).

However, if the health monitoring equipment interacts with a tablet or cellphone that already has the potential to interface with the Internet via the Cloud, the entire network would be significantly more expensive. This is due to the fact that most individuals now have access to these modern information and communication gadgets, which have also decreased in price significantly. Moreover, the system may be made M2M (machine-to-machine) and IoT (Internet of Things) compliant. This chapter goes over the implementation of this sort of healthcare surveillance system (ECG, 2023).

Each sensor has different needs for data quantity or size and bitrate in a health monitoring system. To get a credible and trustworthy result, it must measure the health parameter. One difficult task is concurrently gathering intelligence from several sensors. Making data from sensors discrete correctly is necessary in order to

 DOI: 10.1201/9781032686745-9

transmit it to the data generator via a shared channel with fixed bandwidth (Paschou et al., 2013). Every detector must correctly gather input while adhering to the parameter's suitable bitrate, and the data must all be supplied to the microcontroller without distortion or redundancy in order for the system for medical surveillance to be accurate (Rodrguez et al., 2010). This chapter proposes a programming technique that prevents any interference between several detectors and the ensuing data leakage. The two factors that matter when determining the sensor data schedule are the pulse width necessary when evaluating an attribute and the amount of data quantity per specimen required when detecting an attribute.

While factors, especially if they involve image data along with sound, require much lower specimen rates but have much larger data lengths per sample, echocardiography, Lexicon, Signals Were Recorded, RR, and other linear measurements mean increased signal processing techniques that have shorter records lengths per specimen.

This chapter proposes a rescheduling method that prevents any interference between different sensors and the ensuing data loss. Three elements are critical when choosing sensor data scheduling and measuring a parameter: (i) the sampling rate, (ii) sample size, and (iii) the quantity of specimen or data length. When compared to parameters involving images (such as palpable images and other microscopic pictures) and sound (such as heart and lung sounds), graph-based parameters (such as electrocardiograms, electroencephalograms, electromyograms, and respiration rates) require higher sampling rates but have shorter data lengths per sample.

As a result, we want to provide every value the same importance when delivering health data across a common channel and allocate a specific window of duration. If the sensor characteristic information cannot be compressed inside the scheduled intervals, the data must be divided into several bits that do. The remainder of the paper is organized as shown in what follows. Section 9.2 discusses the Internet of Things and its possible applications in the healthcare sector. The architecture of a healthcare system based on the Internet of Things is then proposed within section 9.3. The problem of continuously gathering information via several wellness detectors is discussed in section 9.4, along with a management approach. Section 9.5 discusses how effective the scheduling technique is with a simple example. Lastly, we give a path for further research in Section 9.6 as we wrap up the article.

## 9.2 INTERNET OF THINGS

The phrase "internet of things" describes a network of real-world and online gadgets that operate in smart settings and link and interact with one another in consumer, interpersonal, and physical environments. The Internet of the Future (ITU, 2015), when everything is connected, could be seen as this. In the network, each object is assigned a special identification. This enables remote device access across the network anytime and everywhere. Smart, ubiquitous, and constantly connected environments are created when IoT-enabled products interact with humans, communicate with one another, and access information through the Internet (Khang, Abdullayev, & Hahanov et al., 2024).

The Internet of Things (IoT) also enables machine-to-machine (M2M) connectivity, allowing devices to be controlled both by other machines and by the Internet. When machines take over, this might alter how technology is utilized since it would remove the barriers that prevent people from connecting with digital systems. The vast amounts of important data that computers can track monitors throughout the globe supply would take years for a person to acquire. IoT brings the ideas of distributed computing and the Internet of Things to life by enabling everyday objects like automobiles, highways, heart rate monitors, and meds-shaped cameras in our digestive tracks, signs that adjust to motorists, freezers, and even cattle equipped with sensors to communicate with humans and assist them in every step. The next section emphasizes the use of IoT in the healthcare sector (Khang & Rana et al., 2023).

## 9.3 IoT IN HEALTHCARE

A patient connected to IoT-enabled medical equipment for remote monitoring is sometimes referred to as a "virtual patient" in the digital era. The virtual patient's physiological circumstances mirror those of the real patient exactly. A doctor can only check on a patient a few times per day, yet medical crises can arise at any time. Continuous monitoring of health data becomes necessary. Because of a patient's capacity to be accessed by other devices and the Internet, thanks to the Internet of Things, their health may be continuously monitored (Bisoi et al., 2013). This makes it possible for serious illnesses to be identified early on, allowing for the implementation of effective measures.

IoT may also be used to gather medical records. Machines are capable of producing statistical data relating to health conditions. It is feasible to collect data more quickly, in large quantities, and without errors than human approaches could possibly manage. Remote health data can be used for illness surveillance, risk mapping, and statistics generation (Beck et al., 2000). This section discusses an approach for connecting to the Internet of wellness tracking. Multiple sensors attached to a person make up a system for keeping track of health. These sensors connect with an information-gathering and analysis equipment. One possibility for the information collector and analysis device is a smartphone or specialist device (Vrushank et al., 2023).

The information unit must gather data from each sensor using a predetermined sample rate in order to build the Human Body Awareness Association (Chen et al., 2011; Patel et al., 2010). As an aggregating unit in our architecture, we employed an Arduino microcontroller, and protothreads were used for scheduling. Our health monitoring system's processing center is a portable computer. The Arduino aggregator communicates with the data processing unit using wired USB serial connections or short-range wireless communication technologies, including router, Internet, LoRaWAN, and ZigBee applications.

The information gathered from the collector unit is processed by the data processing unit, sometimes known as a portable computer. The information might also be used to create interesting features for users, such as interactive graphs and

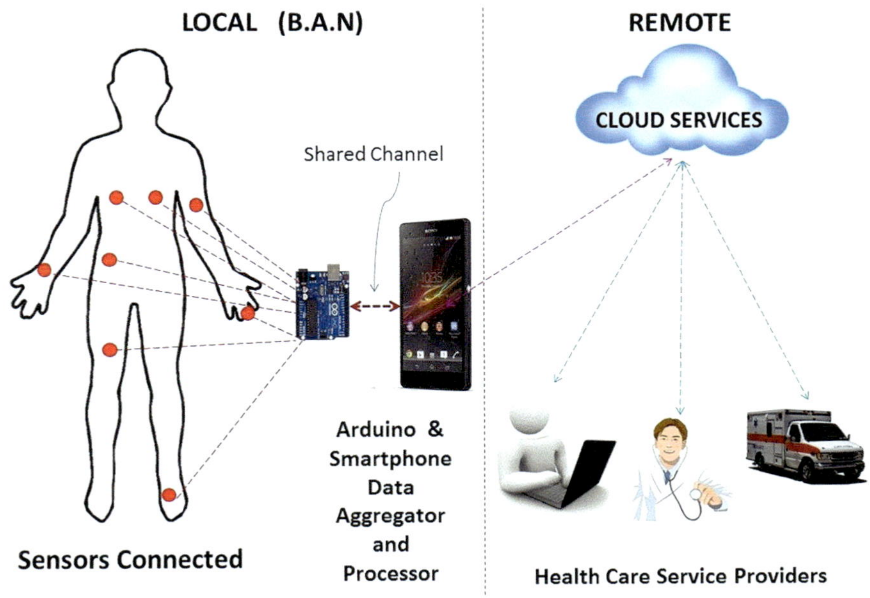


**FIGURE 9.1** The layout of the health monitoring system.

charts (including variables such as an ECG monitoring data graph). By using this tool, patients may obtain crucial medical advice from their doctors and set alarms or reminders for appointments and medications that must be taken on time.

There are two components to the system: local and remote, as shown in Figure 9.1. Data can be saved and sent to distant suppliers, such as urgent care doctors, including careers, thanks to the remote component. Input via detectors linked to a patient is gathered by the neighboring component. Furthermore, software analyzes the gathered raw data to deliver knowledge that experts and medical professionals can understand.

## 9.4 CREATE A FRAMEWORK FOR MONITORING HEALTH

### 9.4.1 Open-Source Hardware

A data microcontroller open-source hardware is employed with the ability to enable the Internet of Things quickly. An Arduino board includes a 16 MHz ceramic resonator, it has 32,000 of portable storage, and two kilobytes of memory. For connecting various sensors and actuators, it features 14 electronic pins and six analog interfaces. This kind of project and other Bluetooth sensory web systems benefit greatly from its high processing capacity and ability to link to a variety of sensors and communication devices. It speaks of an Arduino-powered wireless sensor network. The open-source hardware is linked to a portable information handling and interaction device through a fixed bandwidth serial connection. Given that the Arduino and the handheld data handling device share a channel, each sensor's communication across this shared channel should be handled separately.

### 9.4.2 Sensor

The SPO2 Sensor is also known as a pulse oximeter. This sensor offers unobtrusive tools that capture numerous essential physical characteristics of the human body, known as health sensors. All of the system's sensors are discussed in this section. Upon request from the open-source hardware-based information collector device, the sensor records a specific property value and communicates it back to the data aggregator. Some of the sensors that have been employed in the system are shown in Figure 9.2.

Additionally, the pulse rate is measured. An ECG sensor measures the power supply and contractions in the coronary artery. An airway detector, also known as a respiration detector, tracks the patterns of rate of breathing variations that may indicate serious functional disturbance. The subject is a vital medical tool over quickly identifying a lack of oxygen and insomnia.

- **Temp Sensor**: This sensor measures a person's temperature.
- **Blood Pressure Cuff**: This instrument measures artery blood pressure. The pulse value and diastolic value, which indicate the level of fluid in blood vessels during cardiac contraction and heart dilation, respectively, are the two values provided by this measurement. The human body's status, including being in a position, seated, lying flat, and other positions, is determined by its internal motion detector. There are several illnesses where it is crucial to pay attention to the body's movements. In one case, it could be helpful in determining the neurological patient. This sensor can also detect dizziness or tumbling, making it crucial for elderly people. GSR detector measures the electric conductivity and stiffness of the outermost layer of skin, as it varies with the amount of moisture in the skin. Since the sympathetic nervous system influences sweat glands, intense emotional states alter the skin's

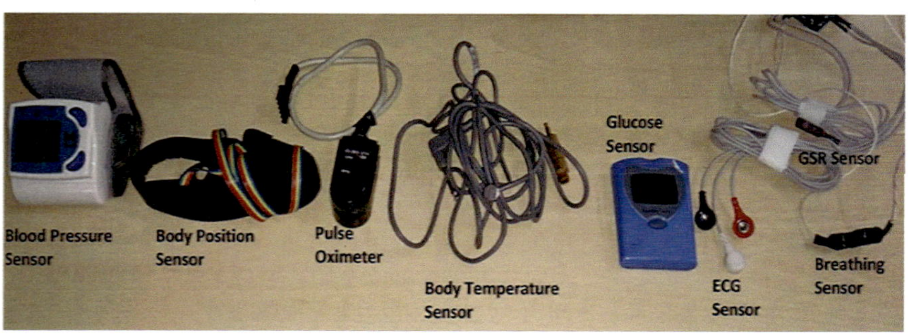


**FIGURE 9.2** Detectors for wellness tracking.

resistance to electricity and conductance. This sensor assists in identifying both emotional and physical arousal.

- **Glucometer**: A glucose detector, it estimates the blood's estimated glucose concentration. A sensor called an electromyogram (EMG) measures the nerve impulses of muscles in the body both at relaxation and when they are contracting. This is used to identify kinesiological anomalies, quantify low back pain, identify neuromuscular illnesses, and examine the biological mechanisms that influence human motion. Additionally, it can aid in the detection of medical anomalies, activation levels, recruitment patterns, and motor control issues. The sensors mentioned previously are used by this healthcare system. But a lot more detectors might be included within this remote surveillance network if advised to do so by qualified medical personnel.

### 9.4.3 Connection for Application

Figure 9.3 depicts a screenshot of the application. All of the sensor values that have been obtained from the data aggregator are displayed on the interface's left side. It comprises a picture of a patient who is wearing sensors. Next to each individual sensor in the image, the sensor's value is presented. Sensor data visualization is given meaning in this manner.

An Android app has also been developed. It can be used by any smartphone or tablet running Android that has a wireless connection. The sensors are connected to the Arduino, and the code communicates with them over a wireless network. Additionally, this program displays an electrocardiogram visualization, heart rate charts, body temp, blood pressure, O2 saturation, and arterial pressure, as shown in Figure 9.4.

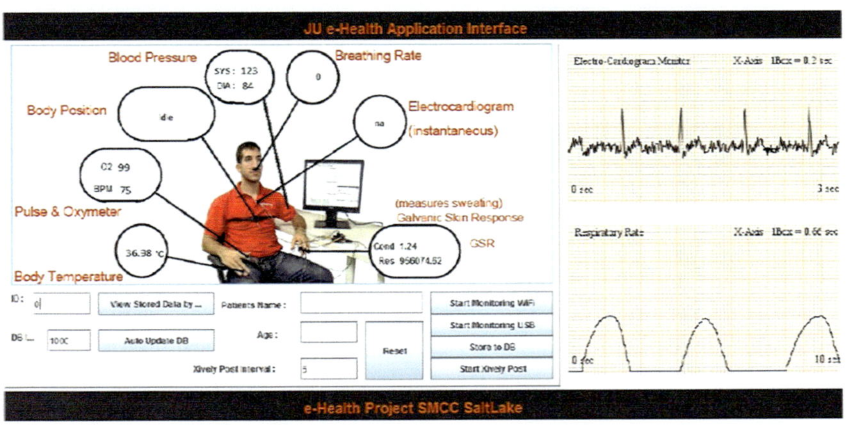


**FIGURE 9.3** Connection for application.

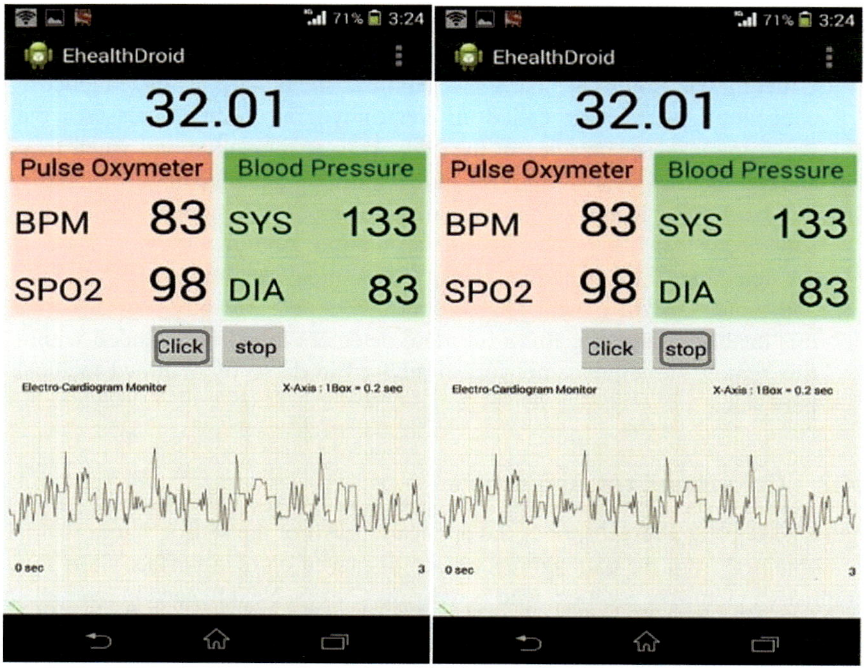


FIGURE 9.4 Android app UI.

## 9.5 ACQUIRING INFORMATION FROM SENSORS

The data gathered by the detectors in the wellness tracking equipment is transmitted via an individual conventional interface between the CPU and the data accumulator module. To produce a trustworthy and dependability-oriented result, these two factors need to be taken into consideration. Input must consistently flow across the common link to every data analysis module to keep up with the specimen rate (Hahanov & Khang et al., 2022).

The sampling rate is faster for measures like the electrocardiogram (ECG), electroencephalogram (EEG), electromyogram (EMG), respiratory rate (RR), and other graph-based metrics, but the data length per sample is less. Although there is still a huge amount of data in each sample, sampling rates for parameters like visuals (such as micro pictures) and sound (containing variables like cardiac and respiratory sounds) are significantly lower. Every sensing device should perform accurate readings while keeping to the prescribed frequency of samples for the parameter. Additionally, there should be no data loss or overlap when sending it to the data processor. In order to prevent data loss while using an established communication channel, sensor data from several sensors must be interleaved. It should be put into practice in a way that ensures every specimen from all sensors is collected and that results are given within the allotted period. In this case, our main goal is to offer a suitable method of linking data across the shared channel (Khang, 2024).

Health metrics that depend on time have a very limited tolerance for delays. The latency and sample rate should be kept constant to preserve the integrity and significance of the data. As a result, a data interleaving technique is used to distribute the obtainable memory across the sensors, allowing each to preserve its testing frequency, delay, and input size. Bc is the overall communication channel high frequency (in bit values per sec). One or more slots may be created out of the bandwidth. The objective is to split the bandwidth between a number of such positions. Data Size = Slotd for 1 millisecond, the needed rate of sampling as well as the information duration for a sensor, are represented by Slot, fi, Si, and Ldi, respectively. Si, Ti = Sensor cycle times or lengths. LdiMax is short for maximum data length. In an 115200bps bandwidth, the single sensor's maximum data length is provided by Equation 9.1:

$$\text{SlotdXTi} = \text{LdiMax (Condition 1)} \tag{9.1}$$

Slotd = Bc/(10008), in Bytes, calculates the data size for each millisecond slot. (Condition 2)

From useful execution experience, it is expected that the absolute data transmission (Bc) of the correspondence channel is 115200 pieces/sec. In this way, applying Condition 2, information size per opening becomes as Equation 9.2:

$$\text{Slotd} = 14 \text{ Bytes.} \tag{9.2}$$

We know in Equation 9.3,

$$\text{Time period} = 1/\text{f} \tag{9.3}$$

where we can measure time period or cycle length and f = recurrence. We can observe two instances right now to see how our technique works.

### 9.5.1 Scenario 1

A single detector, designated S1, is connected through a passive line. Accept that the required information length (Ld1) for the detected boundary is 25 Bytes, and the anticipated examination rate (f1) is 125 Hz. The time duration for S1 is T1 = 8 milliseconds based on Condition 3. It indicates that we receive eight slots, each of 14 Bytes. To keep up with the necessary information stream, openings anticipated for the information length of the sensor S1 should be saved every eight ms. With the set testing rate from Condition 1, we can compute the maximum allowable information length (Ld1Max) for this sensor as Equation 9.4.

$$\text{Ld1Max} = 14 \times 8, \text{ or } 112 \text{ bytes. (Condition 4)} \tag{9.4}$$

The S1 sensor data may be appropriately obligated within the cable transmission frequency because

Ld1 Ld1Ma9. Sensor S1 needs a pair of holes of length Slot, over instance, 14 Bytes, since Ld1 = 25 Bytes. Subsequently, there are six empty areas between each pair of samples. There are 84 free Bytes (6 x 14).

### 9.5.2 Scenario 2

Subsequently, the primary means of communication is expanded to include a second sensor (S2), which has a number of criteria. For S2, the data dimension (Ld2) is equal to 300 Bytes, and the scrutinizing frequency (f2) is equal to 10 Hz. The time period, T2, is equal to 100 milliseconds as a result of Condition 3 being carried out. This will allow us to keep delivering data from sensor S2 each one hundred ms at the current rate.

Considering scenario 1, we get the following maximal informative amount: for every millisecond, Ld2Max is 14 times 100, or 1400 Bytes. Currently, a few recognized knowledge evaluations from sensor S1 are supposed to be delivered within this 100 ms time period for sensor S2 when transferring information from the two sensors across the same channel since S1 has a greater scrutinizing velocity. The amount of tests from S1 that will be included in S2 during one sample period is as follows: (Condition 4) The following criterion defines the available data transfer for sensor S2:Ld2Actual = Ld2Max (f1/f2)X(2XSlotd) (Condition 5).

From Condition 5, it is possible to calculate the available broadcast ability: Ld2Actual = 1400 ((2X14) X12) = 1064 Bytes. When looking at scenario 1, we saw that the most extreme 84 Bytes may be allotted between two samples from sensor S1 for delivering data from the additional sensor S2. Then, data from S1 ought to be provided. Then, further data from S1 must be sent. After that, 84 more Bytes are available, and S2 data may be delivered. As a result, data from the 02 sensors may be combined, as shown in Table 9.1.

For S2, a large information length of 300 Bytes is required. In order to maintain the required example pace of S1, the information produced by S2 should be divided into three parts, each of which should be 84 Bytes in size. The remaining 48 Bytes can then be required in the subsequent free opening. Therefore, we design the sensors such that lengthy information cannot be divided into smaller portions and necessitate the opening of saved information from another sensor.

## 9.6 DISCUSSION AND RESULTS

In order to validate the planning procedure, we employed two detectors as a demonstration within the IoT-enabled assessment of satisfaction paradigm. Electrocardiogram shows a significant occurrence incidence but an insufficient amount of knowledge. There is a low example rate and high material quantity heat within the system level.

Since the electrocardiogram (ECG) detector demands a speed of, for instance, 125 Hz, we actually want to deliver the ECG data every 8 ms. Given that the two sensors use the same channel, it is now required that the data from the inside temperature

**TABLE 9.1**
**Arranging for Medical Treatment**

| Data Size Per Millisecond for Bandwidth 115200 Bit/s | Sensor 1: Sample Rate 125 Hz and Data Size 25B | Sensor 2: Sample Rate 10Hz and Data Size 300B |
|---|---|---|
| 1 —— 14 Bytes | 25 Bytes | |
| 2 —— 14 Bytes | 25 Bytes | |
| 3 —— 14 Bytes | | 84 Bytes |
| 4 —— 14 Bytes | | 84 Bytes |
| 5 —— 14 Bytes | | 84 Bytes |
| 6 —— 14 Bytes | | 84 Bytes |
| 7 —— 14 Bytes | | 84 Bytes |
| 8 —— 14 Bytes | | 84 Bytes |
| 9 —— 14 Bytes | 25 Bytes | |
| 10 —— Bytes 14 | 25 Bytes | |
| 11 —— Bytes 14 | | 84 Bytes |
| 12 —— Bytes 14 | | 84 Bytes |
| 13 —— Bytes 14 | | 84 Bytes |
| 14 —— Bytes 14 | | 84 Bytes |
| 15 —— Bytes 14 | | 84 Bytes |
| 16 —— Bytes 14 | | 84 Bytes |
| 17 —— Bytes 14 | 25 Bytes | |
| 18 —— Bytes 14 | 25 Bytes | |
| 19 —— Bytes 14 | | 84 Bytes |
| 20 —— Bytes 14 | | 84 Bytes |
| 21 —— Bytes 14 | | 84 Bytes |
| 22 —— Bytes 14 | | 84 Bytes |
| 23 —— Bytes 14 | | 84 Bytes |
| 24 —— Bytes 14 | | 84 Bytes |
| 25 —— Bytes 14 | 25 Bytes | |
| 26 —— Bytes 14 | 25 Bytes | |
| 27 —— Bytes 14 | | 48 Bytes |
| 28 —— Bytes 14 | | 48 Bytes |
| 29 —— Bytes 14 | | 48 Bytes |
| 30 —— Bytes 14 | | 48 Bytes |
| 31 —— Bytes 14 | | |
| 32 —— Bytes 14 | | |

content sensor be shared amongst both samples. However, if the body's internal heat level signal is not separated between the ECG sensor instances, this information will overlap with the ECG information, and the translation of the information at the processing unit will be distorted, as shown in Table 9.1.

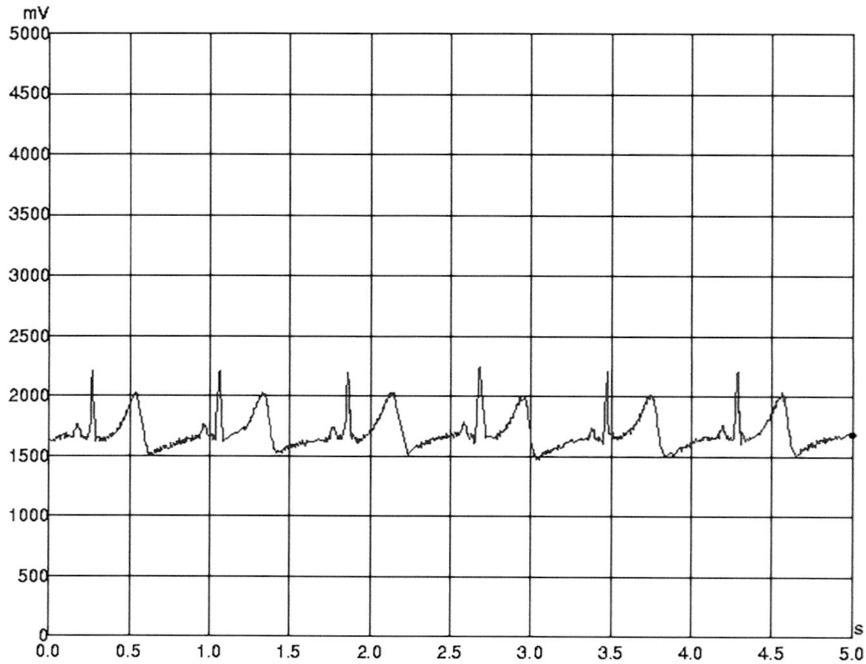


**FIGURE 9.5** Data obtained after using our suggested technique.

The ECG tests are not delayed at that point, and the ECG is faithfully decoded at the data performing unit of service, considering that we figure out the free openings throughout each instance from the ECG sensor and subsequently break down the information from the internal heat level sensor as indicated by the free spaces between the ECG tests as Figure 9.5.

## 9.7 CONCLUSION

We have shown that by incorporating what is available according to the required testing rate and excluding larger information with the largest permitted information size, it is possible to maintain the inspection rate for a number of sensors while ensuring a high-quality exchange of data and effective use of data transfer capacity. For the sensors to operate successfully, an illness tracking system has to satisfy the inspection frequency and duration specifications of each detector (Khang, Abdullayev & Hrybiuk et al., 2024).

## REFERENCES

Beck R. L., Bradley M. L., Wood B. L. "Remote Sensing and Human Health: New Sensors and New Opportunities", *Emerging Infectious Diseases* 6.3 (2000): 217. www.ncbi.nlm.nih.gov/pmc/articles/PMC2640871/

Bisoi S., Bhunia S. S., Roy S., Mukherjee N. "iSENSE: Intelligent Sensor Monitoring Services with Integrated WSN Testbed", *Procedia Technology* 10 (2013): 564–571. www.sciencedirect.com/science/article/pii/S2212017313005586

Chen M. et al. "Body Area Networks: A Survey", *Mobile Networks and Applications* 16.2 (2011): 171–193. https://link.springer.com/article/10.1007/s11036-010-0260-8

ECG (2023). www.meds.queensu.ca/central/modules/ECG/normal_ecg.html

Hahanov V., Khang A., Litvinova E., Chumachenko S., Hajimahmud V. A., Alyar V. A. "The Key Assistant of Smart City—Sensors and Tools", in *AI-Centric Smart City Ecosystems: Technologies, Design and Implementation* (1st ed., vol. 17, p. 10) (2022). CRC Press. https://doi.org/10.1201/9781003252542-17

ITU. *The Internet of Things, ITU Internet Reports 2005* (2015). www.itu.int/internetofthings/

Khang A. *AI and IoT-Based Technologies for Precision Medicine* (2024). IGI Global Press. ISBN: 9798369308769. https://doi.org/10.4018/979-8-3693-0876-9

Khang A., Abdullayev V. A., Hahanov V., Vrushank S. *Advanced IoT Technologies and Applications in the Industry 4.0 Digital Economy* (1st Ed.) (2024). CRC Press. https://doi.org/10.1201/9781003434269

Khang A., Abdullayev V. A., Hrybiuk O., Shukla A. K. *Computer Vision and AI-Integrated IoT Technologies in Medical Ecosystem* (1st Ed.) (2024). CRC Press. https://doi.org/10.1201/9781003429609

Khang A., Rana G., Tailor R. K., Hajimahmud V. A. *Data-Centric AI Solutions and Emerging Technologies in the Healthcare Ecosystem* (2023). CRC Press. https://doi.org/10.1201/9781003356189

Mirzoev D. T. *IEEE Standard for Local and Metropolitan Networks, Part 15.4: Low-Rate Wireless Personal Area Networks (LRWPANs)* (2014). IEEE Computer Society STD. https://arxiv.org/abs/1404.2345

Paschou M. et al. "Health Internet of Things: Metrics and Methods for Efficient Data Transfer", *Simulation Modelling Practice and Theory* 34 (2013): 186–199. www.sciencedirect.com/science/article/pii/S1569190X12001232

Patel M., Wang J. "Applications, Challenges, and Prospective in Emerging Body Networking Area Technologies", *Wireless Communications, IEEE* 17.1 (2010): 80–88. https://ieeexplore.ieee.org/abstract/document/5416354/

Rani S., Chauhan M., Kataria A., Khang A. "IoT Equipped Intelligent Distributed Framework for Smart Healthcare Systems", *Networking and Internet Architecture* 2 (2021): 30. https://doi.org/10.48550/arXiv.2110.04997

Rodrguez C. C. G., Riveill M. *e-Health Monitoring Applications: What About Data Quality?* (2010). https://citeseerx.ist.psu.edu/document?repid=rep1&type=pdf&doi=1ad7ca1b54b349ea839016bd99b981ba1e16548e

Vrushank S., Vidhi T., Khang A. "Electronic Health Records Security and Privacy Enhancement Using Blockchain Technology", in *Data-Centric AI Solutions and Emerging Technologies in the Healthcare Ecosystem* (1st Ed., p. 1) (2023). CRC Press. https://doi.org/10.1201/9781003356189-1

# 10 Cardiovascular Disease Detection Using Deep Learning and Nature-Inspired Optimization Algorithm

*Bhakti Kaushal, Roohum Jegan, Smitha Raveendran, Gajanan Birajdar K., and Mukesh Patil D.*

## 10.1 INTRODUCTION

As per the fact sheet produced by WHO, the cause of the majority of global deaths is cardiovascular diseases (CVDs). In 2019, around 17.9 million people died because of CVDs, and these are estimated to be 32% of all deaths globally. Out of these, stroke and heart attack caused 85% of the deaths (WHO, 2023). In lower- and middle-income countries, more than three-quarters of people die due to CVDs. In 2019, it was estimated that around 17 million premature deaths (under the age of 70) occurred due to non-communicable diseases. Out of these, 38% occurred due to CVDs. The prevention of CVDs can be accomplished by addressing behavioral risk factors like lifestyle diseases, including unhealthy diet with the use of tobacco or alcohol and physical inactivity, giving rise to obesity.

It is essential to understand the basic structure of the heart, its four chambers, the valves, the blood vessels present near the heart, and the beat to understand what happens during the cardiac cycle. The mitral and tricuspid valves connect the atrium (upper chambers) to the ventricles (lower chambers), and they are called the Atrioventricular valves or AV valves. With the help of mitral and tricuspid valves, the blood is circulated to the left ventricle from the left atrium and to the right ventricle from the right atrium, respectively. They close to prevent a backward flow of blood to the atrium and give rise to the S1 sound ('lub') (Liu et al., 2016).

The aortic valve is present between the left ventricle and the aorta, helping to prevent the backward flow of oxygen-rich blood into the left ventricle. The pulmonary valve connects the right ventricle to the pulmonary trunk, preventing the deoxygenated blood from flowing back toward the right ventricle. The aortic and pulmonary valves are also known as semilunar valves, consisting of three flaps or cusps in the crescent moon shape. These valves close, giving rise to the S2 sound ('dub') (Altuve et al., 2020). The sinoatrial node or SA node, located near the opening of the superior vena cava on the right atrium, contracts faster compared to the heart tissue, and with


DOI: 10.1201/9781032686745-10

its help, the cardiac contractions are set in pace. Hence, it is called the pacemaker (Crumbie, 2023). The electrical activation initiated through the SA node in the form of an impulse leads to the mechanical activity of the circulation of blood, giving rise to the cardiac cycle. The cardiac cycle consists of two phases, i.e., diastole (relaxation phase or heart fills with blood) and systole (contraction phase or heart pumps the blood) (Crumbie, 2023), and it is further divided into four stages of atrial and ventricular components:

- **Atrial Diastole**: When both the AV valves are closed, atrias relaxes and fills with blood. The superior and inferior vena cava brings back the deoxygenated blood from the entire body, and it is filled in the right atrium. The pulmonary veins bring back the oxygen-rich blood from the lungs, and it is filled in the left atrium (Liu et al., 2016).
- **Atrial Systole**: When both the atrias contract, forcing the blood to flow from the atria into the ventricles (Altuve et al., 2020).
- **Ventricular Diastole**: In this stage, the ventricles relax, and the AV valves are opened, resulting in the filling up of blood in the ventricles from the atrias, which accounts for most of the blood in it. Through the venae cavae, a small amount of blood directly flows into the ventricles. So, at the end of this stage, the remaining blood present in the atria is moved to the ventricles.
- **Ventricular Systole**: When both ventricles contract, forcing the blood to flow from the right ventricle to the lungs through the pulmonary trunk and from the left ventricle to the whole body through the aorta (Altuve et al., 2020).

The main cause of the blockages inside the blood vessels is the building up of fatty deposits in them, preventing blood from flowing towards the heart or brain, which might give rise to bleeding that, in turn, causes strokes and heart attacks. The behavioral risk factors may affect an individual immediately by a sudden rise in blood pressure and glucose and by being obese. Some of the common CVDs are:

- **Heart Valve Disease**: It occurs when one or more of the four valves of the heart, namely aortic, mitral, pulmonary, or tricuspid, does not form properly, failing to open or shut completely, causing trouble in blood flow or back towards heart chambers due to a backward leak. The different types of defects of the valves are:
- **Stenosis**: The meaning of stenosis is narrowing. It can cause stiffness in your heart valves, preventing blood flow. Due to stenosis, the pressure on the heart builds up to pump blood through the valves, which results in a reduced supply of oxygen in the body. It is classified into four types, i.e., aortic, tricuspid, pulmonary, and mitral valve stenosis, depending on where the stenosis has arisen (Maganti et al., 2010).
- **Regurgitation**: When the flow of blood through a valve leaks in the opposite direction than normal, particularly the backward flow of blood through any heart valve, it is called regurgitation. Based on where the leak exists, it is classified into aortic, tricuspid, pulmonic, and mitral valve regurgitation (Maganti et al., 2010).

- **Prolapse**: It means falling out of place. Here, the flaps of the mitral valve become enlarged or stretched such that they bulge into the left atrium whenever the heart contracts, resulting in mitral valve prolapse or Barlow syndrome. This prolonged effect of prolapse in the mitral valve might lead to mitral valve regurgitation.
- **Atresia**: It means the absence of an opening or abnormal narrowing of a passage in the body. Atresia can affect any of the valves when they are not formed at all, or the flaps are fused together, resulting in malformation. Depending on which valve is underdeveloped, it is classified into mitral, tricuspid, pulmonary, and aortic atresia. It is a congenital defect and may need surgery soon after the baby is born (Maganti et al., 2010).
- **Coronary Artery Disease**: Over a prolonged period of time, the deposits of cholesterol and fat form plaques on the walls of coronary arteries. The artery becomes narrow due to plaque formation, limiting the blood supply to the heart and other parts of the body. This process is called atherosclerosis, and the fatty deposits or plaque formations are called atheroma. Atherosclerosis weakens the heart muscles with time, and it becomes difficult for the heart to pump blood, which may lead to heart failure.

Due to the previously mentioned CVDs, an individual can die early when CVD is not detected in a timely manner. Hence, to increase the patient's life expectancy, it becomes important to detect these diseases at an early stage so that a proper treatment plan can be made by the doctor. The best and easiest way to detect CVDs is by auscultation, which is a method of listening to heart murmurs or heart sounds using a stethoscope. The fundamental heartbeats consist of S1, systole, S2, and diastole, and an expert can hear them on the chest wall to understand whether the heart is functioning normally or abnormally. These heart murmurs are recorded in time series representations and are called phonocardiogram (PCG) signals (Liu et al., 2016).

The normal and pathological heart sounds or audio recordings are shown in Figure 10.1. The PCG signal recordings are the initial clues and guides to further diagnose heart diseases early. Using these recorded PCG signals, patients with abnormal heart sound recording might be asked to continue the investigation and go for cross-examination by undergoing an electrocardiogram (ECG) or echocardiography. This auscultation method to gather the PCG signals is low-cost, and it is easily portable as it uses a stethoscope (Vyas et al., 2021; Kaushal et al., 2023). That is why it is the best diagnosis method for CVDs, as any individual can have immediate access to it, especially people who live in remote and rural areas where it is difficult to get to a primary health center instantly.

In this work, a cardiovascular disease detection algorithm has been proposed that makes use of time-frequency representations (Mistry et al., 2023), three transfer learning models, a manta ray foraging optimization, and a KNN classifier for classifying normal and pathological PCG signals. An open-access database of heart sound recordings, the PhysioNet 2016 Challenge database, is utilized in this algorithm (Liu et al., 2016). In the initial step, the PCG signal acquired from the database is converted into IIR-CQT spectrograms, i.e., time-frequency image representations (Kaushal et al., 2022; Birajdar et al., 2022). These images are applied to the three

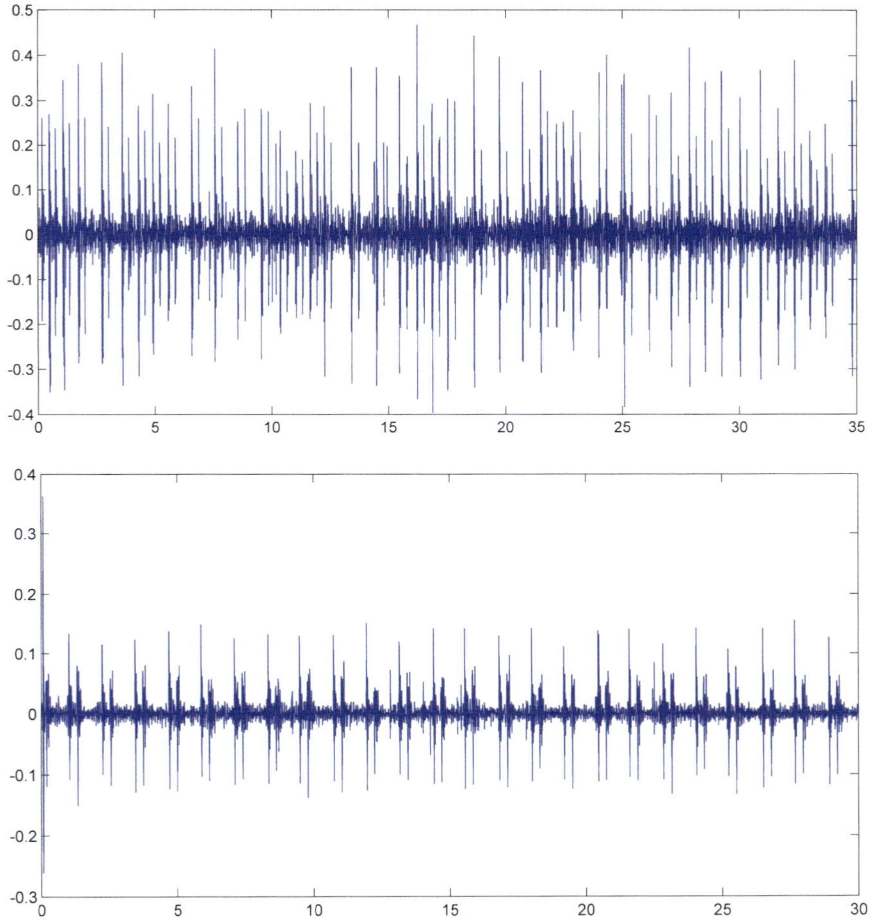

**FIGURE 10.1** (Top) Normal heart sound signal. (Bottom) Pathological heart sound signal.

deep learning models, i.e., ResNet-50, GoogleNet, and Inception-V3, for feature extraction. The deep features are given to the manta ray foraging optimization algorithm to discard the redundant features, and finally, the KNN classifier is used for classification.

The three deep learning architectures, namely, ResNet-50, GoogleNet, and Inception-V3, are explored in this work, and their experimental results are compared using a KNN classifier. To minimize the deep features obtained using the previously mentioned transfer learning models and to determine the most prominent features, the Manta ray foraging optimization algorithm is used for feature selection.

The book chapter is organized as follows: Section 10.2 reviews the literature, Section 10.3 presents the pre-processing techniques, Section 10.4 explains the proposed algorithm, Section 10.5 elaborates on the feature extraction, feature selection, and classification techniques used in this work, Section 10.6 discusses the experimental results, and Section 10.7 concludes the chapter.

## 10.2 LITERATURE SURVEY

In recent years, a lot has already been done using transfer learning models for pattern classification, object detection, disease detection, and classification. Some of the most common architectures are AlexNet, VGG-16, ResNet-50, Inception-V3 (Gaur et al., 2023), etc.

Oh et al. (2020) suggested a WaveNet deep learning model for multi-class heart sound classification of various heart valve diseases. A total of 1,000 recordings, with 200 recordings in each class from the Yaseen and Kwon dataset, were acquired. The best overall accuracy of 97% for multi-class and the highest accuracy of 98.20% for normal class was achieved using a 10-fold cross-validation scheme. Chien et al. (2020) suggested a deep learning-based convolutional autoencoder architecture that compresses the PCG signals to detect cardiovascular diseases using telecare applications at remote sites. In this architecture, seven convolutional layers are present in the encoder that is located in rural areas to collect the patient's data. The decoder consists of the corresponding seven convolutional layers used to decompress the feature maps located at remote hospitals where doctors use the reconstructed signal. They have used the DLUTHS Database in their proposed work. The technique turned out to be better at compression, and the ratio of compression obtained is 32 using this architecture.

To detect heart valve diseases and classify them, Giorgio et al. (2022) proposed a method that employs pre-processing and segmentation of PCG signals, feature extraction, and classification. In the pre-processing stage, the PCG signal is denoised using a fourth-order Butterworth band-pass filter, and a seventh-order Daubechies wavelet was used to obtain 5th-level detail coefficients of the wavelet transform. After that, the Shannon energy envelope is extracted using the Hanning window with a window size of 80 samples to perform nonlinear energy weighting where medium-level energy occurrence and high-level peaks are featured and preserved. The fast Fourier transform (FFT) is applied to the Shannon energy envelope for segmentation. Thirteen features were extracted from each PCG signal, out of which six were retained by employing feature correlation as a feature reduction technique. A combinational circuit was adopted to classify PCG signals to obtain an accuracy of 99.6%.

Al-Issa and Alqudah (Al-Issa et al., 2022) used combined CNN and LSTM components and augmented as well as non-augmented datasets for deep feature extraction and classification of heart sound signals. The accuracy produced by this proposed method using augmented and non-augmented datasets for multi-class problems was 99.87% and 98.5%, respectively. An accuracy of 93.76% was produced using the PhysioNet 2016 challenge dataset for binary class problems in their work. Ma et al. (2023) proposed a method based on de-noising and segmentation to extract time-frequency features combined further with deep learning features. The segmentation of heart sound signals was done using the double-threshold adaptive method. The XGBoost was utilized, which uses a majority voting algorithm to detect heart sounds of three classes, namely, normal, congenital heart disease (CHD), and congenital heart disease—Pulmonary arterial hypertension (CHD-PAH). An accuracy of

88.61% is achieved by the proposed method. Zeng et al. (2023) used Teager–Kaiser energy operator (TKEO) and rational dilation wavelet transform (RDWT) to extract discriminant features. They acquired the PCG signals from the Yaseen and Kwon dataset. They used one-dimensional (1D) convolutional neural networks (CNN) for binary and multi-class classification of heart sound recordings. They have accomplished an overall accuracy of 98.10% for this proposed work.

For the diagnosis of cardiovascular diseases, Ismail and Ismail (Ismail et al., 2023) suggested chirplet Z transform (CZT), spectrogram generation, and round-based transfer learning. Using the chirplet Z transform, they have collected high-resolution spectral contents from a narrow spectral range. They utilized the Kaiser window to generate a spectrogram from the CZT-based spectra. Finally, the round-based transfer learning approach was used to minimize the computational cost. It is observed that more than 98% accuracy was obtained using this approach.

Chen et al. (2023) suggested a method built using a deep neural network model to extract features on raw data without any segmentation to train and classify abnormal heart sound signals to detect cardiovascular diseases. They used two databases, i.e., the PhysioNet 2016 challenge dataset and the Yaseen and Kwon dataset. The feature vector was reduced using principal component analysis (PCA). In their proposed method, 99.61% accuracy for binary and 99.44% accuracy for multi-class classification was achieved using 10-fold cross-validation and multi-layer perceptron as a classifier. Ahmad et al. (2023) proposed an approach to detect congenital heart diseases that used two databases with 583 and 23 heart sound recordings acquired from a local dataset and a public dataset taken from Michigan University, respectively. The datasets were down-sampled to 8KHz, and a band-pass filter was employed for pre-processing the PCG signals. The signals were segmented with four-second duration, and pitch-shifting was employed for data augmentation. The features were passed to a 1D-CNN, and the classification accuracy of 98.56% is achieved from this proposed work.

The binary classification of heart sound signals of healthy or pathological patients using 1D- convolutional neural networks was proposed by Hussain et al. (Hussain et al., 2023). The PhysioNet 2016 dataset with 3,240 heart sound signals was used, comprised of 2,575 normal and 665 abnormal signals. As the dataset exhibits variable length problems with an uneven distribution of normal and abnormal signals, the PCG signals were divided into an '8' second fixed-length window after pre-processing and de-noising it. Then, the pitch shifting and signal rolling data augmentation techniques were applied. The feature extraction and classification were performed using 1D-CNN. This approach yields an accuracy of 95.45%. To differentiate and classify healthy and pathological heart signals, Jamil and Roy (Jamil et al., 2023) proposed three different frameworks taking into consideration both one-dimensional and 2D PCG signals. The MFCC and LPCC features were extracted from 1D PCG signals, and various D-CNN features were extracted from 2D PCG signals. The particle swarm optimization (PSO) and genetic algorithm (GA) were employed for feature selection, and a vision transformer was employed to enhance the classifier's performance. It was observed that the mean average accuracy $Acc$ and $F1$-score of 99.3% and 99% were achieved, respectively.

Bhardwaj et al. (2023) proposed the time-frequency representation method that employs analytical Morlet continuous wavelet transform (CWT) scalograms for the detection of valvular heart diseases (VHD). They used 2D-convolutional neural networks, and the DL visualization techniques, such as occlusion and DDIs, were employed to interpret the CNN model. They have utilized the PhysioNet 2016 database for binary classification and the Yaseen and Kwon database for multi-class classification of VHDs. The multi-class classification earned the highest accuracy of 99.6% and overall accuracy of 98.32% with fivefold cross-validation techniques. The binary classification earned an accuracy of 93.07% for the proposed method.

For the detection of cardiac pathologies in subjects based on PCG signals, Harimi et al. (2023) proposed a Cytex-inspired transform that converts one-dimensional PCG signals into 2D textured images. The four pre-trained deep convolutional neural networks (DCNN), namely, AlexNet, VGG16, Inception-V3, and ResNet50, were used along with data augmentation, hyper-parameter optimization, and drop-out techniques. The data of a total of 2,868 labeled samples were recorded, out of which 2,249 samples were healthy and 619 samples were unhealthy. The F1 score, accuracy, sensitivity, and specificity of 92.06%, 94.53%, 87.75%, and 96.37% were achieved, respectively. The automated prediction framework to classify normal and abnormal heart sounds was suggested by Devi et al. (2023).

The PhysioNet 2016 challenge for the classification of heart sound database was utilized. The features were obtained using continuous wavelet transform (CWT) coefficients (or Scalogram images), and the features were fed to K-Nearest Neighbor, Support Vector Machine, and AlexNet classification models. The AlexNet outperformed the other two models with 98.11% accuracy, 96.20% sensitivity, and 98.73% specificity. Prabhakar and Won (Prabhakar et al., 2023) recommended two methods for the classification of PCG signals. The first strategy employs non-negative matrix factorization (NMF), with two approaches merged with genetic programming (GP) for optimization, i.e., brain-storming (BS) and advanced brain-storming (ABS), and some machine learning classifiers.

The second strategy employs three dimensionality reduction techniques, namely, Kernel–Principal component analysis (K-PCA), Laplacian Eigenmaps (LE), and maximum variance unfolding (MVU) with Fuzzy C-means (FCM) clustering and advanced sine-cosine (ASC) for optimization and some machine learning classifiers. Compared to the second, the first strategy provided a high classification accuracy of 95.39% with the SVM classifier (Rana et al., 2021).

Binary, as well as multi-class detection of four types of heart valve diseases (HVD) present in the heart sounds, was proposed by Maity et al. (2023) using time-frequency representations as input features, i.e., spectrogram, scalogram, and log-mel spectrogram for feature extraction and YAMNet transfer learning model for classification. An accuracy of 92.23% was obtained for binary classification, and overall accuracy, sensitivity, and specificity of 99.83%, 99.59%, and 99.90% were obtained for multi-class classification to detect four types of HVD, respectively. Riccio et al. (2023) employed a technique for detecting abnormal heartbeats using the PhysioNet 2016 challenge heart sound database. This method does not require any de-noising or segmentation steps, and the 1D PCG signal is transformed into 2D color images based on the fractal theory that exploits Partitioned Iterated Function Systems (PIFS). The selected features were fed to the deep CNN, and a modified Accuracy (MAcc) of 0.85 was achieved. Table 10.1 illustrates the various methods present in the literature for cardiovascular disease detection algorithms.

**TABLE 10.1**
**The Existing Cardiovascular Disease Detection Algorithm with Various Feature Extraction, Feature Selection, and Classification Methods and the Datasets Utilized with the Accuracy Achieved by Them**

| Author | Feature Extraction Method | Feature Reduction Method | Classification/Deep Learning Model | Database | Accuracy/ Score |
|---|---|---|---|---|---|
| Oh et al. (2020) | – | – | WaveNet | Yaseen and Kwon dataset | 97%—Multi-class, 98.20%—Normal |
| Chien et al. (2020) | – | – | Deep convolutional autoencoder | Dalian University of Technology heart sounds database (DLUTHSDB) | 32- Compress Ratio |
| Al-Issa et al. (2022) | CNN | – | LSTM | PhysioNet 2016, augmented and non-augmented datasets | 93.76%—Binary, 99.87%—Augmented, 98.5%—Non-Augmented |
| Ma et al. (2023) | Time-frequency features | – | XGBoost | – | 88.61% |
| Zeng et al. (2023) | Teager–Kaiser energy operator (TKEO) and rational dilation wavelet transform (RDWT) | – | CNN | Yaseen and Kwon Dataset | 98.10%—Multi-class |
| Ismail et al. (2023) | Chirplet Z transform (CZT) | – | Round-based transfer learning | PASCAL and Yaseen and Kwon (Y-18) Dataset | >98% |
| Chen et al. (2023) | DNN | PCA | MLP | PhysioNet 2016—Binary Yaseen and Kwon—Multi-class | 99.61%—Binary, 99.44%—Multi-class |
| Ahmad et al. (2023) | – | – | CNN | Local dataset and public dataset from Michigan university | 98.56% |

(Continued)

**TABLE 10.1 (*Continued*)**
**The Existing Cardiovascular Disease Detection Algorithm with Various Feature Extraction, Feature Selection, and Classification Methods and the Datasets Utilized with the Accuracy Achieved by Them**

| Author | Feature Extraction Method | Feature Reduction Method | Classification/Deep Learning Model | Database | Accuracy/ Score |
|---|---|---|---|---|---|
| Hussain et al. (2023) | CNN | – | CNN | PhysioNet 2016 | 95.45% |
| Jamil and Roy (2023) | MFCC and LPCC features | Particle swarm optimization (PSO) and genetic algorithm (GA) | D-CNN | Yaseen and Kwon | 99.3%—Mean Average Accuracy *Acc*, 99% — *F*1-score |
| Bhardwaj et al. (2023) | Analytical Morlet continuous wavelet transform (CWT) scalograms | – | CNN | PhysioNet 2016—Binary Yaseen and Kwon—Multi-class | 93.07%—Binary, 98.32%—Multi-class |
| Harimi et al. (2023) | Cytex-inspired transform | – | ResNet50 | PhysioNet 2016 | 94.53% |
| Devi et al. (2023) | CWT coefficients (or scalograms) | – | AlexNet | | |
| Prabhakar and Won (2023) | Non-Negative Matrix Factorization (NMF) | Brain-storming with genetic programming (BS-GP) and advanced brain-storming (ABS-GP) | Support Vector Machine (SVM) classifier | PhysioNet 2016 | 95.39% |
| Maity et al. (2023) | Time-frequency representations | – | YAMNet Model | PhysioNet 2016—Binary Yaseen and Kwon—Multi-class | 92.23%—Binary, 99.83%—Multi-class |
| Riccio et al. (2023) | Partitioned Iterated Function Systems (PIFS) based on fractal theory | – | Deep CNN | PhysioNet 2016 | 0.85—Modified Accuracy |

## 10.3 PRE-PROCESSING TECHNIQUES

The heart sound recordings that are acquired from the PhysioNet 2016 database are affected by signals arising due to fluctuations in breathing, noise generated due to the movement of a stethoscope, signals from intestinal activity, and noise from the background. These noise signals prevent the classification of PCG signals into abnormal and normal classes (Kaushal et al., 2023). Pre-processing helps to remove the unwanted noise content from the PCG signals and enables the spectrogram to generate time-frequency image representations (Rani et al., 2021).

## 10.4 PROPOSED ALGORITHM

A cardiovascular disease detection method based on a deep transfer learning model and a nature-inspired optimization algorithm is presented in this chapter. The block diagram of the proposed cardiovascular disease detection and classification algorithm is shown in Figure 10.2, and the proposed algorithm is shown in Algorithm 10.1.

### 10.4.1 Heart Sound Signal Acquisition

The PhysioNet/CinC Challenge 2016 database was utilized to acquire the heart sound signal recordings for performing the experiments. The first block in the block schematic, as shown in Figure 10.2, exhibits the acquisition of the heart sound signals (Maganti et al., 2010). The dataset comprises heart sound recordings from varied time durations of five seconds to 120 seconds collected from healthy and pathological subjects. Step A in algorithm 1 explains this block.

### 10.4.2 Time-Frequency Visual Representation

The second block in the block diagram explains the constant-Q transform (IIR-CQT) visual time-frequency representation of the heart sound audio signals.

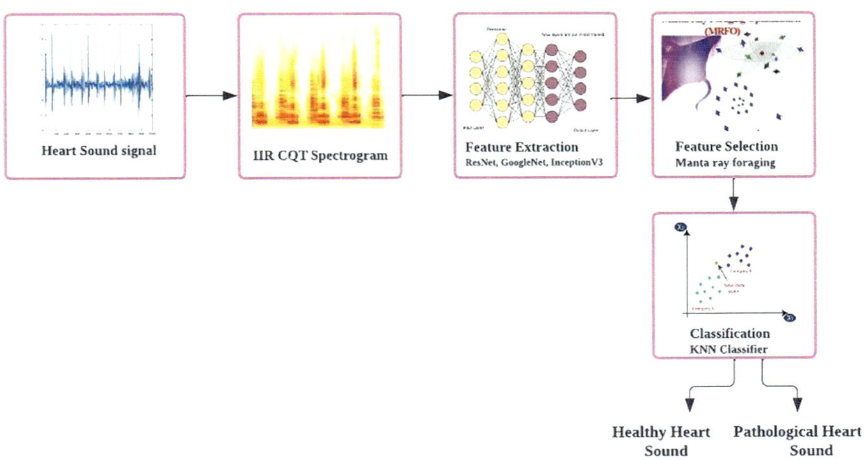


**FIGURE 10.2** The block diagram of the proposed cardiovascular disease detection.

These representations reveal visual patterns that help to distinguish between healthy and pathological heart sound signals. IIR-CQT spectrogram representation is better than the conventional spectrograms. Steps b, c, and d in Algorithm 10.1 describe this block.

### 10.4.3 Feature Extraction Using Deep Learning Models

The third block shown in the block diagram shows the process of feature extraction using deep learning models. ResNet-50, GoogleNet, and Inception-V3 deep learning models are used for feature extraction. Before the process of feature extraction, IIR CQT spectrogram image augmentation is performed using resizing and rotation operations. The spectrogram images are separated into two tests, training and testing sets, as shown in step e of Algorithm 10.1. A detailed discussion about feature extraction is presented in Section 10.5.

### 10.4.4 Feature Selection and Classification

A biologically inspired Manta ray foraging optimization algorithm is utilized for feature selection in this work. The fourth block elucidates the feature selection that results in low-dimension feature vector. The manta ray algorithm effectually delivers the most discriminating optimized feature subset, hence improving the detection accuracy. Somersault foraging is used to get the best fit, find the relevant features, and discard the redundant features. Step g in Algorithm 10.1 explains the manta ray foraging algorithm. The selected features are given to the KNN classifier for detection. The classifier classifies the PCG signals as healthy or pathological. Performance parameters are evaluated to determine the performance of the system. Steps h and i explain the feature selection and classification process.

## 10.5 FEATURE EXTRACTION, FEATURE SELECTION AND CLASSIFICATION

In the field of cardiovascular medicine, routine management of complex conditions like heart attacks, complex arrhythmias, sudden cardiac arrest, cardiovascular diseases, and congenital heart diseases is very important. Making effective predictions and using the data to treat individual patients requires integrating the data from numerous sources. In recent years, diagnoses of heart anomalies using computer-aided tools and PCG signals have gained significant importance. Computer-aided techniques offer robust and accurate diagnoses compared to traditional methods (Chen et al., 2023). Detection of cardiovascular diseases using PCG signals involves steps like pre-processing, feature extraction, and feature selection for the classification of abnormal sounds. Deep learning techniques have shown considerable efficiency in anomaly detection by improving classification performance. As deep learning methods have an end-to-end structure, the feature extraction process is automated (Krittanawong et al., 2019).

Due to time restrictions and computational necessity, we can use the transfer learning concept, which is a powerful method in deep learning. Transfer learning uses pre-trained models that are tailored to suit the requirements by altering the softmax layer (final layer) to optimize the results. Transfer learning is advantageous because of the reduced time required for training and the superior performance of the neural network. Pre-trained are built as a series of layers, and the layers convert the activation function using a differentiable function. In all the pre-trained networks, the architecture places the layers with the input layer as the first layer, followed by the convolution layer and ReLU pooling layer, and finally, the fully connected layer.

The input layers take the images as input, which are resized as per the architecture of the neural network. The calculation of neuron outputs depending on the weights and regions is done in the CNN layer. The output size of the CNN layer depends on the width, height, and number of filters used. ReLU is a piecewise linear activation function that transforms the weighted input into the corresponding output. The pooling layer aids in the dimension reduction of the generated feature maps. These layers control the computations handled by the network by reducing the parameters to be learned by the network. It performs the down-sampling operation. The last layer, or the fully connected layer, multiplies the input from the pooling layer by a weighted matrix and adds a bias vector. The fully connected layer (FC) layer connects all the neurons available in the previous layer.

## ALGORITHM 10.1: THE PROPOSED ALGORITHM FOR CARDIOVASCULAR DISEASE DETECTION USING DEEP LEARNING AND MANTA RAY FORAGING OPTIMIZATION ALGORITHM.

```
Input data to the algorithm -
X = total number of heart sound audio samples in the dataset
Y = number of time-frequency visual representation (spectro-
gram) samples in the dataset.
m=size of image
P= Size of Population
K=5
d=dimension
Results obtained from the algorithm -
accuracy, precision, sensitivity, gmean, specificity, and F1
score
for i ← 1 to X do
   segment 1, segment 2, . . . , segment n ← divide the audio
   signal into length of '5' seconds each.
end for
for j ← 1 to Y do
   I[x,y] ← convert the audio samples into IIR-CQT spectrograms.
   I[m,m] ← downscale the spectrogram images
   Save the downscaled IIR-CQT spectrogram images dataset.
```

```
end for
[Training(), testing()] ← divide the dataset into training and
testing samples.
Feature extraction ← input the IIR-CQT spectrogram images into
ResNet-50, GoogleNet, Inception-V3 - deep learning models
Feature selection← Manta ray foraging optimization algorithm
(somersault foraging)
for j=1 to P do
```

$$sf_j^d(w+1) = sf_j^d(w) + s(\partial_1 sf_{best}^d - \partial_2 sf_j^d(w)$$

```
    Compute the fitness of each individual f(sfjdw+1 if
```

$$f(sf_j^d(w+1) < f(sf_{best}^d)$$

then $sf_{best}^d = sf_j^d(w+1)$

```
end for
Classification ← selected features given as input to KNN clas-
sifier and identifies the input PCG test signal as healthy or
pathological. Set K.
Accuracy, precision, sensitivity, gmean, specificity, and F1
score ← calculate the performance evaluation parameters.
```

Transfer learning helps in the automatic extraction of features. Neural networks can learn the important features from the images, which helps discover a good collection of features that can be used as input to the classification stage.

Three transfer learning models, ResNet-50, GoogleNet, and Inception-V3, are utilized for feature extraction in this work. Resnet Residual Network (ResNet) is a Convolutional Neural Network (CNN) architecture that is designed to support hundreds or thousands of convolutional layers. ResNet provides a solution to the vanishing gradient problem, also known as 'skip connections'. Multiple identity mappings are stacked by ResNet, which then skips those layers and reuses the activations from the preceding layer. By reducing the network into fewer layers, skip connections accelerate the initial training. The remaining components of the network, which are considered to be the residual parts, are free to explore the input image's feature space after the network has been retrained. ResNet-50 has 50 convolutional layers, followed by a MaxPool layer and an average pool layer. There are three layered stacks in ResNet-50, and it uses a bottleneck design, which reduces the number of matrix multiplications.

GoogleNet is a 22-layer deep CNN with 27 pooling layers that provides a significant decrease in error rate as compared to AlexNet. It takes input images of the size 224*224, and the softmax layer has 1,000 nodes, which helps in the classification of 1,000 classes. This architecture uses $1 \times 1$ convolutions that help to reduce the weights and biases of the architecture. The model also uses the technique of global average pooling at the end of the network, which helps in the formation of deeper architecture. The average pooling decreases the number of trainable parameters to 0 and leads to an improvement in accuracy (Demir et al., 2019).

Some models have deeper layers to improve performance and accuracy but compromise on the computational cost. Inception Net is heavily engineered and reduces the computational cost compared to other models. It employs numerous techniques to boost performance in terms of speed and precision. The Inception-V3 architecture employs an RMSprop optimizer that limits the oscillations in the vertical direction. This leads to an increase in the learning rate, which helps the algorithm to take larger steps in the horizontal direction, thereby converging faster. Batch normalization in the fully connected layer of the auxiliary classifier. The label smoothing regularization process regularizes the classifier by estimating label drop-out during training. This regularization provides an improvement of 0.2% from the error rate. Inception-V3 uses 7*7 factorized convolution.

### 10.5.1 Manta Ray Feature Selection

For selecting the best features, the Manta Ray Foraging Optimization (MRFO) approach is applied. Chain foraging, cyclone foraging, and somersault foraging are the three main steps of MRFO.

#### 10.5.1.1 Chain Foraging

In chain foraging, manta rays form an orderly line to form a firm chain to catch plankton as food. The ideal location, according to the MRF optimization algorithm, is one with a high concentration of plankton, the primary prey that the manta ray chain consumes. The MRF algorithm adjusts the manta ray's location depending on its optimum location and the manta ray in front of it, with the exception of the first manta ray. The update in chain foraging is as shown in the mathematical Equation 10.1.

$$\{cf_j^d(w+1) = cf_j^d(w) + \partial(cf_{best}^d(w) - cf_j^d(w)) + \alpha\left(cf_{best}^d(w) - cf_j^d(w)\right) j =$$

$$1\ cf_j^d(w) + \partial\left(cf_{j-1}^d(w) - cf_j^d(w)\right) + \alpha\left(cf_{best}^d(w) - cf_j^d(w)\right) \quad j = 2 \ldots.N \quad (10.1)$$

Where $\alpha = 2.\ \partial\sqrt{|log\ log\ \partial)|}$

d represents the dimension, $\alpha$ denotes the learning rate and $cf_j^d(w)$ is jth individual at t time. $\partial$ takes the values in the range [0,1].

#### 10.5.1.2 Cyclone Foraging

When manta rays find the plankton with the highest quantity during foraging, they construct a spiral by creating a link by connecting their heads and tails (Demir et al., 2019). This information helps each manta ray go not only in the direction of the plankton but also in the direction of the manta ray in front of it. The mathematical expression is shown in Equation 10.2.

$$\{cf_j^d(w+1) = cf_j^d(w) + \partial(cf_{best}^d(w) - cf_j^d(w)) + \beta\left(cf_{best}^d(w) - cf_j^d(w)\right) \quad j =$$

$$1\ cf_j^d(w) + \partial\left(cf_{j-1}^d(w) - cf_j^d(w)\right) + \beta\left(cf_{best}^d(w) - \left(cf_j^d w\right)\right) \quad j = 2 \ldots.N \qquad (10.2)$$

$$where\ \beta = 2exp^{\partial} \frac{T-t+1}{T} 2sin(2\pi r)$$

T is the total number of iterations and $\beta$ denotes coefficient of weights

#### 10.5.1.3 Somersault Foraging

Somersault foraging helps manta rays consume more plankton, as in this type of foraging, the movement is random and cyclic (Amin et al., 2022). The position with the highest concentration of plankton is chosen as the point of reference. Each of the manta rays revolves around this reference point and finally somersaults to a new position. The mathematical representation of somersault foraging is shown in Equation 10.3.

$$sf_j^d(w+1) = sf_j^d(w) + s(\partial_1 sf_{best}^d - \partial_2 sf_j^d(w) \quad j = 1 \ldots\ldots N \tag{10.3}$$

$sf$ represents the somersault factor and $\partial_1$ and $\partial_2$ are two arbitrary numbers in the range [0,1].

The IIR-CQT spectrogram images from healthy and abnormal heart sound signals are fed as input to the deep learning models. In this work, three models are used for feature extraction: ResNet-50, GoogleNet, and Inception-V3. The feature extraction produces a large dimension feature vector; hence, the manta ray optimization-based feature selection approach is utilized, as shown in Figure 10.3. The manta ray algorithm effectively delivers the most discriminating optimized feature set that is provided to the KNN classifier for the classification of healthy and pathological heart sounds.

### 10.5.2 Classification

KNN-K nearest neighbor's algorithm is used to store all existing classes and helps to classify new classes with the help of a similarity measurement. KNN is a non-parametric method of classification and has found widespread importance in statistical approximation and pattern recognition (Yadav et al., 2020). Classification of a particular class is based on the majority score of its neighbors, with the class getting allocated to the group that is most common among its K nearest neighbors. The distance is measured by a function defined by the expression, as shown in Equation 10.4.

$$df = \sqrt{\sum_{j=1}^{k} (x_i - k_i)^2} \tag{10.4}$$

## 10.6 EXPERIMENTAL RESULTS AND DISCUSSION

This chapter presents an unsegmented heart sound detection technique using deep transfer learning model feature extraction and a manta ray feature selection algorithm. IIQ-CQT spectrogram images are applied to transfer learning architecture to generate features. In this section, the database, experimental settings, and results are presented. The experimental results are produced on the PhysioNet Challenge 2016

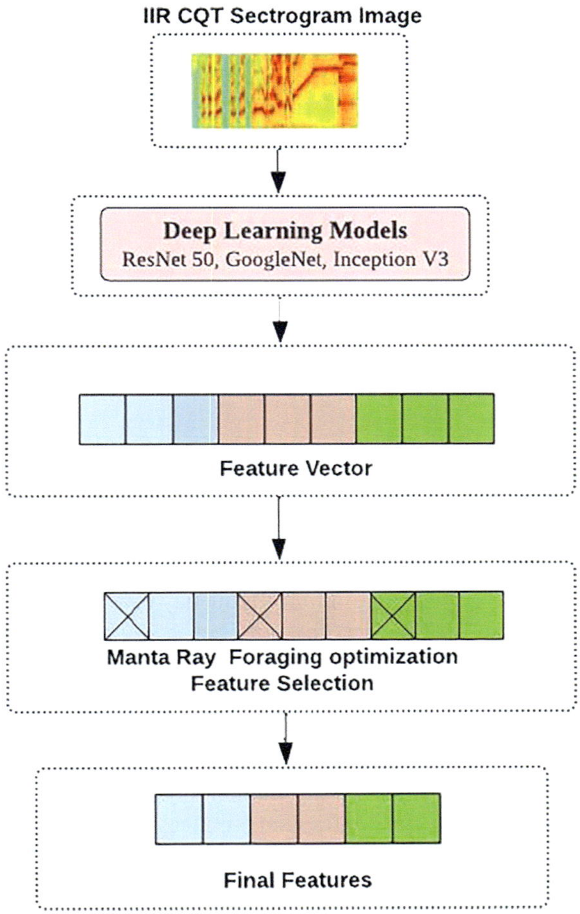


**FIGURE 10.3** Feature selection using the Manta Ray Foraging Optimization algorithm for final feature vector generation.

database (Liu et al., 2016). The PhysioNet Challenge dataset consists of heart sound recordings from varied time durations of five seconds to 120 seconds collected from healthy and pathological subjects.

The original database involves 3,126 heart sound files combined in nine datasets. As the proposed algorithm is based on non-segmented heart sound samples, it does not require a segmentation process of recordings for feature extraction, which reduces the algorithm's complexity. After the pre-processing step, IIR-CQT spectrogram images from healthy pathological samples are generated. IIR-CQT spectrogram images are produced from PCG audio samples of five seconds time duration. For experimentation, 1,182 diseased and 1,186 normal IIR-CQT spectrogram images are generated from the PhysioNet Challenge 2016 database. 80% of randomly selected spectrogram images are employed to obtain training features from deep learning models, and the remaining 20% are for testing features.

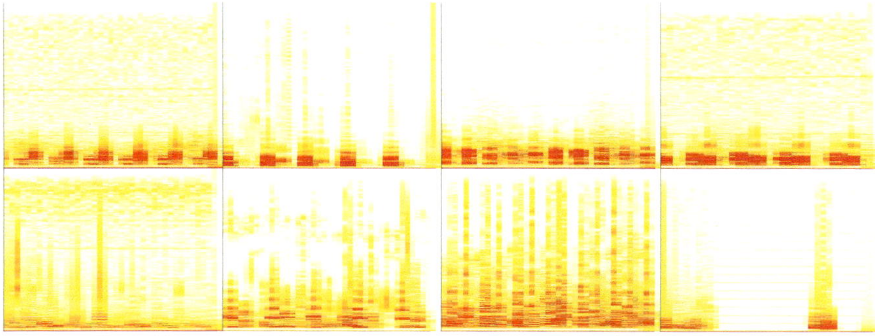

**FIGURE 10.4** The sample healthy and pathological IIR-CQT spectrogram images.

The IIR-CQT spectrogram images from healthy and abnormal heart sound signals are generated. In this step, each healthy and abnormal heart sound is framed for a 5s time duration, retaining the same original sampling frequency. Figure 10.4 depicts healthy and pathological IIR-CQT spectrogram images. The Q-factor of 13 is employed for IIR-CQT spectrogram time-frequency image generation using 4,096 bins. The spatial resolution of the spectrogram images is 875 × 656 pixels. As stated previously, three transfer learning models are compared for the feature extraction process: ResNet-50, GoogleNet, and Inception-V3.

Before the transfer learning feature extraction, the spectrogram image database augmentation process is performed using resizing and rotation operations. A fully connected layer of each transfer learning model is employed for feature extraction with a batch size of 64. The feature extraction produces a large dimension feature set; hence, the manta ray optimization-based feature selection approach is explored. The manta ray algorithm effectively furnishes the most discriminating optimized feature subset, improving detection accuracy. A number of solutions and a maximum number of iteration counts are set as 10 and 100 in manta ray optimization settings. The threshold for manta ray foraging optimization is set as 0.5 with a somersault factor of 2. The effect of the threshold on the detection rate is also analyzed in this study. K is set to 5 in the KNN classifier.

The error rate is employed as the fitness function for the manta ray foraging optimization algorithm. Various performance metrics are utilized for evaluating the proposed algorithm performance: gmean, sensitivity, precision, specificity, accuracy, and F1-measure, and are defined in Equations 10.5–10.10.

$$Sensitivity = \frac{TrPos}{FaNeg + TrPos} \tag{10.5}$$

$$Specificity = \frac{TrNeg}{FaPos + TrNeg} \tag{10.6}$$

$$Accuracy = \frac{TrPos + TrNeg}{FaNeg + TrPos + FaPos + TrNeg} \tag{10.7}$$

$$Precision = \frac{TrPos}{FaPos + TrPos} \tag{10.8}$$

$$F1 - score = \frac{2 \times TrPos}{2 \times TrPos\ FaPos + FaNeg} \tag{10.9}$$

$$gmean = \sqrt{Specificity \times Sensitivity} \tag{10.10}$$

The first set of experimental results is presented without applying the manta ray foraging feature selection algorithm. Tables 10.2–10.4 show accuracy, sensitivity, specificity, precision, F1-score, and gmean with a batch size of 32, 64, and 128 without applying manta ray foraging optimization technique for ResNet-50, GoogleNet, and Inception-V3 transfer learning model, respectively. It can be seen from these tables that GoogleNet features attained the lowest accuracy, whereas Inception-V3 attained a maximum detection accuracy rate of 98.73%.

It is also observed that, in all deep learning models, a batch size of 32 obtained the highest detection accuracy compared to 64 and 128. Average gmean, F1-score,

**TABLE 10.2**
**Performance Measures Obtained Using ResNet-50 Deep Learning Features with Different Batch Sizes without Feature Selection**

| Batch Size | Accuracy | Sensitivity | Specificity | Precision | F1-Score | gmean |
|---|---|---|---|---|---|---|
| 32 | 0.9789 | 0.9788 | 0.9789 | 0.9788 | 0.9788 | 0.9789 |
| 64 | 0.9662 | 0.9492 | 0.9831 | 0.9825 | 0.9655 | 0.9660 |
| 128 | 0.9429 | 0.9322 | 0.9536 | 0.9524 | 0.9522 | 0.9428 |

**TABLE 10.3**
**Accuracy, Sensitivity, Specificity, Precision, F1-Score, and gmean Values Derived from GoogleNet Transfer Learning Features with a Batch Size of 32, 64, and 128 without Applying the Manta Ray Foraging Optimization Technique**

| Batch Size | Accuracy | Sensitivity | Specificity | Precision | F1-Score | gmean |
|---|---|---|---|---|---|---|
| 32 | 0.9704 | 0.9746 | 0.9662 | 0.9664 | 0.9705 | 0.9704 |
| 64 | 0.9662 | 0.9703 | 0.9620 | 0.9622 | 0.9662 | 0.9662 |
| 128 | 0.9577 | 0.9534 | 0.9620 | 0.9615 | 0.9574 | 0.9577 |

**TABLE 10.4**
**Various Performance Parameters Using Features Extracted from Inception-V3 Deep Learning Architecture with Three Different Batch Sizes without Feature Selection**

| Batch Size | Accuracy | Sensitivity | Specificity | Precision | F1-Score | gmean |
|---|---|---|---|---|---|---|
| 32 | 0.9873 | 0.9873 | 0.9873 | 0.9873 | 0.9873 | 0.9873 |
| 64 | 0.9746 | 0.9703 | 0.9789 | 0.9786 | 0.9745 | 0.9746 |
| 128 | 0.9619 | 0.9576 | 0.9662 | 0.9658 | 0.9617 | 0.9619 |

and sensitivity parameters have shown improvement in features extracted from the Inception-V3 model as opposed to GoogleNet and ResNet-50. Inception-V3 is optimized using the branch structure, and two 1-D convolutional kernels are employed, which effectively extract spatial details of the input, resulting in an improved detection rate.

In the next step, experimental results are obtained after applying the manta ray foraging optimization algorithm.

Tables 10.5–10.7 depict different performance measures obtained with different batch sizes and manta ray optimization-based feature selection using ResNet-50, GoogleNet, and Inception-V3 transfer learning models. In all batch sizes and deep learning models, the detection accuracy and other parameters are notably improved.

**TABLE 10.5**
**Performance Measures Obtained Using ResNet-50 Deep Learning Features with Different Batch Sizes with Feature Selection**

| Batch Size | Accuracy | Sensitivity | Specificity | Precision | F1-Score | gmean |
|---|---|---|---|---|---|---|
| 32 | 0.9915 | 0.9915 | 0.9916 | 0.9915 | 0.9915 | 0.9915 |
| 64 | 0.9873 | 0.9873 | 0.9873 | 0.9873 | 0.9873 | 0.9873 |
| 128 | 0.9623 | 0.9748 | 0.9621 | 0.9663 | 0.9662 | 0.9620 |

**TABLE 10.6**
**Accuracy, Sensitivity, Specificity, Precision, F1-Score, and gmean Values Derived from GoogleNet Transfer Learning Features with a Batch Size of 32, 64, and 128 with Manta Ray Foraging Optimization Technique**

| Batch Size | Accuracy | Sensitivity | Specificity | Precision | F1-Score | gmean |
|---|---|---|---|---|---|---|
| 32 | 0.9810 | 0.9873 | 0.9747 | 0.9749 | 0.9811 | 0.9810 |
| 64 | 0.9704 | 0.9703 | 0.9705 | 0.9703 | 0.9703 | 0.9704 |
| 128 | 0.9514 | 0.9534 | 0.9494 | 0.9494 | 0.9514 | 0.9514 |

**TABLE 10.7**
**Various Performance Parameters Using Features Extracted from Inception-V3 Deep Learning Architecture with Three Different Batch Sizes with Feature Selection**

| Batch Size | Accuracy | Sensitivity | Specificity | Precision | F1-Score | gmean |
|---|---|---|---|---|---|---|
| 32 | 0.9958 | 0.9915 | 1.000 | 1.000 | 0.9957 | 0.9958 |
| 64 | 0.9831 | 0.9788 | 0.9873 | 0.9872 | 0.9830 | 0.9831 |
| 128 | 0.9789 | 0.9746 | 0.9831 | 0.9829 | 0.9787 | 0.9788 |

Similar to the first set of experiments, Inception-V3 produced the highest accuracy of 99.58%, whereas ResNet-50 and GoogleNet delivered 99.15% and 98.10% accuracy, respectively.

The manta ray foraging optimization algorithm not only reduces the feature vector dimensions but also improves the sensitivity, accuracy, precision, F1-score, and gmean parameter values. F1-score and gmean are above 99% in Inception-V3, illustrating enhanced performance. Figures 10.5 and 10.6 show the confusion matrix obtained using ResNet-50, GoogleNet, and Inception-V3 deep learning features.

As apparent from these confusion matrices, false positives and false negatives are significantly lowered in Inception-V3 compared to other models. Further, Figures 10.7 and 10.8 depict ROC plots with AUC for normal and abnormal class samples using ResNet-50 and GoogleNet models, respectively.

## 10.7 OPTIMIZATION-BASED FEATURE SELECTION ANALYSIS

As outlined earlier, the proposed algorithm employs a manta ray foraging algorithm for feature selection. The most relevant and discriminating features from the input feature pool are chosen using the manta ray optimization. The detection error rate of the classification model is used as a fitness function. The fitness value is evaluated for each iteration for selecting the important feature subset. Figures 10.9 and 10.10 depict fitness value vs. number of iterations for manta ray optimization using ResNet-50, GoogleNet, and Inception-V3 models.

The threshold value in the manta ray optimization impacts the detection accuracy and other related parameter values. The effect of threshold on these performance metrics is also analyzed in this work. Figures 10.11–10.13 show sensitivity, specificity, precision, F-measure, and average accuracy for ResNet-50, GoogleNet, and Inception-V3 deep learning models when the manta ray optimization threshold is set to 0.5, 0.6, and 0.7. It is observed that a threshold value of 0.5 attains the highest detection rate as compared to 0.6 and 0.7. Accordingly, experiment results are presented using a 0.5 threshold value.

The proposed deep transfer learning and manta ray feature selection algorithm are compared with recent heart sound detection approaches in Table 10.8. For a fair

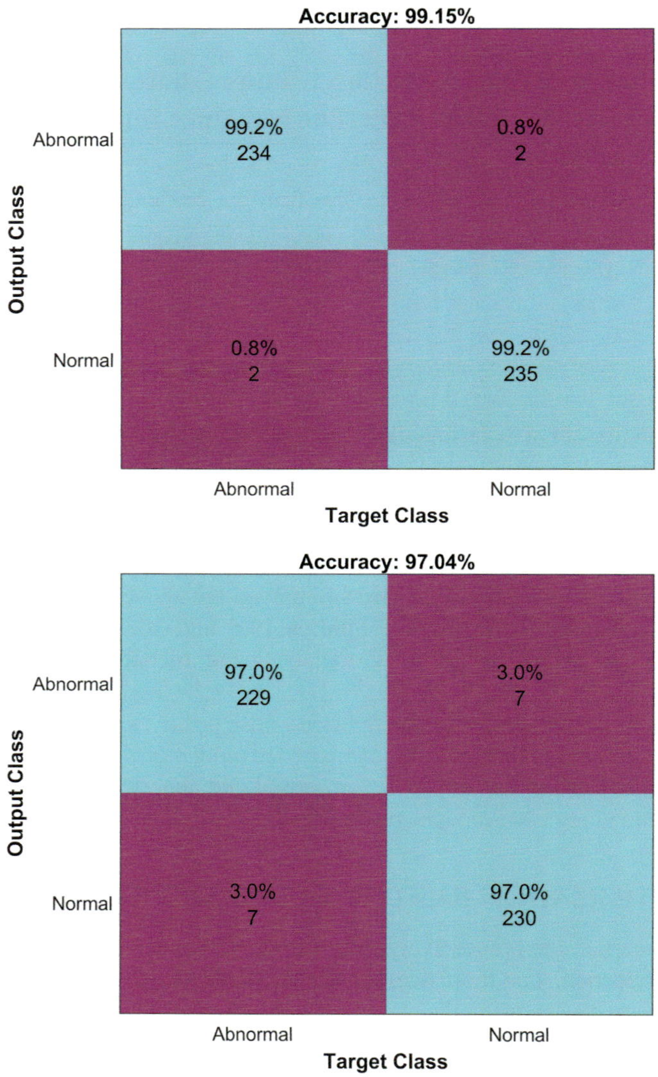


**FIGURE 10.5** The confusion matrix obtained using ResNet-50 and GoogleNet.

comparison, existing algorithms that employed the PhysioNet/CinC Challenge 2016 database for experimental evaluation are considered. As is evident from Table 10.6, the proposed Inception-V3 model-based features result in the highest detection accuracy (Khang, 2024). In Singh et al. (2020), scalogram images are applied to the GoogleNet model, and in Li (2022), MFCC images are fed to ResNet-50 transfer learning architecture, whereas the proposed approach employed IIR-CQT spectrogram images for feature extraction.

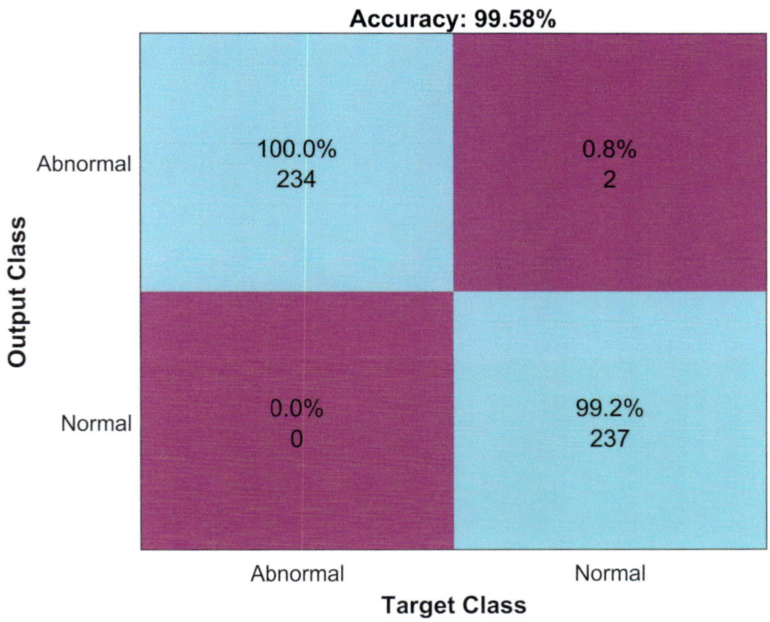


**FIGURE 10.6** The confusion matrix obtained using Inception-V3 deep learning features.

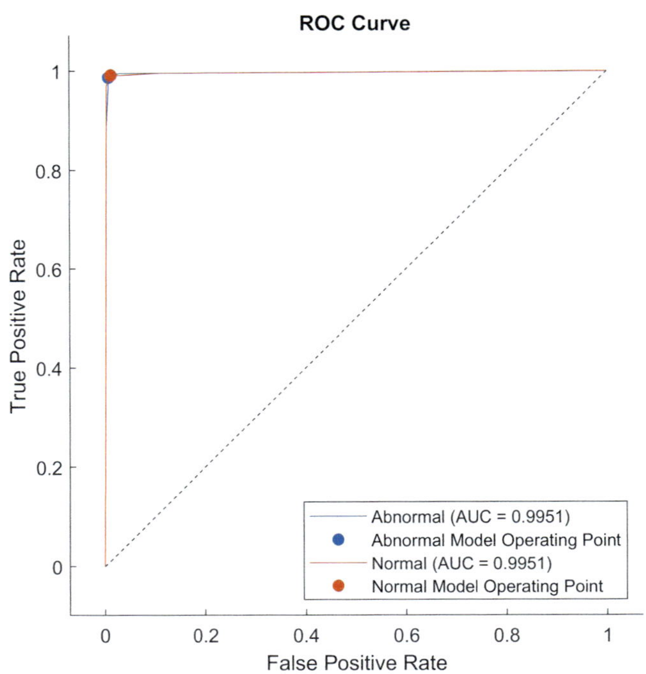


**FIGURE 10.7** ROC plots with AUC for normal and abnormal class samples using ResNet-50 models, respectively.

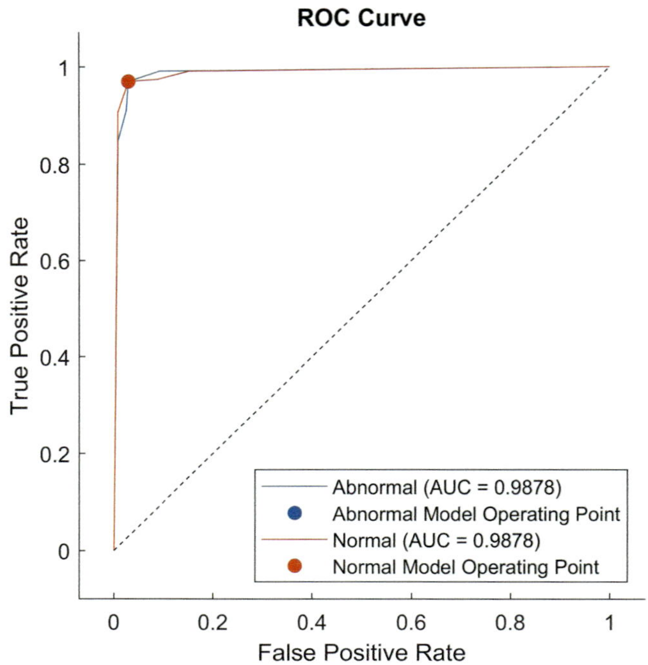


**FIGURE 10.8** ROC plots with AUC for normal and abnormal class samples using GoogleNet models, respectively.

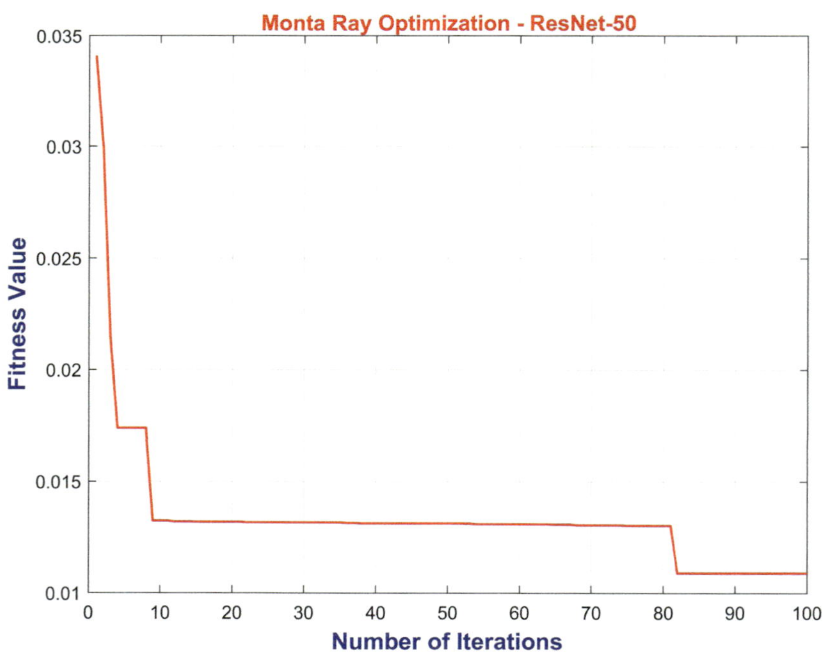


**FIGURE 10.9** The fitness value vs. number of iterations for manta ray optimization using ResNet-50 (top) and GoogleNet (bottom) models.

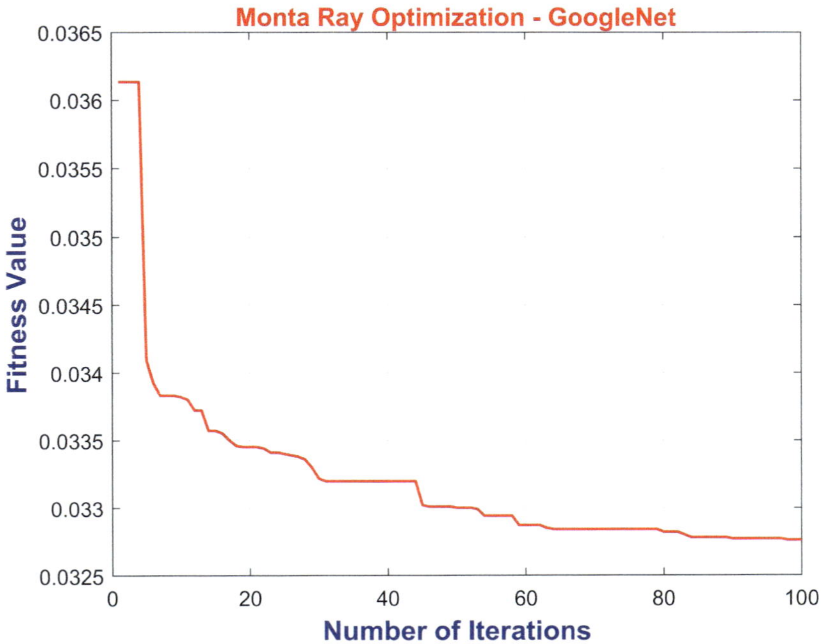


**FIGURE 10.9** *(Continued)*

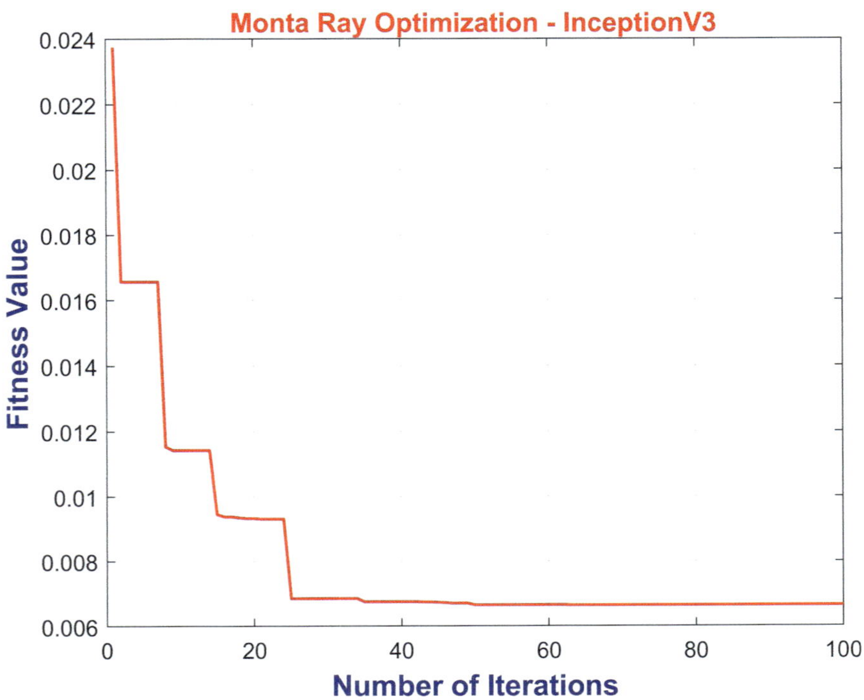


**FIGURE 10.10** The fitness value vs. the number of iterations for manta ray optimization using the Inception-V3 model.

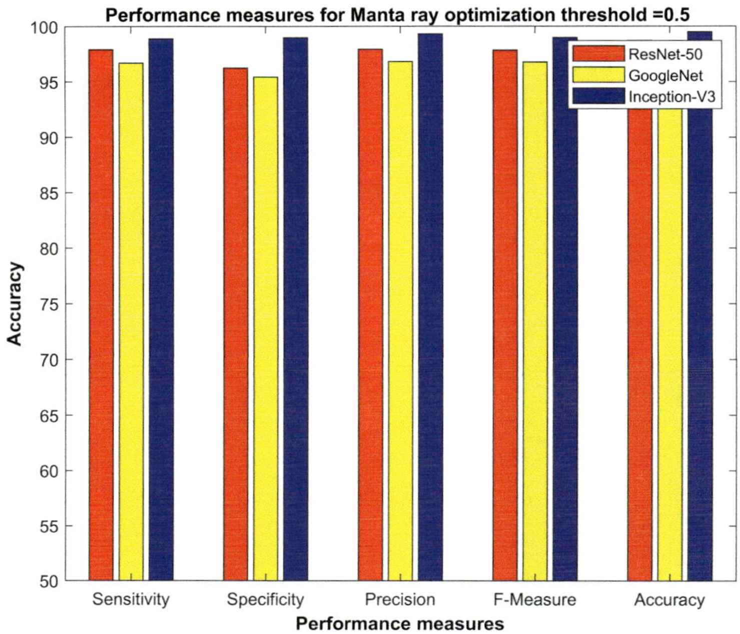


**FIGURE 10.11** Sensitivity, specificity, precision, F-measure, and average accuracy for ResNet-50, GoogleNet, and Inception-V3 deep learning models.

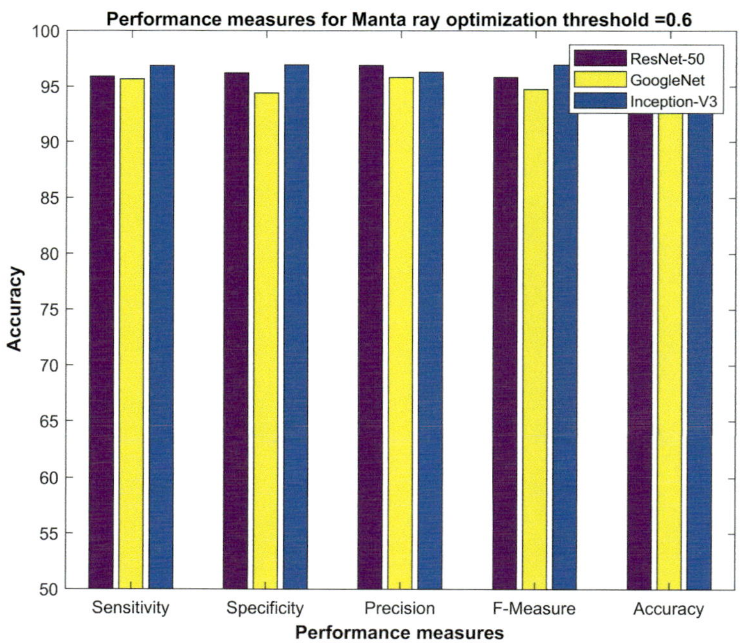


**FIGURE 10.12** Various performance measures for ResNet-50, GoogleNet, and Inception-V3 deep learning models.

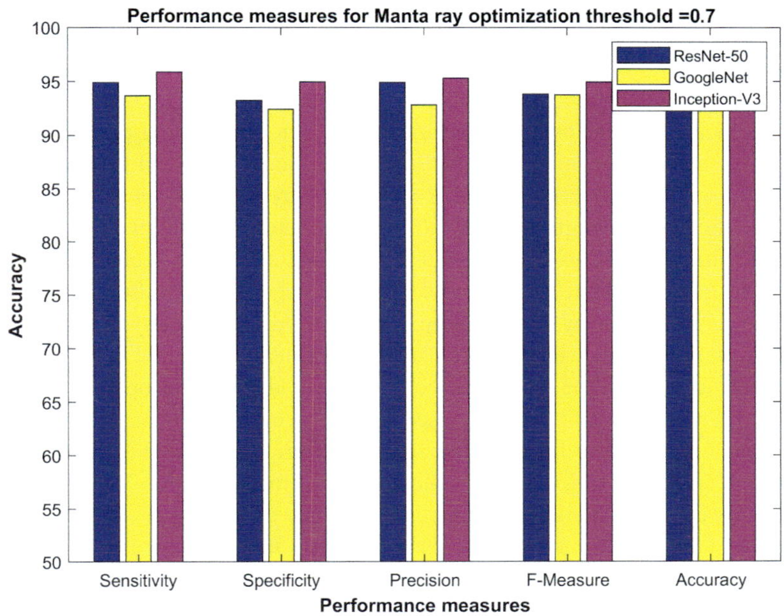


**FIGURE 10.13** Sensitivity, specificity, precision, F-measure, and average accuracy for ResNet-50, GoogleNet, and Inception-V3 deep learning models.

**TABLE 10.8**
**Comparison of the Proposed Heart Sound Detection Algorithm with Existing Techniques.**

| Algorithm | Technique/Features | Database | Classifier | Average Accuracy |
|---|---|---|---|---|
| (Li et al., 2019) | Energy entropy of the wavelet fractal coefficients | PhysioNet/CinC Challenge 2016 | TWSVM | 90.4 |
| (Singh et al., 2020) | 2-D scalogram images | PhysioNet/CinC 2016 Challenge | GoogleNet | 87.96 |
| (Krishnan et al., 2020) | CNN and Feedforward NN | PhysioNet/CinC 2016 Challenge | 1-D CNN | 85.66 |
| (Li et al., 2021) | STFT | PhysioNet/CinC 2016 Challenge | CNN | 87 |
| (Arslan et al., 2022) | VGG16, ResNet-50 and MobileNetV2 | PhysioNet/CinC Challenge 2016 | ML-ELM | 98.9 |
| (Li et al., 2022) | MFCC images | PhysioNet/CinC Challenge 2016 | ResNet-50 | 94.43 |
| Proposed | IIR-CQT spectrogram images | PhysioNet/CinC Challenge 2016 | ResNet-50 | 99.15 |
| Proposed | IIR-CQT spectrogram images | PhysioNet/CinC Challenge 2016 | Inception-V3 | 99.58 |

## 10.8 CONCLUSION

In this work, a time-frequency visual representation-based heart sound detection technique is proposed. Input heart sounds are first converted into IIR-CQT spectrogram images which represent detailed variations between normal and pathological subjects. Three transfer learning models, ResNet-50, GoogleNet, and Inception-V3, are utilized for feature extraction from IIR-CQT time-frequency visual representations. To reduce the feature-length and to minimize computational complexity, a manta ray foraging optimization-based feature subset selection algorithm is employed. Finally, the KNN classifier identifies the input PCG test signal as healthy or pathological data. The classification layer of the deep learning models efficiently extracts complex features, attaining improved detection accuracy (Khang et al., 2023).

The performance of the proposed deep features and manta ray optimization-based technique is assessed using precision, sensitivity, specificity, F1-measure, gmean and average accuracy on the heart sound samples from the PhysioNet challenge 2016 database. It is evident from the experimental results that Inception-V3 transfer learning features attained the highest detection accuracy of 99.58% as compared to resNet-50 and GoogleNet models. It is also observed that the feature subset generated by applying the manta ray foraging optimization algorithm improves the algorithm's performance while reducing the complexity (Khang et al., 2024).

## REFERENCES

Ahmad Z, Zeeshan M, Sohail A, Haris M, Khan MU, Hussain SS, Khan MS. Automatic Detection of paediatric congenital heart diseases from phonocardiogram signals. In *2023 3rd international conference on artificial intelligence (ICAI)*. 2023 Feb 22 (pp. 188–195). IEEE. https://ieeexplore.ieee.org/abstract/document/10136668/

Al-Issa Y, Alqudah AM. A lightweight hybrid deep learning system for cardiac valvular disease classification. *Scientific Reports*. 2022 Aug 22;12(1):14297. www.nature.com/articles/s41598-022-18293-7

Altuve M, Suárez L, Ardila J. Fundamental heart sounds analysis using improved complete ensemble EMD with adaptive noise. *Biocybernetics and Biomedical Engineering*. 2020 Jan 1;40(1):426–439.

Amin J, Sharif M, Mallah GA, Fernandes SL. An optimized features selection approach based on Manta Ray Foraging Optimization (MRFO) method for parasite malaria classification. *Frontiers in Public Health*. 2022 Sep 6;10:969268. www.frontiersin.org/articles/10.3389/fpubh.2022.969268/full

Arslan Ö. Automated detection of heart valve disorders with time-frequency and deep features on PCG signals. *Biomedical Signal Processing and Control*. 2022 Sep 1;78:103929. www.sciencedirect.com/science/article/pii/S1746809422004335

Bhardwaj A, Singh S, Joshi D. Explainable deep convolutional neural network for valvular heart diseases classification using PCG signals. In *IEEE transactions on instrumentation and measurement* 2023 May 8. IEEE. https://ieeexplore.ieee.org/abstract/document/10121470/

Birajdar GK, Raveendran S. Indian language identification using time-frequency texture features and kernel ELM. *Journal of Ambient Intelligence and Humanized Computing*. 2022 Mar 15:1–4. https://link.springer.com/article/10.1007/s12652-022-03781-5

Chen Y, Su B, Zeng W, Yuan C, Ji B. Abnormal heart sound detection from unsegmented phonocardiogram using deep features and shallow classifiers. *Multimedia Tools and Applications*. 2023 Jan 16:1–25. https://link.springer.com/article/10.1007/s11042-022-14315-8

Chien YR, Hsu KC, Tsao HW. Phonocardiography signals compression with deep convolutional autoencoder for telecare applications. *Applied Sciences*. 2020 Aug 24;10(17):5842. www.mdpi.com/2076-3417/10/17/5842

Crumbie, L. *Cardiac cycle*. 2023 July 29. www.kenhub.com/en/library/anatomy/cardiac-cycle

Demir F, Şengür A, Bajaj V, Polat K. Towards the classification of heart sounds based on convolutional deep neural network. *Health Information Science and Systems*. 2019 Dec;7:1–9. https://link.springer.com/article/10.1007/s13755-019-0078-0

Devi KM, Chanu MM, Singh NH, Singh KM. Classification of unsegmented phonocardiogram signal using scalogram and deep learning. *Soft Computing*. 2023 Jul 1:1–3. https://link.springer.com/article/10.1007/s00500-023-08834-1

Gaur NS, Patil MD, Birajdar GK. *Underwater image enhancement using generative adversarial network*. Generative Adversarial Networks and Deep Learning: Theory and Applications 2023 Apr 10. www.google.com/books?hl=en&lr=&id=P_GyEAAAQBAJ&oi=fnd&pg=PT246&dq=Underwater+Image+Enhancement+Using+Generative+Adversarial+Network.+Generative+Adversarial+Networks+and+Deep+Learning:+Theory+and+Applications&ots=r8heXrn98P&sig=dGU1yCyvoLm08d4elenz02NqwJ0

Giorgio A, Guaragnella C, Rizzi M. An effective CAD system for heart sound abnormality detection. *Circuits, Systems, and Signal Processing*. 2022 May;41(5):2845–2870. https://link.springer.com/article/10.1007/s00034-021-01916-1

Harimi A, Ameri MA, Sarkar S, Totaro MW. Heart sounds classification: Application of a new CyTex inspired method and deep convolutional neural network with transfer learning. *Smart Health*. 2023 Jun 24:100416. www.sciencedirect.com/science/article/pii/S2352648323000442

Hussain SS, Ashfaq M, Khan MS, Anwar S. Deep learning based phonocardiogram signals analysis for cardiovascular abnormalities detection. In *2023 international conference on robotics and automation in industry (ICRAI)* 2023 Mar 3 (pp. 1–6). IEEE. https://ieeexplore.ieee.org/abstract/document/10089537/

Ismail S, Ismail B. PCG signal classification using a hybrid multi round transfer learning classifier. *Biocybernetics and Biomedical Engineering*. 2023 Jan 1;43(1):313–334. www.sciencedirect.com/science/article/pii/S0208521623000049

Jamil S, Roy AM. An efficient and robust phonocardiography (PCG)-based valvular heart diseases (VHD) detection framework using vision transformer (VIT). *Computers in Biology and Medicine*. 2023 May 1;158:106734.

Kaushal B, Raveendran S, Patil MD, Birajdar GK. Spectrogram image textural descriptors for lung sound classification. In *Machine learning and deep learning in efficacy improvement of healthcare systems* 2022 May 18 (pp. 109–136). CRC Press. www.researchgate.net/profile/Gajanan-Birajdar/publication/359306672_Spectrogram_Image_Textural_Descriptors_for_Lung_Sound_Classification/links/626815411b747d19c2aa247e/Spectrogram-Image-Textural-Descriptors-for-Lung-Sound-Classification.pdf

Kaushal B, Raveendran S, Patil MD, Birajdar GK. Deep autoencoder neural networks for heart sound classification. In *Artificial intelligence in medical virology*. 2023 Apr 22 (pp. 165–189). Springer Nature. www.google.com/books?hl=en&lr=&id=vPe6EAAAQBAJ

Khang A. *AI and IoT-based technologies for precision medicine*. 2024. IGI Global Press. ISBN: 9798369308769. https://doi.org/10.4018/979-8-3693-0876-9

Khang A, Abdullayev VA, Hrybiuk O, Shukla AK. *Computer vision and AI-integrated IoT technologies in medical ecosystem*. 2024 (1st Ed.). CRC Press. https://doi.org/10.1201/9781003429609

Khang A, Rana G, Tailor RK, Hajimahmud VA. *Data-centric AI solutions and emerging technologies in the healthcare ecosystem*. 2023. CRC Press. https://doi.org/10.1201/9781003356189

Krishnan PT, Balasubramanian P, Umapathy S. Automated heart sound classification system from unsegmented phonocardiogram (PCG) using deep neural network. *Physical and Engineering Sciences in Medicine*. 2020 Jun;43:505–515. https://link.springer.com/article/10.1007/s13246-020-00851-w

Krittanawong C, Johnson KW, Rosenson RS, Wang Z, Aydar M, Baber U, Min JK, Tang WW, Halperin JL, Narayan SM. Deep learning for cardiovascular medicine: A practical primer. *European Heart Journal*. 2019 Jul 1;40(25):2058–2073. https://academic.oup.com/eurheartj/article-abstract/40/25/2058/5366208

Li F, Zhang Z, Wang L, Liu W. Heart sound classification based on improved mel-frequency spectral coefficients and deep residual learning. *Frontiers in Physiology*. 2022 Dec 22;13:1084420. www.frontiersin.org/articles/10.3389/fphys.2022.1084420/full

Li J, Ke L, Du Q. Classification of heart sounds based on the wavelet fractal and twin support vector machine. *Entropy*. 2019 May 6;21(5):472. www.mdpi.com/1099-4300/21/5/472

Li T, Yin Y, Ma K, Zhang S, Liu M. Lightweight end-to-end neural network model for automatic heart sound classification. *Information*. 2021 Jan 26;12(2):54. www.mdpi.com/2078-2489/12/2/54

Liu C, Springer D, Li Q, Moody B, Juan RA, Chorro FJ, Castells F, Roig JM, Silva I, Johnson AE, Syed Z. An open access database for the evaluation of heart sound algorithms. *Physiological Measurement*. 2016 Nov 21;37(12):2181. https://iopscience.iop.org/article/10.1088/0967-3334/37/12/2181/meta

Ma P, Ge B, Yang H, Guo T, Pan J, Wang W. Application of time-frequency domain and deep learning fusion feature in non-invasive diagnosis of congenital heart disease-related pulmonary arterial hypertension. *Methods*. 2023 Jan 1;10:102032. www.sciencedirect.com/science/article/pii/S2215016123000365

Maganti K, Rigolin VH, Sarano ME, Bonow RO. Valvular heart disease: Diagnosis and management. In *Mayo clinic proceedings*. 2010 May 1 (Vol. 85, No. 5, pp. 483–500). Elsevier. www.sciencedirect.com/science/article/pii/S0025619611603376

Maity A, Pathak A, Saha G. Transfer learning based heart valve disease classification from Phonocardiogram signal. *Biomedical Signal Processing and Control*. 2023 Aug 1;85:104805. www.sciencedirect.com/science/article/pii/S1746809423002380

Mistry YD, Birajdar GK, Khodke AM. Time-frequency visual representation and texture features for audio applications: A comprehensive review, recent trends, and challenges. *Multimedia Tools and Applications*. 2023 Mar 16:1–35. https://link.springer.com/article/10.1007/s11042-023-14734-1

Oh SL, Jahmunah V, Ooi CP, Tan RS, Ciaccio EJ, Yamakawa T, Tanabe M, Kobayashi M, Acharya UR. Classification of heart sound signals using a novel deep WaveNet model. *Computer Methods and Programs in Biomedicine*. 2020 Nov 1;196:105604. www.sciencedirect.com/science/article/pii/S0169260720314371

Prabhakar SK, Won DO. Phonocardiogram signal classification for the detection of heart valve diseases using robust conglomerated models. *Expert Systems with Applications*. 2023 Jul 1;221:119720. www.sciencedirect.com/science/article/pii/S095741742300221X

Rana G, Khang A, Sharma R, Goel AK, Dubey AK. *Reinventing manufacturing and business processes through artificial intelligence*. 2021. CRC Press. https://doi.org/10.1201/9781003145011

Rani S, Chauhan M, Kataria A, Khang A. IoT equipped intelligent distributed framework for smart healthcare systems. *Networking and Internet Architecture*. 2021;2:30. https://doi.org/10.48550/arXiv.2110.04997

Riccio D, Brancati N, Sannino G, Verde L, Frucci M. CNN-based classification of phonocardiograms using fractal techniques. *Biomedical Signal Processing and Control*. 2023 Sep 1;86:105186. www.sciencedirect.com/science/article/pii/S1746809423006195

Singh SA, Meitei TG, Majumder S. Short PCG classification based on deep learning. In *Deep learning techniques for biomedical and health informatics*. 2020 Jan 1 (pp. 141–164). Academic Press. www.sciencedirect.com/science/article/pii/B9780128190616000069

Vyas S, Patil MD, Birajdar GK. Classification of heart sound signals using time-frequency image texture features. *Computational Intelligence and Healthcare Informatics*. 2021 Oct 7:81–101. https://onlinelibrary.wiley.com/doi/abs/10.1002/9781119818717.ch5

WHO. *Cardiovascular diseases (CVDs).* Cited 2023 July 29. www.who.int/news-room/fact-sheets/detail/cardiovascular-diseases-(cvds)

Yadav KS, Singha J. Facial expression recognition using modified Viola-John's algorithm and KNN classifier. *Multimedia Tools and Applications.* 2020 May;79(19–20):13089–13107. https://link.springer.com/article/10.1007/s11042-019-08443-x

Zeng W, Su B, Yuan C, Chen Y. Automatic detection of heart valve disorders using Teager-Kaiser energy operator, rational-dilation wavelet transform and convolutional neural networks with PCG signals. *Artificial Intelligence Review.* 2023 Jan;56(1):781–806. https://link.springer.com/article/10.1007/s10462-022-10184-7

# 11 Internet of Things (IoT) Smart Wearable Sensors in Healthcare

*Nidhya M. S., Shaik Bajidvali, Nageswara Rao A. V., and Javeed Md. S.*

## 11.1 INTRODUCTION

Connecting intelligent items (things) to the Internet in an invisible manner is the foundation of the IoT (Internet of Things). This results in a safer and more seamless flow of information between all connected devices and their users. By 2020, when Cisco Frameworks predicts that 50 billion gadgets will be associated with the Web, numerous actual items, like PCs, sensor actuators, and others, can have exceptional addresses and safely move information, from regular exercises to limited clinical records. This multitude of actual articles that contain implanted advancements can be reconciled, rationally associated, and empowered to convey, sense, or communicate with the actual world, as well as among themselves as per the Internet of Things (IoT) (Tuan et al., 2015). The expression "Web of Things" (IoT) alludes to the interconnection of "anything" that might be "whenever, anyplace, utilizing any assistance, and on any organization" (Riazul et al., 2015). Some of the medical applications that make the healthcare industry one of the most appealing to IoT are remote checks of wellbeing, practice programs, ongoing sicknesses, and geriatric considerations.

As a result of studies conducted at MIT's Auto-ID Center in 1999 (Sarma & Brock, 2000), the phrase "Internet of Things" became widely used in the IT industry. "Internet" means "the overall organization of interconnected PC organizations," utilizing a normalized correspondence convention, and "Thing" signifies "an item not exactly recognizable" (SC et al., 2020). Together, these two thoughts structure the premise of the Web of Things (IoT). Because of these thoughts, any lifeless thing might have a Web Convention (IP) address and partake in a cutting-edge setting like a clinic.

IoT can moreover be thought of as "a self-planned strong overall association establishment with standards and interoperable correspondence shows where physical and virtual 'things' have characters, genuine qualities, and virtual characters, and are reliably integrated into the information structure" (Commission et al., 2016). As a matter of fact, IoT alludes to the worldwide organization that is made when savvy objects are connected together utilizing broadened Web innovations, as well as the


DOI: 10.1201/9781032686745-11

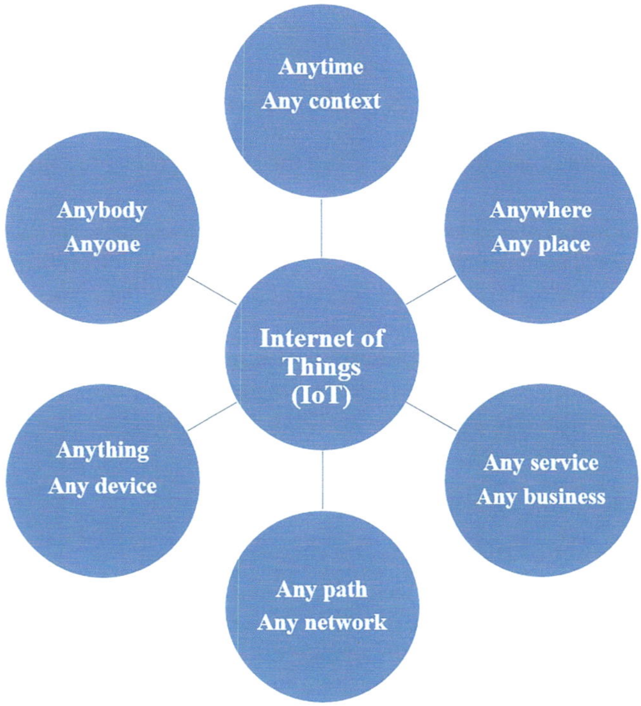


**FIGURE 11.1** Dimensions of the Internet of Things.

set-up of uses and administrations that make the most of these advancements to make new business and market open doors, as shown in Figure 11.1.

## 11.2 HEALTHCARE

A few social issues have become progressively evident in the medical services field (Khang, Abdullayev & Hrybiuk et al., 2024), issues that the IoT might have the option to forestall or battle in the best manner, given that are generally connected with populace development, rustic urbanization, declining birthrate, populace maturing, monetary development, and socially uneven asset usage:

- A lack of disaster preparedness and health management expertise.
- A severe dearth of trained medical professionals and institutional facilities, particularly in rural regions; including
  - A paucity of medical resources;
  - A subpar standard of service;
  - An insufficient healthcare infrastructure.

- An imperfect disease prevention system places an undue cost on the economy, people, families, and the State by failing to satisfy the needs of a national policy to protect citizen health.
- Poor capacity for early illness identification and prevention.

However, there are problems that can be addressed with the aid of IoT:

- Medical image and video data consultation and transmission links.
- The removal of geographical obstacles, allowing for quick clinical reactions.
- IoT-based healthcare with a unified taxonomy for all data types.

Numerous potential uses may be found in the medical industry, one of which is the use of smartphones as a stage for observing clinical pointers that could caution patients about potential health problems (Khang et al., 2022).

## 11.2.1 Healthcare Technologies

### 11.2.1.1 Internet of Things

Internet of Things (IoT)-enabled technologies and devices have several applications in healthcare. A larger role for IoT in healthcare would be beneficial for both patients and professionals. Medical apps for mobile devices and wearable technology that collect health information from patients are two examples of how healthcare IoT is being put to use (Anh et al., 2024). The Internet of Things is used in crisis facilities to follow the whereabouts of patients, clinical gear, and staff. The advancements that can be utilized in IoT-based medical care frameworks are recorded in what follows. Hosted services for further information on how cloud computing may improve healthcare via the Internet of Things (IoT), as well as the most effective method to convey administrations on request through an organization and run tasks to satisfy different requests (Council et al., 2012).

### 11.2.1.2 Grid Computing

Noninvasive detecting and low-power remote correspondence innovations have permitted persistent checking and handling of portable patients using biomedical sensor hubs, permitting the idea of Lattice Registering to be applied to IoT. Regardless of their minuscule size and restricted memory, energy, handling, and correspondence capacities, wearable clinical gadgets can consistently screen imperative markers, including circulatory strain, temperature, Electrocardiogram (ECG), Electromyogram (EMG), and oxygen saturation. (If you want to learn more about grid computing and the Internet of Things, see Hariharasudhan et al., 2012).

### 11.2.1.3 Big Data

The completeness and timeliness of health diagnosis and monitoring may be enhanced by analyzing all available data collected by medical sensors in the healthcare setting and developing appropriate tools (Riazul et al., 2015).

#### 11.2.1.4 Short-Range Networks

Wireless personal area networks (WPANs), wide-area networks (WLANs), wireless local area networks (6LoWPANs), wireless sensor networks (WSNs), and long-range networks, such as cellular networks, must be designed to support the physical architecture of IoT-based healthcare. Communications protocols and technologies, including ultra-wideband (UWB), Bluetooth Low Energy (BLE), Near Field Communication (NFC), and Radio Frequency Identification (RFID), may be used in low-power medical sensor devices. (Riazul et al., 2015). Ambient intelligence due to the human nature of the healthcare network's end users, clients, and consumers (patients or health-conscious persons), ambient intelligence plays an essential role in IoT-based healthcare. Human-Computer Interaction (HCI) is one of these areas. (Riazul et al., 2015).

#### 11.2.1.5 Augmented Reality

The healthcare sector has been revolutionized by augmented reality. This method has many possible restorative purposes. In later years, expanded reality will impact the clinical business, from assisting surgeons to enhancing medical education. In addition to potentially preventing patient deaths, augmented reality has the potential to improve the efficiency and accuracy of many healthcare operations. We will investigate the many ways this remarkable technology is already being put to use in the medical field (Medicalaugmentedreality.com, 2014).

#### 11.2.1.6 Wearables

Wearable medical technologies may serve as markers for patient participation and public health improvement, as stated in (Riazul et al., 2015). The three main advantages of this are linked data, healthcare networks focused on specific populations, and gamification.

### 11.2.2 Healthcare Services

The individual medical services concerns and resident contribution to medical care are areas where Ambient Assisted Living systems may shine. For medical care observing, which is a way IoT may provide help, the AAL frameworks give a biological system of clinical sensors, PCs, remote organizations, and programming applications. It is fundamental to have a devoted IoT administration (Rani et al., 2021).

#### 11.2.2.1 m-Health Things (m-IoT)

Mobile Internet of Things (m-IoT) is characterized as one more thought that matches the functionalities of m-prosperity and IoT for new and inventive future (4G prosperity) applications (Istepanian et al., 2011). As indicated by (Istepanian et al., 2004), m-IoT incorporates the utilization of cell phones, clinical sensors, and communications technology to improve access to healthcare. It is hypothesized that "m-IoT" acclimates a progressive medical services organizing worldview that interfaces the 6LoWPAN with developing 4G organizations for future web based m-wellbeing applications. It is critical to take note of that albeit m-IoT frequently represents the

IoT for medical care administrations, there are specific components intrinsic to the worldwide versatility of partaking organizations that set it apart (Istepanian et al., 2004; Riazul et al., 2015).

#### 11.2.2.2 Adverse Drug Reaction

Adverse drug reactions may occur after a single dosage of a medicine, after repeated dosing, as a result of a drug interaction, or as a side effect of taking many medications (Jara et al., 2010). As an example of a service that may be given by the Internet of Things, consider a network that spans the area surrounding a city, a public hospital, a neighborhood, or a rural region. Energy efficiency and cooperativeness of an Internet of Things platform for healthcare monitoring in rural areas have been shown (Rohokale et al., 2011).

#### 11.2.2.3 Wearable Device Access

With the rise of wireless sensor networks (WSNs), a number of noninvasive sensors have been created for use in healthcare (Chung et al., 2008). In the future, these sensors might use the Internet of Things to provide the same functions. However, wearables may have a number of advantages that are well suited to the Internet of Things framework.

#### 11.2.2.4 Semantic Medical Access

There has been much thought given to the possibility of using semantics and ontologies to facilitate the widespread dissemination of medical knowledge and data (Burgun et al., 1999). IoT healthcare application developers have paid special attention to the promising future of medical ontologies and semantics.

#### 11.2.2.5 Indirect Emergency Healthcare

Inclement weather, transportation (aircraft, ships, trains, and vehicles), and earthen site collapse are all examples of indirect emergencies that may impact healthcare. That is why there is a thing called indirect emergency health care (IEH): it will provide a whole bunch of answers, including how to get hold of resources like databases (Riazul et al., 2015; EPoSS et al., 2010).

#### 11.2.2.6 Embedded Gateway Configuration

Embedded gateway configuration (EGC) administration is a designed door administration that connects network hubs, where patients are associated, to the Web and all the clinical hardware. This kind of gateway service needs certain common integration characteristics, which vary based on the intended use of the installed gateway (Riazul et al., 2015).

#### 11.2.2.7 Embedded Context Prediction

Appropriate mechanisms (ECP) service (Riazul et al., 2015) is one solution to the problem of the structures that each outsider designer might need to develop with suitable instruments. In the field of omnipresent health care, EPoSS (EC: European Communities, 2010) developed such a paradigm.

#### 11.2.2.8 Early Intervention/Prevention

Human activity and health monitoring, including reporting on normal daily activities to a medical facility or loved ones. Internet of Things (IoT) gadgets might give a means of keeping tabs on all those goings-on (Khang et al., 2023).

### 11.2.3 Healthcare Applications

#### 11.2.3.1 Electrocardiogram Monitoring Arrhythmias

Myocardial ischemia and extended QT intervals are only a few examples of the cardiovascular issues that contribute to the estimated 30% of all fatalities reported (Zhang et al., 2013). The electrocardiogram (ECG) measures the electrical action of the heart and gives data about pulses and cadence, as well as other information that can be used to diagnose conditions like arrhythmias, myocardial ischemia, and delayed QT stretches. IoT-based applications for ECG checking may provide the most data and send it to medical professionals (Dash et al., 2002).

#### 11.2.3.2 Electromyography

Electromyography (EMG) is a noninvasive technique used to monitor electrical potentials in muscles; this information has applications in areas as varied as disease and injury diagnosis, functional electrical stimulation, and prosthetic limb control. In Kneisz et al. (2015) and Zhang et al. (2013), we see examples of wireless electromyography (EMG) sensors. In Zhang et al. (2013), a sensor for monitoring EMG and ECG is given; it has four straightforward channels, a chip that uses 19 W (while looking at from one channel), and information transmission at 200 kbps while using 160 W. The device's adaptability stems from its ability to be powered by either radio frequency (RF) power transmission or thermoelectric energy collection.

#### 11.2.3.3 Blood Pressure Monitoring

Preventing issues in the cardiovascular system requires regular blood pressure checks; hence, IoT-based apps may remotely regulate correspondence between a wellbeing post and a wellbeing community (Riazul et al., 2015). Globally, high blood pressure is the leading cause of death and disability. It raises the probability of developing heart disease, cardiovascular issues, stroke, and aneurysms. Since heart rate is such an essential vital sign, keeping an eye on it in real-time might help doctors determine what is wrong. In Aldaoud et al. (2015), the idea of implantable wireless blood pressure sensors is discussed. A sensor capable of measuring blood pressure for the purpose of regulating vascular graft deterioration is provided in Murphy et al. (2013). It is generally agreed that the blood pressure sensor for vascular grafts described in Murphy et al. (2013) represents the current state of the art. The 2.67 mm2 chip of this sensor is held in place by two coils within a vascular graft. The gadget has a sensitivity of 0.176 mmHg and consumes just 21.6 W when digitally digitizing and back-scatting pressure.

#### 11.2.3.4 Body Temperature Monitoring

The human body uses homeostasis to keep systems, such as body temperature, in check or to bring them back to normal functioning after a disturbance. As a critical vital indicator, body temperature must be closely monitored as part of any medical therapy. Embedded in a TelosB device is a temperature sensor that may be used to retrieve temperature fluctuations from the body and report them to a home door-based temperature checking framework through the Internet of Things (Riazul et al., 2015).

#### 11.2.3.5 Oxygen Saturation Monitoring

Beat oximetry is a non-meddlesome and constant checking strategy used to evaluate blood vessel blood oxygen immersion levels. Oxygen saturation monitoring may be facilitated by incorporating a pulse oximeter into an Internet of Things-based application.

#### 11.2.3.6 Medication Management

Medication provides a significant financial and logistical challenge in public health. With the Internet of Things, we now have a whole new method to fix this problem (Riazul et al., 2015).

#### 11.2.3.7 Wheelchair Management

Like the quickening speed of work, the Internet of Things is responding with smart wheelchairs that provide complete automation for handicapped persons. To achieve the goal of prevention and early detection of various lifestyle disorders, the Remote Monitoring and Management Platform of Healthcare Information (RMMP-HI) (Zha et al., 2011) is a framework that can be used in the real world to offer monitoring and management of these conditions. IoT-based networks enable body medical sensors to register, remove, and update data, which they then collect and transmit to an information-sharing focus, which thus spreads the information to clinical staff or emergency clinic offices as indicated by rules, for example, an earnest notification generated from the data (Vrushank et al., 2023).

#### 11.2.3.8 Implantable Devices for Glucose

Glucose oxidase, an enzyme, coats the filament and catalyzes the production of hydrogen peroxide from glucose. Hydrogen peroxide interacts with platinum to release electrons and split into hydrogen and oxygen, producing electricity. This electrical signal is sent wirelessly to a portable reader or smartphone, where an algorithm interprets it as a blood glucose level, as shown in Figure 11.2.

Glucose oxidase, an enzyme that breaks down glucose into hydrogen peroxide, coats the filament. Hydrogen peroxide breaks down into hydrogen, oxygen, and electrons when it combines with platinum. A portable scanner or smartphone receives this signal wirelessly and runs it via an algorithm to get a glucose measurement. After 7–14 days, the accuracy of the reading begins to degrade due to the body's reaction to the filament penetration point and the degradation of the sensor chemistry. Future sensors may be more compact, have a longer battery life, and detect more than just glucose.

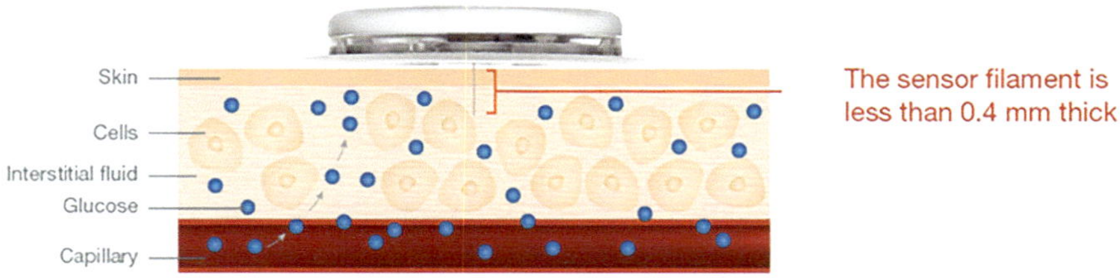


**FIGURE 11.2** Implantable glucose devices.

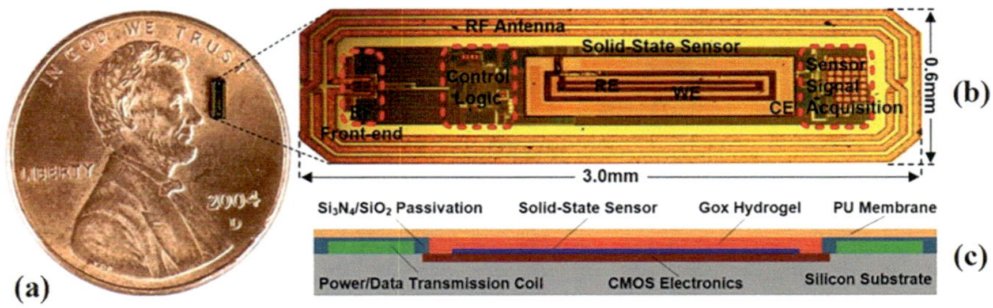


**FIGURE 11.3** (a, b, c) A unique microchip measuring glucose using the same surface chemistry as conventional CGMs.

Experimental sensors the size of a sesame seed were produced in 2019 and implanted just under the skin with the help of a special, user-friendly injector. A unique microchip measuring glucose using the same surface chemistry as conventional CGMs and transmitting the data wirelessly to a wearable receiver like a wristwatch, is the core innovation. When the sensor's useful life is over, the user may remove it by pulling on a thread, as shown in Figure 11.3.

There are a few benefits to reducing the size of the sensor. To begin with, it lessens pain and tissue damage. Suppressing the immune system's foreign-body reaction improves speed, precision, and consistency. Thinner capsules take longer to respond because glucose diffuses through them more quickly.

Furthermore, the absence of wire improves precision and sensitivity by decreasing background noise. Researchers used pigs as a model for human physiology to test their technology. They injected it just below the pigs' abdomen skin and took blood samples via an IV line every 5–10 minutes to test with a home glucose monitor and every 15–20 minutes to test with laboratory equipment. After being implanted, the sensor began gathering data within 10 minutes and continued to do so for weeks. After fast swings in blood glucose levels, the researchers still discovered that its glucose values were consistent with the other devices. This product, not yet on the market, demonstrates miniaturization potential.

### 11.2.3.9 Wearable Enzymatic Fuel Cells

Research into EFCs has shifted away from implantable applications and toward wearable ones due to the difficulties involved with using them. As a result, scientists are looking into other physiological fluids than blood to use in EFCs as shown in Figure 11.4.

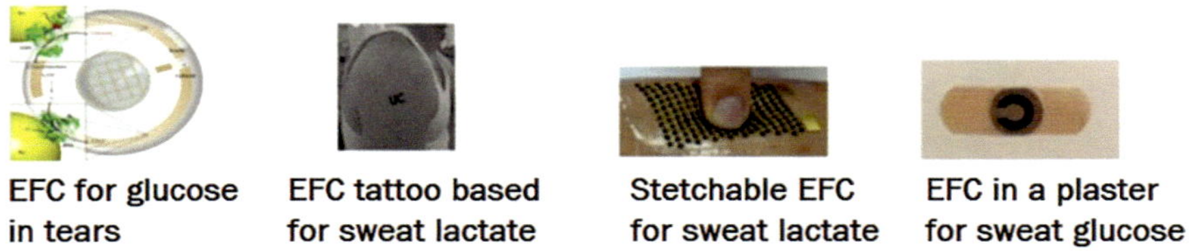


**FIGURE 11.4** The current state of wearable EFCs (Mohammadifar et al., 2017; Falk et al., 2012; Bandodkar et al., 2017).

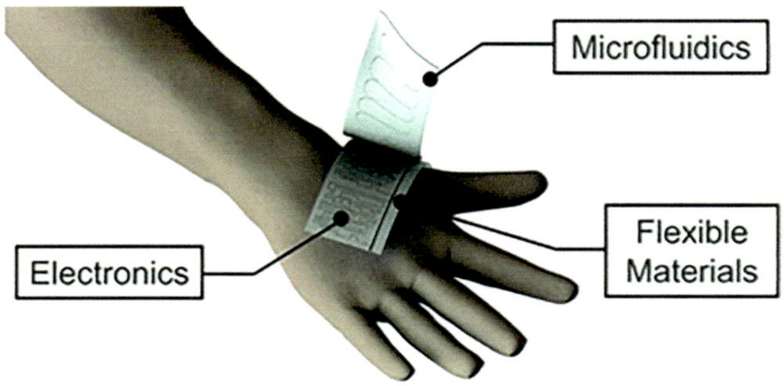


**FIGURE 11.5** Sweat analysis.

#### 11.2.3.10 Gait Analysis

High manufacturing costs, operating energy consumption, or inadequate analysis approaches that hardly include machine learning or apply suboptimal models necessitating enormous datasets for training are the primary limitations of current wearable electronics of gait analysis (Zhang et al., 2020). Cost-effective triboelectric intelligent socks were created to wirelessly transmit sensory data gathered from the wearer's feet. Self-sufficient socks with built-in functionality may also serve as wearable sensors, providing users with data on their identities, physical activities, and health conditions (Vrushank et al., 2023).

As a further response to the problem of inefficient analysis methods, we propose a profound learning model with a beginning-to-end structure on the socks signals for the stride examination, which yields an ID exactness of 93.54% across 13 members and a recognition precision of 96.67% across five particular human exercises. In light of a legitimate concern for commonsense application, we utilize a virtual planning of the actual signs accumulated through the socks to make a computerized human framework for use in sports checking, medical care, ID, and expected future shrewd home applications (Eswaran & Khang, 2024).

#### 11.2.3.11 Microfluid Wearable

The created flexible microfluidic wearable technologies have allowed for a variety of bio-sensing applications, such as in situ sweat metabolites measurement, vital signs monitoring, and gait analysis, by capitalizing on such microfabrication and liquid manipulation capabilities, as shown in Figure 11.5.

## 11.3 CONCLUSION

Sensors in IoT have a wide range of uses in monitoring and predicting the prescribed threshold and are intimated to the base station or sink node. It is highly risk for an individual to visit a hospital for small issues. There are a number of IoT technologies applied in the medical field as wearable devices to monitor patients. In this chapter, we analyzed a number of wearable devices, such as biocompatible flexible sensors and biodegradable flexible sensors, to monitor elderly people, patients, and athletes (Khang, Abdullayev & Hahanov et al., 2024).

IoT devices applied in healthcare, technologies used to predict the health of a patient, and normal persons using IoT were evaluated. Healthcare services like monitoring glucose, sweat for athletes, EMG, pressure, and wheelchair management were analyzed. IoT is one technology that will efficiently help normal people and mingle with the medical field to save human life in various ways (Rath et al., 2024).

## REFERENCES

Aldaoud A., Laurenson C., Rivet F., Yuce M.R., Redouté J. Design of an inductively powered implantable wireless blood pressure sensing interface using capacitive coupling. *IEEE/ASME Transactions on Mechatronics*. 2015;20(1):487–491. https://ieeexplore.ieee.org/abstract/document/6822620/

Anh P.T.N., Hahanov V., Triwiyanto, Ragimova N. A., Rashad İ., Abdullayev V.A., Abuzarova, V.A. AI models for disease diagnosis and prediction of heart disease with artificial neural networks. In *Computer vision and AI-integrated IoT technologies in medical ecosystem* (1st Ed.). 2024. CRC Press. https://doi.org/10.1201/9781003429609-9

Bandodkar A.J., You J.-M., Kim N.-H., Gu Y., Kumar R., Mohan A.M.V., Kurniawan J., Imani S., Nakagawa T., Parish B. et al. Soft, stretchable, high power density electronic skin-based biofuel cells for scavenging energy from human sweat. *Energy & Environmental Science*. 2017;10:1581–1589. https://pubs.rsc.org/en/content/articlehtml/2017/ee/c7ee00865a

Burgun A., Botti G.M.F., Beux P.L. Sharing knowledge in medicine: Semantic and ontologic facets of medical concepts. In *Proceedings of IEEE international conference systems, man, and cybernetics (SMC)* (pp. 300–305). 1999. IEEE.

Chung W.-Y., Lee Y.D., Jung, S.J. A cooperative Internet of Things (IoT) for rural healthcare monitoring and control. In *A wireless sensor network compatible wearable u-healthcare monitoring system using integrated ECG, accelerometer and SpO2* (pp. 1529–1532). 2008. https://ieeexplore.ieee.org/abstract/document/5940920/

Commission: Internet of things strategic research roadmap. 2009. www.internet-ofthingsresearch.eu/pdf/IoT_Cluster_Strategic_Research_ Agenda_2009.pdf [Online; accessed 18 Jan 2016]

Council, C.S.C. *Impact of cloud computing on healthcare*. 2012. www.academia.edu/download/54646512/IRJET-V3I5590.pdf

Dash P.K. Electrocardiogram monitoring. *Indian Journal of Anaesthesia*. 2002; 46:251–260. https://journals.lww.com/ijaweb/Abstract/2002/46040/ELECTROCARDIOGRAM_MONITORING.2.aspx

EC: European Communities. *Internet of things in 2020*. 2010. www.umic.pt/images/stories/publicacoes2/Internet-of-Things_in_2020_EC-EPoSS_Workshop_Report_2008_v3.pdf [Online; accessed 18 Jan 2016]

Eswaran U., Khang A. AI-aided computer vision in health care system. In *Computer vision and AI-integrated IoT technologies in medical ecosystem* (1st Ed.). 2024. CRC Press. https://doi.org/10.1201/9781003429609-8

Falk M., Andoralov V., Blum Z., Sotres J., Suyatin D.B., Ruzgas T., Arnebrant T., Shleev S. Biofuel cell as a power source for electronic contact lenses. *Biosensors and Bioelectronics*. 2012; 37:38–45. www.sciencedirect.com/science/article/pii/S0956566312002461

Hariharasudhan Viswanathan E.K.L., Pompili D. Mobile grid computing for data and patient-centric ubiquitous healthcare. In *The first IEEE workshop on enabling technologies for smartphone and internet of things (ETSIoT)*. 2012. https://ieeexplore.ieee.org/abstract/document/6311263/

Istepanian R.S., Hu S., Philip N.Y., Sungoor A. *The potential of internet of m-health things "m-IoT" for non-invasive glucose level sensing*. Conference of the IEEE Engineering in Medicine and Biology Society. 2011. https://ieeexplore.ieee.org/abstract/document/6091302/

Istepanian R.S.H., Zhang Y.T. Guest editorial introduction to the special section on m-health: Beyond seamless mobility and global wireless health-care connectivity. In *IEEE transactions on information technology in biomedicine* (pp. 405–414). 2004. https://ieeexplore.ieee.org/abstract/document/1362649/

Jara A.J., Belchi F.J., Gomez-Skarmeta A.F. A pharmaceutical intelligent information system to detect allergies and adverse drugs reactions based on internet of things. In *Proceedings IEEE international conference pervasive computer communication workshops (PERCOM Workshops)* (pp. 809–812). 2010. https://ieeexplore.ieee.org/abstract/document/5470547/

Khang A. Material4Studies. In *Material of computer science, artificial intelligence, data science, IoT, blockchain, cloud, metaverse, cybersecurity for studies*. 2021. www.researchgate.net/publication/370156102_Material4Studies

Khang A., Abdullayev V.A., Hahanov V., Vrushank S. *Advanced IoT technologies and applications in the industry 4.0 digital economy* (1st Ed.). 2024. CRC Press. https://doi.org/10.1201/9781003434269

Khang A., Abdullayev V.A., Hrybiuk O, Shukla AK. *Computer vision and AI-integrated IoT technologies in medical ecosystem* (1st Ed.). 2024. CRC Press. https://doi.org/10.1201/9781003429609

Khang A., Ragimova N.A., Hajimahmud V.A., Alyar V.A. Advanced technologies and data management in the smart healthcare system. In *AI-centric smart city ecosystems: Technologies, design and implementation* (1st Ed., vol. 16, p. 10). 2022. CRC Press. https://doi.org/10.1201/9781003252542-16

Khang A., Rana G., Tailor R.K., Hajimahmud V.A. *Data-centric AI solutions and emerging technologies in the healthcare ecosystem*. 2023. CRC Press. https://doi.org/10.1201/9781003356189

Kneisz L., Unger E., Lanmuller H., Mayr W. In vitro testing of an implantable wireless telemetry system for long-term electromyography recordings in large animals. *Artificial Organs*. 2015;39(10):897–902. https://onlinelibrary.wiley.com/doi/abs/10.1111/aor.12626

Kumar S., Padmashree S., Jayalekshmi R. Correlation of salivary glucose, blood glucose and oral candidal carriage in the saliva of type 2 diabetics: A case-control study. *Contemporary Clinical Dentistry*. 2014; 5:312–317. www.ncbi.nlm.nih.gov/pmc/articles/PMC4147805/

Medicalaugmentedreality.com, I.S. *How augmented reality can bridge the gap in healthcare?* 2014. www.augmentedrealitytrends.com/augmented-reality/healthcare-industry.html [Online; accessed 18 Jan 2016]

Mohammadifar M., Cho E., Choi S. *A self-powered sensor patch for glucose monitoring in sweat*. Proceedings of the 2017 IEEE 30th International Conference on Micro Electro Mechanical Systems (MEMS), Las Vegas, NV, USA (pp. 366–369). 22–26 Jan 2017. https://ieeexplore.ieee.org/abstract/document/7863417/

Murphy OH, Bahmanyar MR, Borghi A, McLeod CN, Navaratnarajah M, Yacoub MH, et al. Continuous in vivo blood pressure measurements using a fully implantable wireless SAW sensor. *Biomedical Microdevices*. 2013;15(5):737–749. https://link.springer.com/article/10.1007/s10544-013-9759-7

Rani S., Chauhan M., Kataria A, Khang A. IoT equipped intelligent distributed framework for smart healthcare systems. *Networking and Internet Architecture*. 2021; 2:30. https://doi.org/10.48550/arXiv.2110.04997

Rath K.C., Khang A., Roy D. The role of internet of things (IoT) technology in industry 4.0. In *Advanced IoT technologies and applications in the industry 4.0 digital economy* (1st Ed.). 2024. CRC Press. https://doi.org/10.1201/9781003434269-1

Riazul Islam S.M., Kwak D, Kwak K.S. The internet of things for health care: A comprehensive survey. In *IEEE access*. 2015. https://ieeexplore.ieee.org/abstract/document/7113786/

Rohokale V.M., Prasad N.R.P., Prasad R. *A cooperative internet of things (IoT) for rural healthcare monitoring and control*. 1st International Conference on Wireless Communication, Vehicular Technology, Information Theory and Aerospace & Electronic Systems Technology (Wireless VITAE) (pp. 1–6). 2011. https://ieeexplore.ieee.org/abstract/document/5940920/

Sarma S., Brock, K.A. *The networked physical world*. 2000. http://cocoa.ethz.ch/downloads/2014/06/None_MIT-AUTOID-WH-001.pdf

Tuan N.G., Rahmani A.M., Tenhunen H. Fault tolerant and scalable IoT based architecture for health monitoring. In *IEEE access*. 2015. https://ieeexplore.ieee.org/abstract/document/7133626/

Vrushank S., Khang A., Internet of medical things (IoMT) driving the digital transformation of the healthcare sector. In *Data-centric AI solutions and emerging technologies in the healthcare ecosystem* (1st Ed., p. 1). 2023. CRC Press. https://doi.org/10.1201/9781003356189-2

Vrushank S., Vidhi T., Khang A. Electronic health records security and privacy enhancement using blockchain technology. In *Data-centric AI solutions and emerging technologies in the healthcare ecosystem* (1st Ed., p. 1). 2023. CRC Press. https://doi.org/10.1201/9781003356189-1

Zha W.O., Wang C.W., Nakahira Y. Medical application on IoT. In *International conference on computer theory and applications (ICCTA)* (pp. 660–665). 2011. www.google.com/books?hl=en&lr=&id=HrCI4ZyuZL0C&oi=fnd&pg=PA1&dq=.+In:+International+Conference+on+Computer+Theory+and+Applications+&ots=i_HnLRhYrL&sig=mjOY3yzjnlFGv8iF999NDgoHUfI

Zhang J., Hodge W., Hutnick C., Wang X. Noninvasive diagnostic devices for diabetes through measuring tear glucose. *Journal of Diabetes Science and Technology*. 2011; 5:166–172. https://journals.sagepub.com/doi/abs/10.1177/193229681100500123

Zhang Y. et al. A batteryless 19 μW MICS/ISM-band energy harvesting body sensor node SoC for ExG applications. *IEEE Journal of Solid-State Circuits*. 2013;48(1):199–213. https://ieeexplore.ieee.org/abstract/document/6399579/

Zhang Z, He T, Zhu M. et al. Deep learning-enabled triboelectric smart socks for IoT-based gait analysis and VR applications. *NPJ Flexible Electronics*. 2020;4:29. www.nature.com/articles/s41528-020-00092-7

# 12 Preventing Sepsis in ICU by Analyzing Patients with Big Data Using Tableau Application

*Seenu Raj, Baishali Patra, Shahistha Jabeen Hashim, Supratim Dasgupta, and Dinesh Kumar*

## 12.1 PROBLEM STATEMENT

With one in three hospitalizations resulting in death attributed to sepsis, this study aims to analyze biomarkers and other factors associated with sepsis in hospital settings. By examining patients who develop sepsis during their ICU stay and utilizing a large dataset, the study aims to gain crucial insights that can support healthcare providers in improving patient outcomes and enhancing overall healthcare delivery (Rani et al., 2021).

## 12.2 INTRODUCTION

Sepsis is a condition where the immune system responds abnormally to an infection, posing a serious threat to life. It is a leading cause of death in the United States and has been identified as the most expensive medical condition to treat. Every year, an estimated 1.7 million adults are affected by sepsis in the United States, and nearly one in three hospitalizations resulting in death is linked to sepsis (Matot and Sprung, 2001). Given its significant impact on the US healthcare system, examining the onset of sepsis in the hospital is crucial. The following are the parameters examined in the study population.

### 12.2.1 GLUCOSE

Metabolic derangement is a prominent feature during sepsis, involving various pathophysiological changes. Among these metabolic alterations, hyperglycemia stands out as a significant factor. Elevated blood glucose levels, characteristic of hyperglycemia, play a crucial role in these conditions. They can adversely affect the immune response, impair organ function, and contribute to poor outcomes. Recognizing the significance of hyperglycemia in sepsis highlights the need for targeted interventions to manage glucose levels and mitigate its detrimental effects (Hirasawa et al., 2009).


DOI: 10.1201/9781032686745-12

### 12.2.2 White Blood Cells (WBC)

WBC count is widely utilized to assess infection. In the case of sepsis, WBC levels can manifest as either leukocytosis (elevated count) or leukopenia (reduced count). However, a significant number of septic patients fall within the range of normal WBC without exhibiting extreme values (Farkas, 2020).

### 12.2.3 Partial Thromboplastin Time (PTT)

In patients with sepsis, the activation of the coagulation system and subsequent consumption of clotting factors often lead to prolonged PTT (Gando et al., 2016).

### 12.2.4 Hemoglobin

Low hemoglobin levels are common in sepsis and can be caused by reduced red blood cell (RBC) production due to systemic inflammation and increased RBC destruction from hemolysis and bleeding. Low hemoglobin levels can further impair tissue oxygenation by decreasing arterial oxygen concentration (Jung et al., 2019).

### 12.2.5 Liver-Related Parameters

The liver, the largest gland in the human body, is essential for maintaining metabolic and immunological balance. It performs over 200 functions, including detoxification, storage, energy production, nutrient processing, hormone regulation, and blood clotting. Due to its crucial role, the liver's proper functioning is vital for the survival of individuals experiencing severe conditions like sepsis. Studies have demonstrated that liver dysfunction and failure, especially in the context of sepsis, significantly contribute to disease progression and mortality, underscoring the liver's critical importance in overall patient outcomes (Yan et al., 2014). The liver parameters analyzed included bilirubin direct, bilirubin total, lactate, phosphate, and alkaline phosphatase.

### 12.2.6 Renal-Related Parameters

Sepsis is a significant risk factor for Acute Kidney Injury (AKI), accounting for 26% to 50% of AKI cases. Sepsis-associated AKI tends to be more severe and carries a higher mortality risk than non-septic AKI. While AKI complicates the short-term management of sepsis patients, it also increases the likelihood of long-term complications, including the development of chronic kidney disease (CKD), kidney failure requiring replacement therapy (KFRT), and increased short- and long-term mortality (Flannery et al., 2021). The kidney parameters analyzed included blood urea nitrogen, creatinine, chloride, and potassium.

### 12.2.7 Cardiovascular System-Related Parameters

Persistent systemic inflammation resulting from infections, including sepsis, is strongly linked to cardiovascular disease. The inflammatory response triggered by the infection can lead to endothelial dysfunction, increased oxidative stress, and dysregulation of the immune system, all of which contribute to the development and progression of cardiovascular disorders. Additionally, the inflammatory mediators released during sepsis can directly damage the heart muscle, leading to myocardial dysfunction and heart failure (Mankowski et al., 2019). The heart-related parameters analyzed were blood pressure, mean arterial pressure, heart rate, body temperature, and troponin.

### 12.2.8 Acute Respiratory Distress Syndrome

ARDS is a devastating complication of severe sepsis. Sepsis and ARDS have similar underlying mechanisms characterized by inflammation and endothelial dysfunction (Stapleton et al., 2005). In addition, patients with sepsis-induced ARDS have higher case fatality rates than patients with other risk factors of ARDS (Stapleton et al., 2005).

### 12.2.9 Acid-Base Disturbances

Sepsis patients often display a wide spectrum of acid-base disorders, among which metabolic acidosis is frequently encountered. The occurrence of metabolic acidosis in these patients is linked to higher morbidity and mortality rates within the ICU. Moreover, it is noteworthy that certain individuals may present with simultaneous irregularities involving both metabolic acidosis and alkalosis (Szrama et al., 2016). Acid-base disturbances were studied by Arterial Blood Gas analysis, base excess, and bicarbonate analysis.

### 12.2.10 Sequential Organ Failure Assessment (SOFA)

The SOFA scale is a valuable tool utilized across various medical disciplines, including ICU. It enables the evaluation of disease severity and prognosis in patients with multiple organ failure, providing a dynamic reflection of organ function changes over time. By assessing key organ systems, SOFA aids in identifying the extent of organ dysfunction and guides appropriate treatment strategies. In the context of sepsis, the SOFA score plays a crucial role in assessing disease progression and informing clinical decision-making (Liu et al., 2022).

## 12.3 METHODOLOGY

### 12.3.1 Data Source

In this study, the dataset used for analysis was obtained from physionet.org. PhysioNet is a renowned online repository for physiological data and related resources that provides access to a wide range of datasets contributed by researchers and institutions worldwide.

### 12.3.2 Data Analysis

In this study, data analysis was carried out utilizing the software tool Tableau version 2022.2. Tableau is a widely recognized and powerful data visualization tool that enables users to connect to various data sources, explore data, create interactive visualizations, and generate insightful reports and dashboards.

### 12.3.3 Identification of Sepsis Patients

Sepsis patients were identified based on the criteria based in Table 12.1.

### 12.3.4 Definition of Hospital-Onset Sepsis

Hospital-onset sepsis is defined as sepsis that emerges 48 hours or more after a patient's admission to a hospital. The patients who had sepsis at the time of admission to the hospital were labeled as "Present on Admission" (POA) and were not a part of this study.

### 12.3.5 Parameters Analyzed

The cut-offs used for the parameters included in our analysis are listed in Table 12.2.

**TABLE 12.1**
**Identification of Sepsis (Faix, 2013)**

| Criteria for SIRS |
|---|
| **Two or more of the following are required:** |
| Body Temperature > 38°C or < 36°C |
| Heart Rate > 90 beats per minute |
| Respiratory Rate > 20 beats per minute (or arterial $pCO_2$ <32 mm Hg, indicating hyperventilation) |
| WBC Count > 12.0 x $10^9$/L (or <4.0 x $10^9$/L) |
| **Sepsis = Infection + SIRS** |
| **Severe Sepsis = Sepsis + Evidence of Organ Dysfunction** |

**TABLE 12.2**
**Study Parameters and Their Abbreviations and Ranges**

| Parameters | Abbreviation | Ranges |
|---|---|---|
| Base excess | BE | -2 to +2 mEq/L |
| pH | pH | 7.35–7.45 |
| Bicarbonate | HCO3 | 22 to 26 mEq/L |
| Lactate | [La−]b | 4.5 to 19.8 mg/dL |

*(Continued)*

**TABLE 12.2 (*Continued*)**
**Study Parameters and Their Abbreviations and Ranges**

| Parameters | Abbreviation | Ranges |
|---|---|---|
| Alkaline Phosphatase | ALP | 44 to 147 IU/L |
| Aspartate Aminotransferase | AST | 8–33 Micro Liter |
| Phosphate | PO4 | Adults: 2.8 to 4.5 mg/dL<br>Children: 4.0 to 7.0 mg/dL |
| Potassium | K | Normal: 3.5–5 mEq/L<br>Hypokalemia: <3.5 mEq/L<br>Hyperkalemia: >5 mEq/L |
| Chloride | Cl | Normal: 96–106 mmol/L<br>Hypochloremia: <96 mmol/L<br>Hyperchloremia: >106 mmol/L |
| Blood Urea Nitrogen | BUN | 6–24 mg/dL |
| Creatinine | Cr | Males: 0.7–1.3 mg/dL<br>Females: 0.6–1.1 mg/dL |
| Bilirubin | Br | Bilirubin Direct: 0.1–0.3 mg/dL<br>Bilirubin Total: 0.3–1.0 mg/dL |
| Glucose | BG | Normal: <140 mg/dL<br>Prediabetes: 140 — <200 mg/dL<br>Diabetes: >=200 mg/dL |
| Partial Thromboplastin Time | PTT | 25–35 seconds |
| Hemoglobin | Hb | Males: 13.2–16.6 g/dL<br>Females: 11.6–15.0 g/dL |
| Mean Arterial Pressure | MAP | 70–100 mm Hg |
| Blood Pressure | BP | Systolic BP:<br>Normal: <120 mm Hg<br>Prehypertension: 120–140 mm Hg<br>Hypertension: >140 mm Hg<br>Diastolic BP:<br>Normal: <80 mm Hg<br>Prehypertension: 80–90 mm Hg<br>Hypertension: >90 mm Hg |
| Heart Rate | HR | 60–100 beats per minute |
| Body Temperature | BTR | 98.6°F (37 °C)<br>Range: 97°F (36.1°C)—99°F (37.2°C) |
| Troponin | TropT | 0 and 0.04 ng/mL |
| Partial Carbon Dioxide | PaCO2 | 38 to 42 mm Hg (5.1 to 5.6 kPa) |
| End Tital Carbon Dioxide | EtCO2 | 35–45 mmHg |
| Respiratory Rate | RR | 12–18 breaths/minute |
| Oxygen Saturation | Sa02/SpO2 | Normal: 94–99%<br>Under oxygenated: <90%<br>Fatal: <70% |
| Sequential Organ Failure Assessment | SOFA | The total score of SOFA ranges from 0–24<br>SOFA score > =2 + presence of infection indicates sepsis |
| Arterial Blood Gas | ABG | pH: 7.35–7.45<br>PaCo2: 35–45 mm Hg<br>HCO3: 22–26 mEq/L |

## 12.4 RESULTS AND DISCUSSION

### 12.4.1 Demographics

In our dataset, we had a total of 40,336 patients. Among them, 426 patients had sepsis at the time of admission, while the remaining patients were non-sepsis cases at POA. Out of the non-sepsis patients, 2,506 individuals developed sepsis after staying in the hospital for 48 hours or more, known as onset sepsis patients. Among the onset sepsis patients, there were 1,018 males (40.6%) and 1,488 females (49.4%). The onset sepsis patient count by age and gender is depicted in Figure 12.1.

### 12.4.2 Glucose

Among patients who developed hospital-onset sepsis, a significant proportion of 30% exhibited hyperglycemia, while 42% had prediabetes, as seen in Figure 12.2. These findings suggest a potential association between sepsis development and disturbances in glucose regulation. The prevalence of hyperglycemia in sepsis cases aligns with existing research, emphasizing its common occurrence.

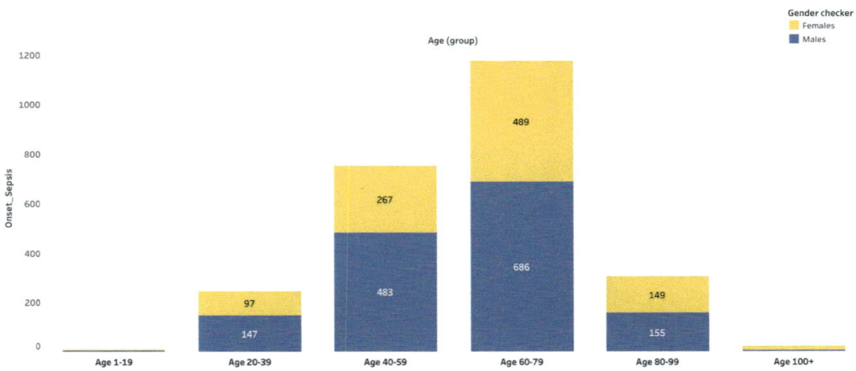


**FIGURE 12.1** Onset sepsis patient count by age and gender.

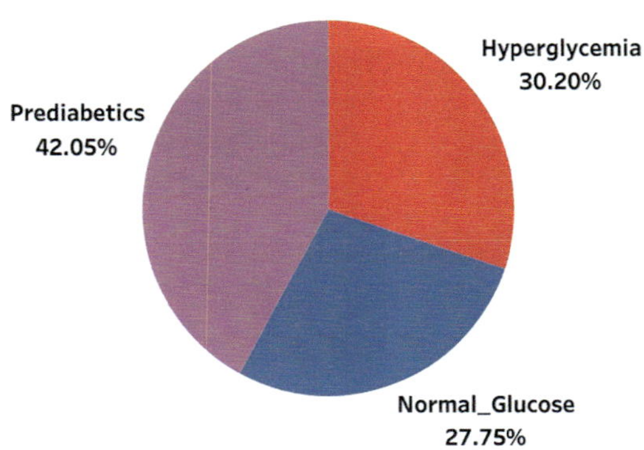


**FIGURE 12.2** Glucose analysis in onset sepsis patients.

### 12.4.3 WBC

In our analysis, we observed leukocytosis in 992 males and 678 females, indicating an abnormally high white blood cell count associated with immune response. Leukopenia was found in 147 males and 89 females, as shown in Figure 12.3. These findings highlight varying immune responses in male and female sepsis patients. Leukocytosis is commonly linked to infections and inflammation, while leukopenia may suggest immune suppression or underlying conditions. Monitoring white blood cell counts helps assess immune response severity and guide interventions.

### 12.4.4 Partial Prothrombin Time

Among the total onset sepsis patients, 33.8% exhibited high Partial Thromboplastin Time (PTT) levels, while 12.2% had low PTT levels, as shown in Figure 12.4. PTT is a laboratory test used to assess blood clotting function. In sepsis, abnormalities in clotting mechanisms are common, and both increased and decreased PTT levels can

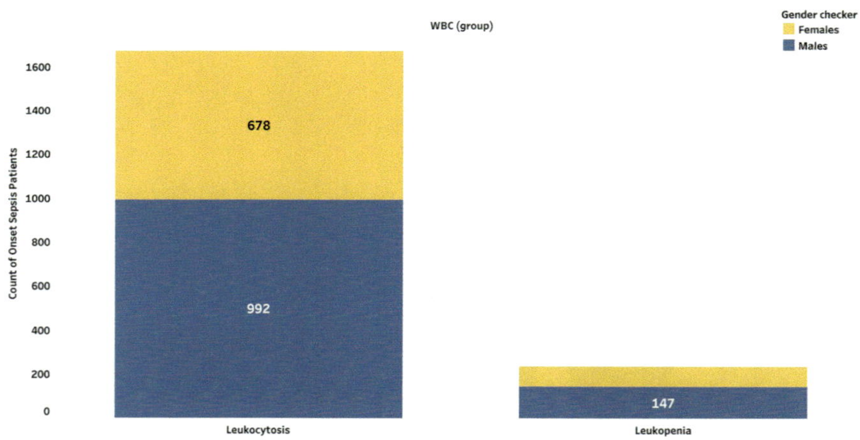


**FIGURE 12.3** Abnormal WBC levels in onset sepsis patients.

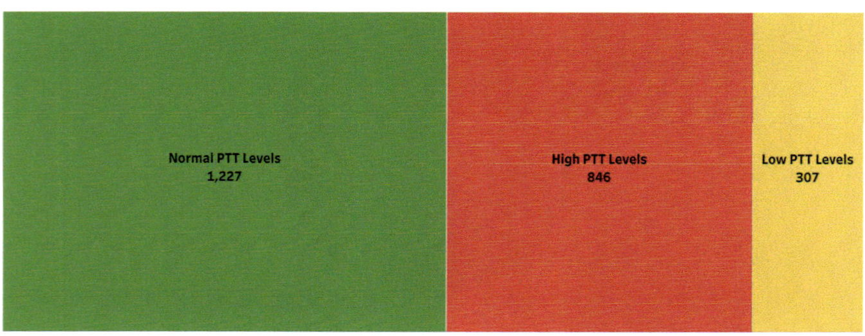


**FIGURE 12.4** Partial prothrombin time in onset sepsis patients.

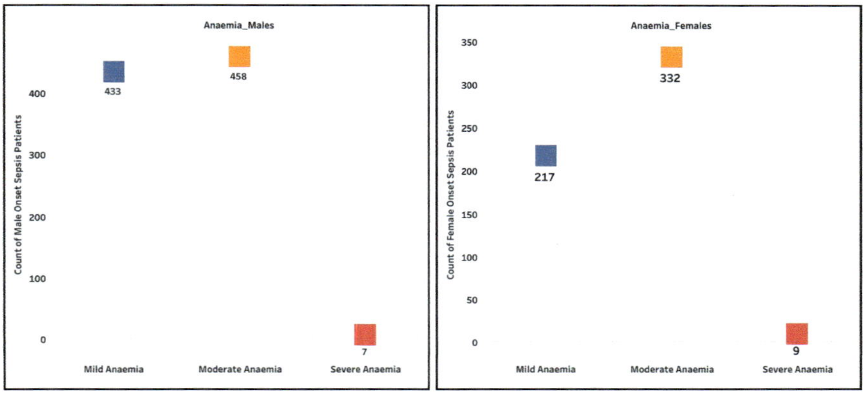


**FIGURE 12.5** Anemia severity in onset sepsis patients.

occur. By closely observing PTT, healthcare providers could identify any abnormalities in blood clotting, and prompt intervention could possibly prevent the onset or progression of sepsis.

### 12.4.5 Hemoglobin

Our analysis of onset sepsis patients found varying degrees of anemia in both male and female individuals. Among males, 433 had mild anemia, 458 had moderate anemia, and seven had severe anemia. Among females, 217 had mild anemia, 332 had moderate anemia, and nine had severe anemia, as shown in Figure 12.5. Anemia, characterized by low red blood cell or hemoglobin levels, can significantly impact oxygen transport and tissue perfusion, exacerbating the effects of sepsis. The severity of anemia can vary and may reflect the overall disease progression and physiological response in sepsis patients. By closely monitoring hemoglobin, medical staff can identify any abnormalities in oxygen-carrying capacity and could potentially prevent the onset (Khang et al., 2023).

### 12.4.6 Combination of Anemia with Other Abnormal Biomarkers

Among the anemic patients in our study, 41 individuals displayed a combination of hyperglycemia (high blood sugar levels), hypertension (high blood pressure), and abnormal white blood cell (WBC) count, as shown in Table 12.3. These findings suggest a potential correlation between anemia and these specific physiological abnormalities in the context of sepsis.

### 12.4.7 Cardiovascular System Related Biomarkers

#### 12.4.7.1 Heart Rate, Body Temperature, and Blood Pressure

Among the onset sepsis patients in our study, a total of 547 males and 426 females exhibited a combination of high heart rate, high systolic blood pressure, high diastolic

**TABLE 12.3**
**Association of Anemia with Other Abnormal Biomarkers**

| Gender | Count of Onset Sepsis Patients with Anemia, Abnormal WBC, Hyperglycemia, Hypertension |
|---|---|
| Males | 21 |
| Females | 20 |
| Total | 41 (1.6%) |

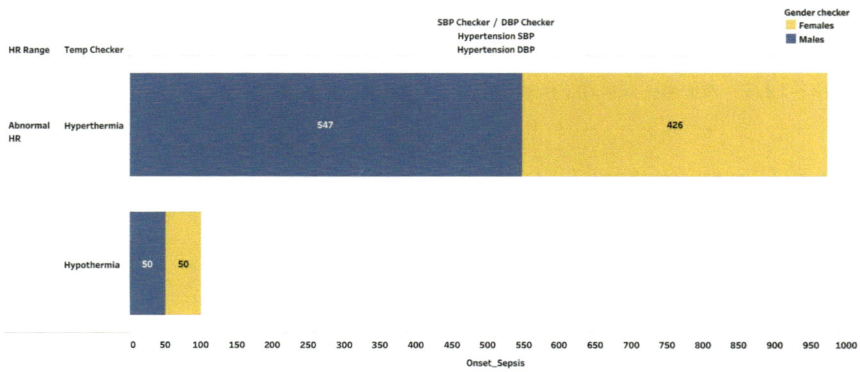


**FIGURE 12.6** Abnormalities in heart rate, body temperature, and hypertension.

blood pressure, and hyperthermia. These physiological abnormalities indicate the presence of a systemic inflammatory response commonly observed in sepsis. The concurrent elevation of heart rate, systolic and diastolic blood pressure, and hyperthermia in these patients suggest a state of heightened physiological stress and inflammation. These findings contribute to our understanding of the clinical presentation and severity of sepsis in both male and female patients, as shown in Figure 12.6.

### 12.4.7.2 Mean Arterial Pressure

In the age group of 40–80, both males and females exhibit high (>100 mmHg) and low (<65 mmHg) mean arterial pressure (MAP). However, males tend to have higher MAP levels than females (Figure 12.7). High MAP in this age group suggests an increased risk of heart attack, while low MAP indicates the potential for sepsis and internal bleeding. Regular monitoring of mean arterial pressure (MAP) may be crucial in the hospital setting to prevent sepsis. By closely monitoring MAP, healthcare providers can identify any deviations from the normal range and intervene promptly to maintain adequate tissue perfusion, prevent hypotension, and reduce the risk of sepsis development (Khang et al., 2022). This proactive approach may allow for timely interventions, such as fluid resuscitation or administration of vasoactive medications, as shown in Figure 12.7.

Among the patients with onset sepsis, 52 individuals exhibited high mean arterial pressure (MAP) and low oxygen saturation levels. Interestingly, there was a

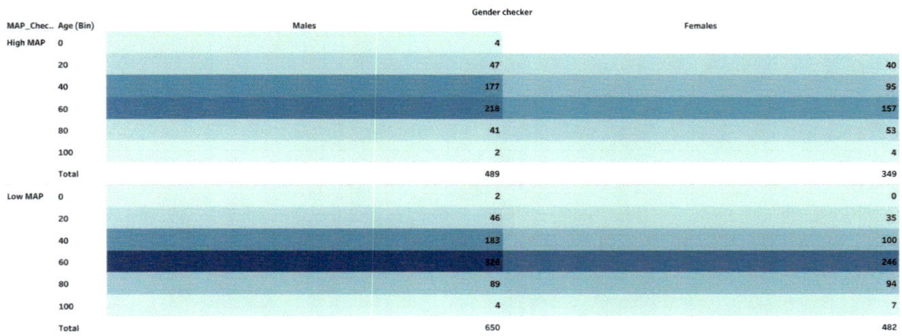


**FIGURE 12.7** Mean arterial pressure in onset sepsis patients.

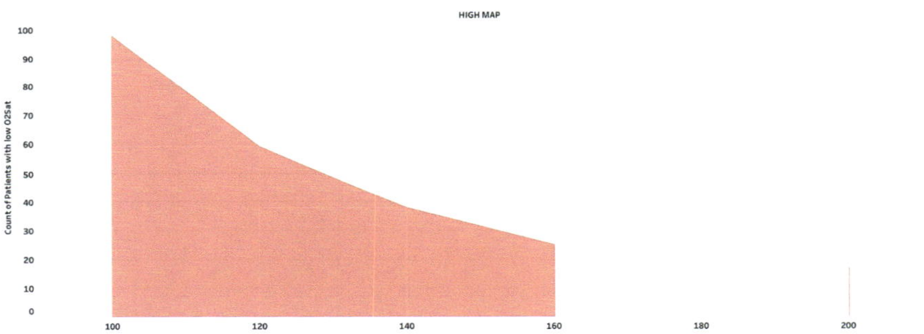


**FIGURE 12.8** Onset sepsis patients with high MAP and low O2 saturation.

noticeable trend where the number of patients with low oxygen saturation decreased as the mean arterial pressure increased. This finding suggests a potential inverse relationship between oxygen saturation and mean arterial pressure in patients with onset sepsis. It implies that higher mean arterial pressure values may be associated with improved oxygen saturation levels, as shown in Figure 12.8.

#### 12.4.7.3 Troponin

Elevated troponin levels were observed in 252 males and 187 females among our study participants. Notably, the highest number of cases with elevated troponin levels was found in the age group of 60–80 years. Troponin is a cardiac biomarker that indicates damage to the heart muscle, such as in cases of myocardial infarction or heart failure. The findings suggest a higher prevalence of cardiac injury in older individuals within the onset sepsis population, as shown in Figure 12.9.

### 12.4.8 Liver-Related Biomarkers

#### 12.4.8.1 Lactate, ALP, and Phosphate

Sepsis can impact liver function and disrupt the balance of phosphorus in the body, leading to changes in these biomarkers. The specific pattern of ALP and phosphate levels can vary depending on the individual patient and the underlying factors

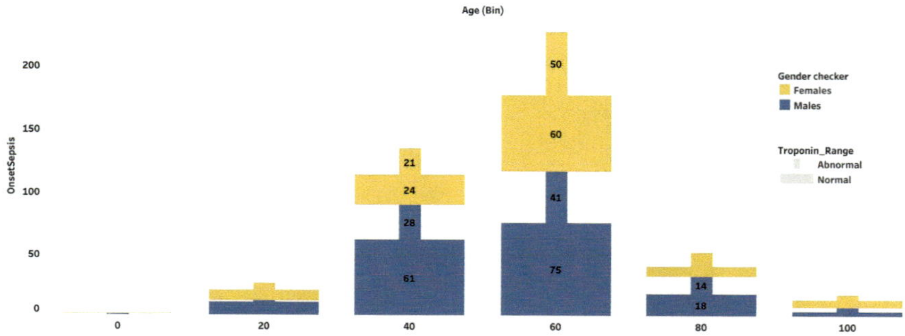


**FIGURE 12.9** Troponin analysis in onset sepsis patients.

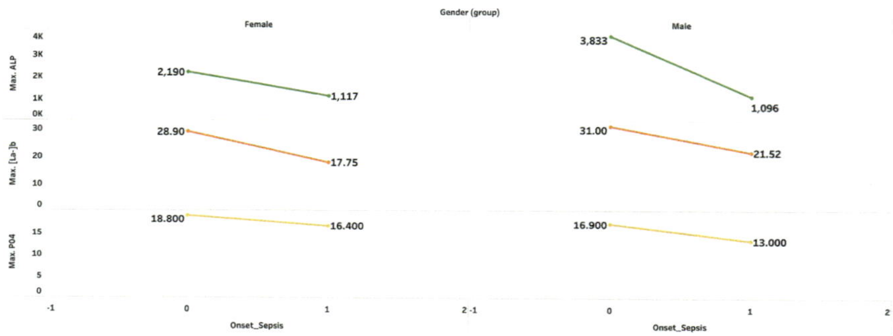


**FIGURE 12.10** Maximum levels of lactate, ALP, and phosphate in onset sepsis patients.

contributing to sepsis. In our dataset, when patients transitioned from non-sepsis to sepsis, there was a notable decrease in the maximum levels of lactate, ALP, and phosphate, as shown in Figure 12.10.

#### 12.4.8.2 Bilirubin Direct and Bilirubin Total Levels

The transition from non-sepsis to sepsis resulted in a significant increase in the levels of both direct and total bilirubin, as shown in Figure 12.11. These findings are consistent with previous studies, further supporting the observed relationship between sepsis development and elevated bilirubin levels. By closely monitoring bilirubin, hospital workers may identify any abnormalities in liver function and make timely interventions that may prevent the onset or progression of sepsis.

#### 12.4.8.3 Elevation of Liver Parameters

Among the onset sepsis patients, 508 individuals (20.2%) exhibited elevated levels of at least one of the following biomarkers: bilirubin total, bilirubin direct, alkaline phosphatase (ALP), or aspartate transaminase (AST), as shown in Figure 12.12. Additionally, 29 patients demonstrated abnormal values for all four biomarkers, indicating more severe liver involvement. Monitoring these biomarkers is crucial for assessing liver function and identifying potential complications. Identifying and

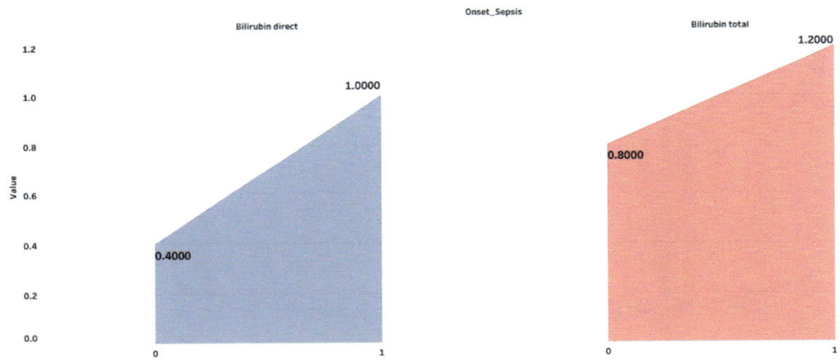


**FIGURE 12.11** Bilirubin direct and bilirubin total levels in patients transitioning to onset sepsis.

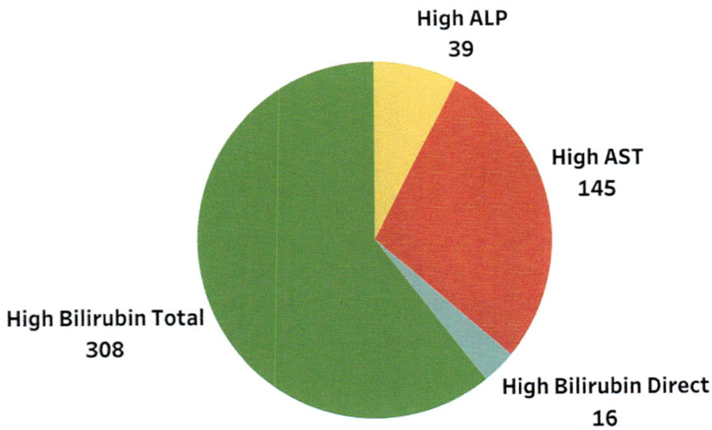


**FIGURE 12.12** Abnormal liver parameters in onset sepsis patients.

addressing abnormal biomarker levels promptly can aid in optimizing patient care and improving outcomes in sepsis patients.

### 12.4.9 Renal-Related Biomarkers

#### 12.4.9.1 Potassium

Among the 2,506 patients who developed onset sepsis, a subset of 176 individuals was found to have hypokalemia, indicating lower than normal potassium levels. Additionally, 124 patients exhibited hyperkalemia, which refers to higher-than-normal potassium levels. However, it is worth noting that the majority of onset sepsis patients had potassium levels within the normal range, as shown in Figure 12.13. This suggests that while some patients experienced abnormal potassium levels, a significant proportion maintained potassium levels within the expected range. Monitoring

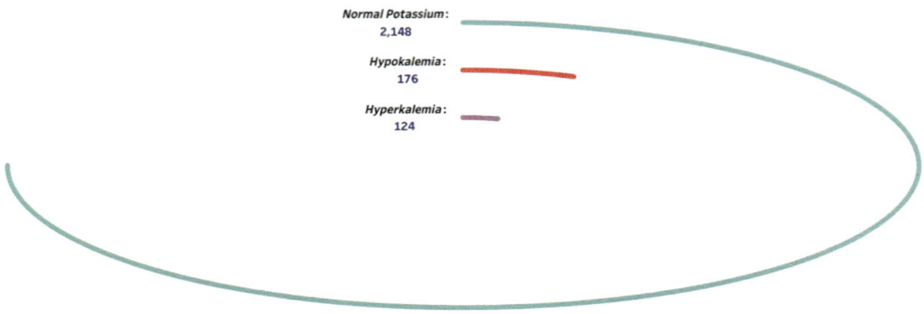


**FIGURE 12.13** Potassium analysis using radial bar chart.

and managing potassium levels in sepsis patients, particularly those with hypokalemia or hyperkalemia, can be crucial in ensuring appropriate electrolyte balance and optimizing patient care.

#### 12.4.9.2 Chloride

Among the patients in our study, 34% exhibited hyperchloremia, indicating higher than normal chloride levels, while 3% had hypochloremia, indicating lower than normal chloride levels, as shown in Figure 12.14. These findings highlight the prevalence of electrolyte imbalances in the study population. Hyperchloremia can be associated with various conditions such as dehydration, kidney dysfunction, and certain medications, while hypochloremia may be linked to fluid losses, metabolic alkalosis, or other underlying factors. Monitoring and managing chloride levels in onset sepsis patients is crucial for maintaining electrolyte balance.

#### 12.4.9.3 Creatinine

Among the onset sepsis patients, 400 individuals had hypocreatinemia (lower than normal creatinine levels), while 1,008 patients had hypercreatinemia (higher than normal creatinine levels). Notably, the highest occurrence of both hypocreatinemia and hypercreatinemia was observed in the age group of 60–80 years. These findings suggest that renal function, indicated by creatinine levels, can be affected in onset sepsis patients, with a significant number experiencing abnormal creatinine levels. Early detection of elevated creatinine levels can prompt timely actions and appropriate management strategies to prevent the progression and complications of sepsis as Figure 12.15.

#### 12.4.9.4 Correlation between BUN and Creatinine Levels

In onset sepsis patients, there was a strong correlation between blood urea nitrogen (BUN) and creatinine levels in both genders. This correlation was demonstrated by a high R-squared value of 0.88, indicating that approximately 88% of the variation in creatinine levels could be explained by changes in BUN levels. The observed correlation was statistically significant, as indicated by a p-value of less than 0.0001, as shown in Figure 12.16.

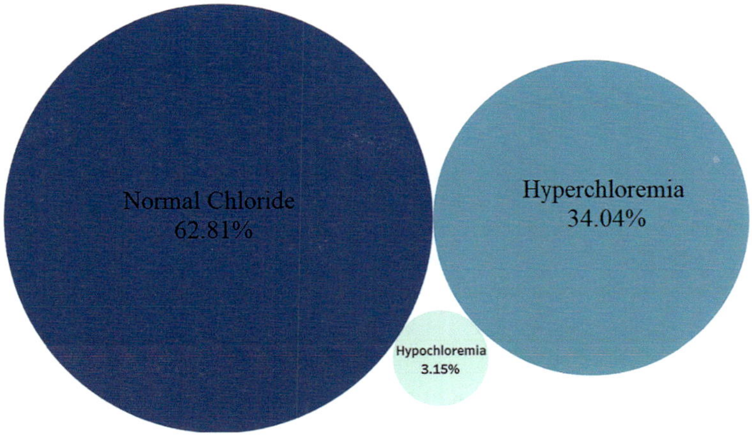


**FIGURE 12.14** Distribution of onset sepsis patients by blood chloride levels.

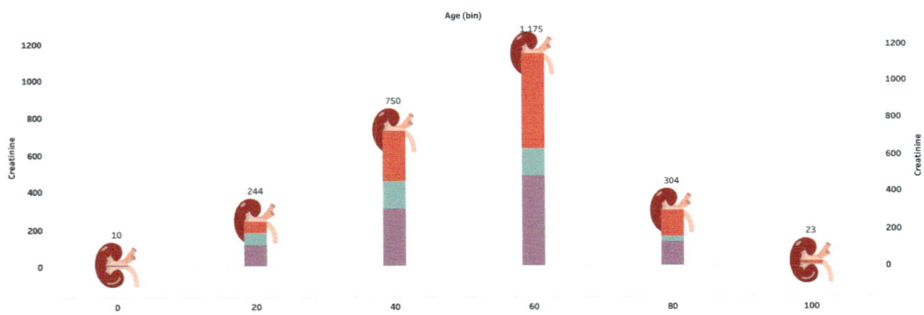


**FIGURE 12.15** Age-wise analysis of creatinine levels.

#### 12.4.9.5 Acute Kidney Injury

In our study, a significant proportion of males (67%) and females (32%) exhibited abnormal kidney biomarkers, indicating the presence of acute kidney injury (AKI). Notably, the age group of 60–80 had the highest number of AKI cases. These findings highlight the prevalence of AKI in sepsis patients, particularly among older individuals, as shown in Figure 12.17.

### 12.4.10 Lungs-Related Biomarkers

#### 12.4.10.1 End Tital Carbon Dioxide

EtCO2 values of less than 35 have been identified as a screening tool to predict mortality and severe sepsis in potentially septic patients. Our analysis revealed that the onset sepsis population, comprising both genders aged 40 and above, exhibited lower EtCO2 levels, as shown in Figure 12.18.

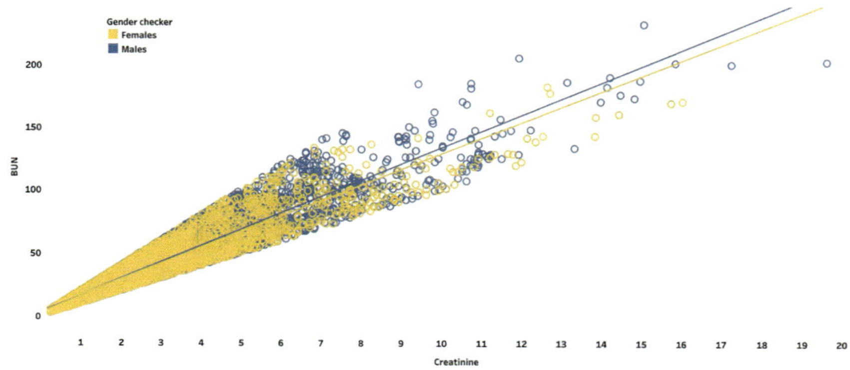


**FIGURE 12.16** Correlation between BUN and creatinine levels in onset sepsis patients.

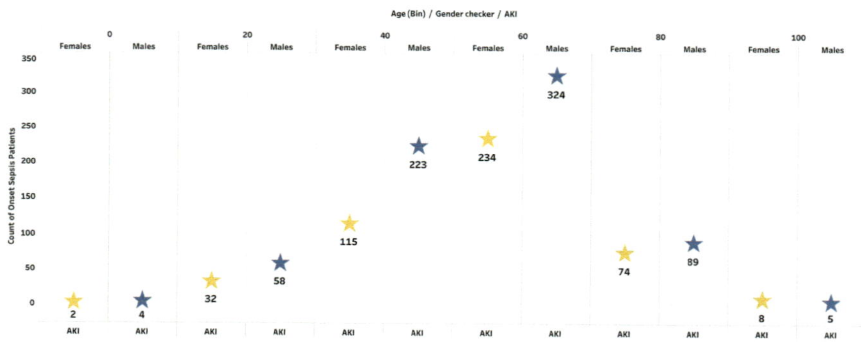


**FIGURE 12.17** Patients with abnormal levels of Acute Kidney Injury parameters.

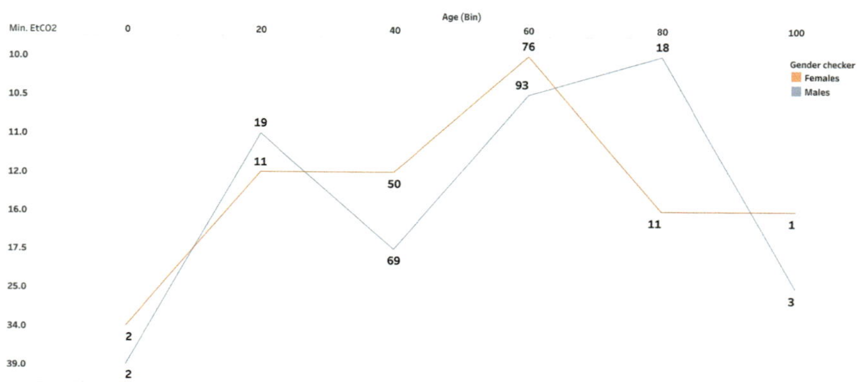


**FIGURE 12.18** EtCO2 in onset sepsis patient's age and gender wise.

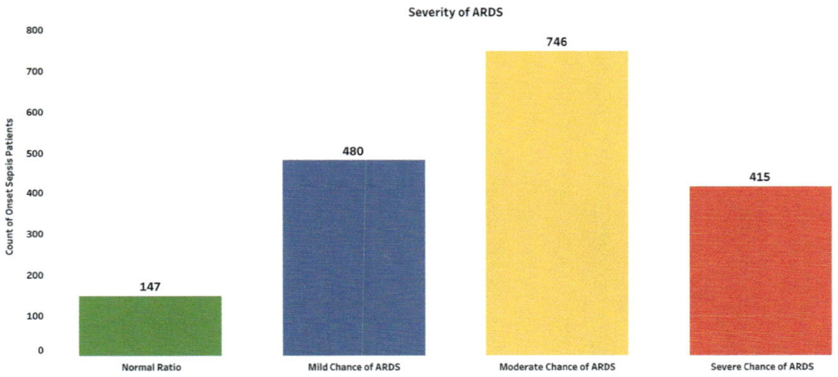


**FIGURE 12.19** ARDS severity in onset sepsis patients.

**TABLE 12.4**
**Prediction of Mortality by ARDS Severity Levels (ARDS, 2012)**

| ARDS Severity | PàO/FiO2 | Mortality |
|---|---|---|
| Mild | 200–300 | 27% |
| Moderate | 100–200 | 32% |
| Severe | < 100 | 45% |

#### 12.4.10.2 Acute Respiratory Distress Syndrome Severity

Among the onset sepsis patients in our study, 480 individuals were classified as having a mild chance of developing Acute Respiratory Distress Syndrome (ARDS), while 746 patients had a moderate chance, and 415 patients had a severe chance of ARDS, as shown in Figure 12.19.

ARDS is a potentially life-threatening condition characterized by severe respiratory distress and lung inflammation. The higher the ARDS risk, the greater the likelihood of experiencing respiratory complications and associated mortality, as shown in Table 12.4. Prompt recognition of ARDS is crucial in improving patient outcomes.

### 12.4.11 Acid-Base Disturbances

#### 12.4.11.1 Base Excess and Bicarbonate

Based on correlation analysis, a strong positive relationship exists between base excess and bicarbonate levels in onset sepsis patients, observed in both males and females. The R-squared value (0.75) indicates that 75.17% of bicarbonate level variation can be explained by base excess (p-value <0.0001), as shown in Figure 12.20.

#### 12.4.11.2 Arterial Blood Gas Analysis

Among the onset sepsis patients in our study, 113 individuals exhibited abnormal arterial blood gas (ABG) values, indicating disturbances in their acid-base balance.

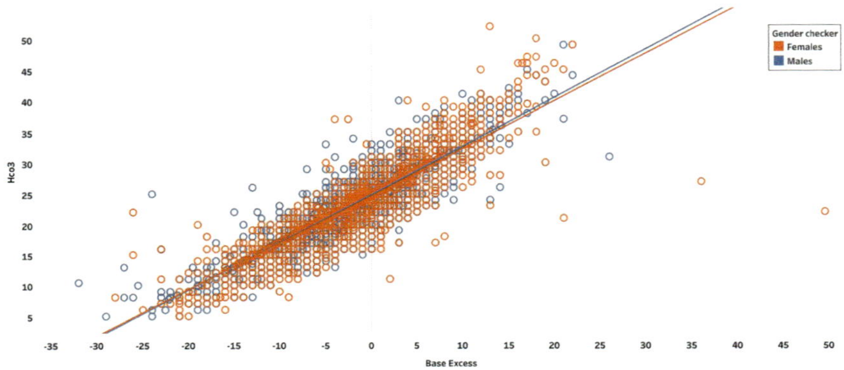


**FIGURE 12.20** Correlation between base excess and bicarbonates in onset sepsis patients.

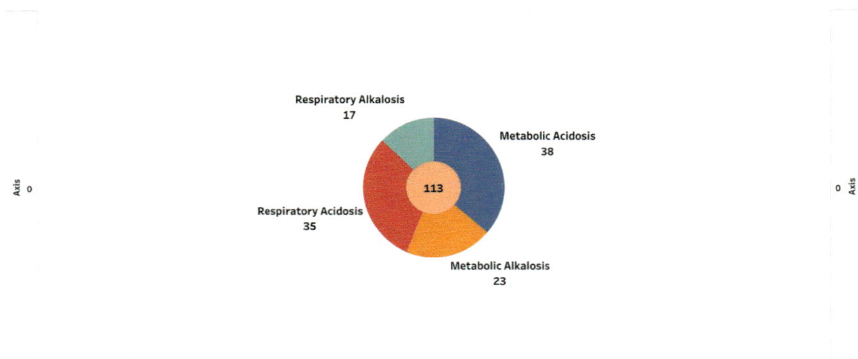


**FIGURE 12.21** ABG analysis in onset sepsis patients.

Further analysis revealed the specific types of acid-base imbalances present in these patients. Among the group with abnormal ABG, 35 patients showed respiratory acidosis, characterized by an excess of carbon dioxide in the blood due to impaired lung function. Additionally, 17 patients had respiratory alkalosis, indicating low carbon dioxide levels caused by hyperventilation. Furthermore, 38 patients displayed metabolic acidosis, which occurs when there is an excess of acid or a deficit of bicarbonate in the body. Lastly, 23 patients had metabolic alkalosis, characterized by an excess of bicarbonate in the blood, as shown in Figure 12.21.

### 12.4.11.3 Compensation Mechanism

We observed different levels of compensation for acid-base imbalances. Among the patients, 33 individuals exhibited uncompensated acid-base disturbances, indicating an imbalance without any compensatory mechanisms. Additionally, 62 patients showed partial compensation, where the body's compensatory mechanisms were initiated but not fully effective in restoring balance. On the other hand, 268 patients displayed full compensation, suggesting that the body successfully restored the acid-base balance through compensatory mechanisms, as shown in Figure 12.22.

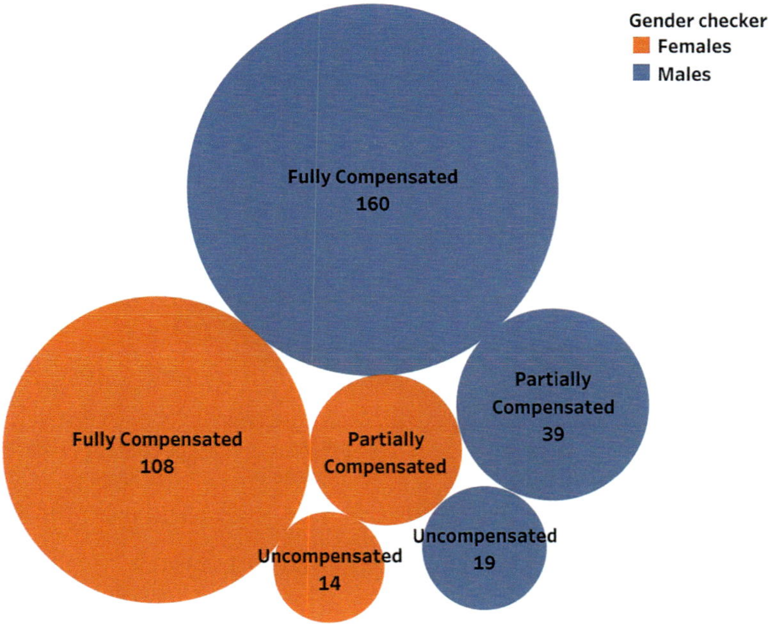


**FIGURE 12.22** Compensation mechanism.

### 12.4.12 SOFA Score

The SOFA score is based on six different scores for the respiratory, cardiovascular, hepatic, coagulation, renal, and neurological systems, each scored from 0 to 4, with higher scores indicating worsening organ dysfunction (Lambden et al., 2019), as shown in Table 12.5.

Among the onset sepsis patients, 127 individuals were found to have a SOFA score of 2 or above. The age group of 68–80 had the highest number of patients with elevated SOFA scores. Thus, the SOFA score is a useful tool for evaluating organ dysfunction in sepsis patients, as shown in Figure 12.23.

## 12.5 CONCLUSION

In conclusion, this study has provided valuable insights highlighting the micro-analysis of parameters in hospital-induced sepsis patients. The analysis of biomarkers, such as leukocytosis, leukopenia, elevated troponin levels, abnormal kidney biomarkers, abnormal liver biomarkers, and deranged ABG values, has provided a deeper understanding of the pathophysiological changes occurring in these patients (Khang, 2024).

Furthermore, the study has identified important factors associated with the onset of sepsis, such as metabolic derangement, coagulation activation, and low hemoglobin levels. The results emphasize the need for early detection, accurate monitoring,

**TABLE 12.5**
**The Criteria for Assessment of the Sequential Organ Failure Assessment (SOFA) Score**

| | SOFA Score | | | | |
|---|---|---|---|---|---|
| **Biomarker** | **0** | **1** | **2** | **3** | **4** |
| Respiratory system- $PaO_2/FiO_2$ (mmHg) | >400 | <400 | <300 | <200 with respiratory support | <100 with respiratory support |
| Nervous system- Glasgow Coma Scale | 15 | 13–15 | 10–12 | 6–9 | <6 |
| Cardiovascular system- Mean arterial pressure (MAP) | MAP > 70 mmHg | MAP < 70 mmHg | Dopamine ≤5 μg/kg/min | Dopamine >5 μg/kg/min | Dopamine >15 μh/kg/min |
| Liver- Bilirubin (mg/dl) [μmol/L] | <1.2 (<20) | 1.2–1.9 [20–32] | 2.0–5.9 [33–101] | 6.0–11.9 [102–204] | >12.0 [>204] |
| Coagulation- Platelets $\times 10^3$/ml | >150 | <150 | < 100 | < 50 | < 20 |
| Kidneys- Creatinine (mg/dl) [μmol/L] | <1.2 [<110] | 1.2–1.9 [110–170] | 2.0–3.4 [171–299] | 3.5–4.9 [300–440] | >5.0 [>440] |

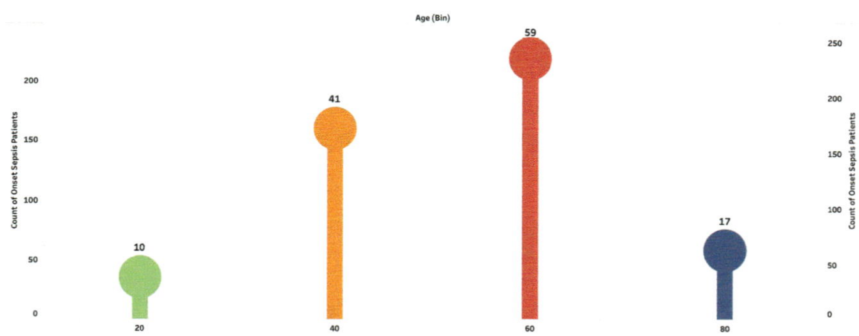


**FIGURE 12.23** SOFA score of 2 and above in onset sepsis patients by age.

and prompt intervention to improve patient outcomes. The study interprets that if healthcare professionals can monitor these biomarkers at regular intervals in the ICU and treat them promptly, the chances of sepsis development may decrease. Thus, this study contributes to the existing knowledge on the onset of sepsis and provides a foundation for further research and advancements in the field (Khang, 2024).

## REFERENCES

The ARDS Definition Task Force*. (2012). Acute respiratory distress syndrome: The Berlin definition. *JAMA*, 307(23), 2526–2533. doi:10.1001/jama.2012.5669

Faix, J. D. (2013). Biomarkers of sepsis. *Critical Reviews in Clinical Laboratory Sciences*, 50(1), 23–36. doi:10.3109/10408363.2013.764490

Farkas, J. D. (2020). The complete blood count to diagnose septic shock. *Journal of Thoracic Disease*, 12(Suppl 1), S16. doi:10.21037/jtd.2019.12.63

Flannery, A. H., Li, X., Delozier, N. L., Toto, R. D., Moe, O. W., Yee, J., & Neyra, J. A. (2021). Sepsis-associated acute kidney disease and long-term kidney outcomes. *Kidney Medicine*, 3(4), 507–514. doi:10.1016/j.xkme.2021.02.007

Gando, S., Levi, M., & Toh, C. H. (2016, June 2). Disseminated intravascular coagulation. *Nature Reviews Disease Primers*, 2, 16037. doi:10.1038/nrdp.2016.37. PMID: 27250996.

Hirasawa, H., Oda, S., & Nakamura, M. (2009, September 7). Blood glucose control in patients with severe sepsis and septic shock. *World Journal of Gastroenterology*, 15(33), 4132–4136. doi:10.3748/wjg.15.4132. PMID: 19725146; PMCID: PMC2738808.

Jung, S. M., Kim, Y. J., Ryoo, S. M., & Kim, W. Y. (2019). Relationship between low hemoglobin levels and mortality in patients with septic shock. *Acute and Critical Care*, 34(2), 141–147. doi:10.4266/acc.2019.00465

Khang, A. (2024). *AI and IoT-based technologies for precision medicine*. IGI Global Press. ISBN: 9798369308769. doi:10.4018/979-8-3693-0876-9

Khang, A., Abdullayev, V. A., Hrybiuk, O., & Shukla, A. K. (2024). *Computer vision and AI-integrated IoT technologies in medical ecosystem* (1st Ed.). CRC Press. doi:10.1201/9781003429609

Khang, A., Ragimova, N. A., Hajimahmud, V. A., & Alyar, V. A. (2022). Advanced technologies and data management in the smart healthcare system. In *AI-centric smart city ecosystems: Technologies, design and implementation* (1st Ed., vol. 16, p. 10). CRC Press. doi:10.1201/9781003252542-16

Khang, A., Rana, G., Tailor, R. K., & Hajimahmud, V. A. (2023). *Data-centric AI solutions and emerging technologies in the healthcare ecosystem*. CRC Press. doi:10.1201/9781003356189

Lambden, S., Laterre, P. F., Levy, M. M. et al. (2019). The SOFA score—development, utility, and challenges of accurate assessment in clinical trials. *Critical Care*, 23, 374. doi:10.1186/s13054-019-2663-7

Liu, C., Suo, S., Luo, L., Chen, X., Ling, C., & Cao, S. (2022, August 10). SOFA score in relation to sepsis: Clinical implications in diagnosis, treatment, and prognostic assessment. *Computational and Mathematical Methods in Medicine*, 2022, 7870434. doi:10.1155/2022/7870434. PMID: 35991153; PMCID: PMC9385349.

Mankowski, R. T., Yende, S., & Angus, D. C. (2019). Long-term impact of sepsis on cardiovascular health. *Intensive Care Medicine*, 45, 78–81. doi:10.1007/s00134-018-5173-1

Matot, I., & Sprung, C. L. (2001). Definition of sepsis. *Intensive Care Medicine*, 27(14), S3–S9.

Rani, S., Chauhan, M., Kataria, A., & Khang, A. (2021). IoT equipped intelligent distributed framework for smart healthcare systems. *Networking and Internet Architecture*, 2, 30. doi:10.48550/arXiv.2110.04997

Stapleton, R. D., Wang, B. M., Hudson, L. D., Rubenfeld, G. D., Caldwell, E. S., & Steinberg, K. P. (2005, August). Causes and timing of death in patients with ARDS. *Chest*, 128(2), 525–532. doi:10.1378/chest.128.2.525. PMID: 16100134.

Szrama, J., & Smuszkiewicz, P. (2016). An acid-base disorders analysis with the use of the Stewart approach in patients with sepsis treated in an intensive care unit. *Anaesthesiology Intensive Therapy*, 48(3). doi:10.5603/AIT.a2016.0020

Yan, J., Li, S., & Li, S. (2014). The role of the liver in sepsis. *International Reviews of Immunology*, 33(6), 498–510. doi:10.3109/08830185.2014.889129

# 13 Revolutionizing Healthcare with IoT
## *Connecting the Dots for Better Patient Outcomes*

*Sangeetha Rangasamy, Kavitha Rajamohan, Debanjan Basu, Kenneth John Menezes, and Ayushya Chongder*

## 13.1 INTRODUCTION

Healthcare involves medical services to prevent, diagnose, and treat illnesses, including preventative care and long-term services. Collaboration between patients, healthcare professionals, and organizations is essential to provide high-quality, patient-centered care. IoT refers to the network of devices, sensors, and objects that are connected to the Internet, allowing them to communicate with each other and collect and transmit data. IoT technology provides capabilities such as identification, communication, services, computing, sensing, and data transfer. These functions enable various applications in healthcare and other fields. IoT allows for remote patient monitoring, smart home automation, and real-time tracking of objects, people, and animals. The technology's ability to collect, transmit, and analyze data facilitates better decision-making and improved patient outcomes.

Healthcare Internet of Things (HIoT) refers to the integration of Internet of Things (IoT) technologies into healthcare systems to enhance the efficiency of healthcare delivery. In healthcare, IoT technology can be used to gather data from various sources, such as medical devices, wearables, and mobile apps, and analyze that data to provide insights into patient health and wellness. HIoT is revolutionizing the way healthcare is delivered, making it more patient-centered, efficient, and cost-effective (Vrushank et al., 2023). HIoT helps resolve security concerns in healthcare by providing secure data transmission and storage, preventing unauthorized access to medical equipment, and providing real-time alerts to healthcare professionals in case of security breaches. This improves the security and reliability of healthcare data, building trust and improving patient care (Khang, 2024).

## 13.2 ELEMENTS OF HIoT

Knowing the underlying components of HIoT is crucial for comprehending its function and usefulness, as shown in Figure 13.1.


DOI: 10.1201/9781032686745-13

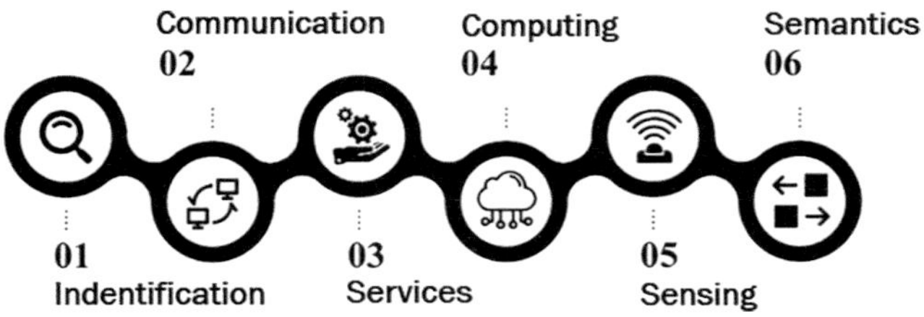


**FIGURE 13.1** Elements of HIoT.

### 13.2.1 Identification

The process of identification involves declaring one's identity and subsequently authenticating the data's validity (Porkodi et al., 2014). This is crucial in systems comprising interconnected components to ensure their proper functioning, and identifiers play a vital role in achieving this objective. Identifiers serve as distinct patterns utilized to identify entities within IoT examples. For instance, in smart home automation, each connected device, such as thermostats, lights, and door locks, possesses a unique identifier. This identifier allows the system to differentiate between the devices and assign specific commands or actions to each one. Similarly, in industrial IoT applications, sensors embedded in machinery are assigned unique identifiers to track their performance, detect anomalies, and trigger maintenance alerts.

In healthcare IoT, medical devices, patients, healthcare providers, and healthcare institutions are identified through unique patterns or identifiers, enabling accurate monitoring, integration, and secure data exchange. Identifiers play a crucial role in establishing connections and managing the vast network of entities within IoT systems, ensuring efficient and effective operation. Their selection depends on the specific application and requirements (Aqeel-Ur-Rehman et al., 2013). In the context of the Healthcare Internet of Things (HIoT), it is essential to identify both objects and users for electronic interactions. Identification facilitates the connection, relationship, and remote management of countless objects via the Internet (Van & Bassi, 2012).

Proper identification is of utmost importance in healthcare to ensure effective and efficient healthcare delivery. It enables the identification of medical devices, patients, healthcare providers, healthcare institutions, and clinical data, enabling accurate tracking, monitoring, and integration. This, in turn, facilitates the association of patient records with the correct individuals, secures communication among care providers, and prevents data breaches. Effective identification processes lead to improved patient outcomes and streamlined healthcare delivery.

### 13.2.2 Communication

The HIoT involves leveraging Internet connectivity to establish communication and data exchange between interconnected devices, eliminating the need for human intervention (Bkheet & Agbinya, 2021). HIoT encompasses various communication types, including Human to Machine (H2M), Machine to Machine (M2M), Machine to Human (M2H), and Human to Human (H2H). IoT protocols like Bluetooth, Wi-Fi, and ZigBee are employed to ensure secure data exchange.

The success of IoT in healthcare relies heavily on effective communication elements, which have specific requirements such as range, power consumption, security, and privacy. To overcome challenges and enhance communication capabilities in the healthcare industry, research teams worldwide are exploring innovative communication methods, aiming to enable seamless communication anytime, anywhere, through any media and mode. Artificial intelligence (AI), machine learning (ML), and business analytics further contribute to optimizing HIoT operations, analyzing large datasets, and deriving meaningful insights for improved healthcare outcomes.

### 13.2.3 Services

IoT services in the healthcare industry mainly consist of identity-related services, information aggregation services, collaborative-aware services, and ubiquitous services. Identity-related services involve unique identifiers, authentication mechanisms, and secure communication protocols to ensure object identity validity. Additionally, these services encompass access control, authorization, and identity management, which are essential for maintaining the integrity and security of IoT deployments, ultimately enhancing reliability and functionality (Marques & Garcia et al., 2017; Hema et al., 2018).

- Information aggregation services collect, summarize, and process all the information from objects and send it back to the application.
- Collaborative-aware services turn the collected information into a decision and send appropriate responses to the devices.
- Ubiquitous services provide collaborative-aware services immediately to anyone at any time and place.

Other application-based services include cloud platforms, analytics, visualization, predictive maintenance, remote monitoring, automation, and system integrations. Cloud platforms host and manage IoT services like data storage and processing. Analytics extract insights from IoT data. The visualization displays IoT data quickly. Predictive maintenance predicts equipment failure. Remote monitoring allows remote control of IoT devices. Automation enables devices to perform actions based on predefined rules or data analysis. Integrations provide a comprehensive solution. These services aim to improve patient monitoring and decision-making and provide real-time responses.

### 13.2.4 Computing

In the computation step of HIoT, valuable information is extracted through processing procedures, which can be enhanced by AI, ML, and business analytics.

Hardware and software platforms like Arduino, Raspberry Pi, and Intel Galileo are utilized, while cloud computing enables real-time processing of big data and knowledge extraction for end-users. Sensors play a vital role in computation, removing unnecessary information. In healthcare IoT, computational elements include wearable devices, mobile devices, Electronic Health Records (EHRs), Clinical Decision Support Systems (CDSSs), remote patient monitoring, telemedicine, and big data analytics for pattern identification in patient health data. AI, ML, and business analytics further optimize these processes by enabling advanced data analysis, predictive modeling, and actionable insights for improved healthcare outcomes.

### 13.2.5 Sensing

In the Healthcare Internet of Things (HIoT), sensing involves collecting data from the environment using a range of sensors such as actuators, RFID tags, smart sensors, and wearable sensors (Hema et al., 2018; Shaown et al., 2019). The collected data is then stored in databases, remote locations, local systems, or the cloud. Artificial intelligence (AI) and machine learning (ML) techniques can be applied to analyze this vast amount of healthcare IoT data. AI and ML algorithms can identify patterns, detect anomalies, and provide insights for improving patient care, treatment outcomes, and operational efficiency (Rana et al., 2021).

Furthermore, businesses can leverage this data to develop innovative healthcare services, personalize patient experiences, and optimize resource allocation. AI, ML, and business applications play a significant role in harnessing the potential of healthcare IoT data to drive advancements in healthcare delivery and improve patient outcomes.

### 13.2.6 Semantics

The Internet of Things (IoT) is a system of devices and technologies that enable users to perform tasks, and the integration of AI and ML presents significant business opportunities. Semantics, acting as the brain of the IoT system, extracts knowledge from machines, utilizes resources, and makes decisions to respond to devices (Hema et al., 2018). In this context, AI and ML techniques can be employed to analyze and derive insights from the vast amount of data generated by IoT devices. Semantic Web technologies like RDF and OWL play a crucial role in organizing and structuring this data (Shaown et al., 2019).

Wireless networks such as Wi-Fi and cellular networks facilitate data transmission between IoT devices and other systems, while cloud computing provides a centralized platform for data storage and processing. Additionally, middleware and APIs enable seamless communication and data exchange, creating opportunities for businesses to leverage AI, ML, and IoT for improved efficiency and innovation. Table 13.1 shows a brief summarization of the elements of IoT that are used in the Healthcare Industry.

**TABLE 13.1**
**Summarization on Elements of IoT**

| Elements | Description | Technologies |
|---|---|---|
| Identification | Responsible for device identification | Ecode, Ucode, IPv4 and IPv6 |
| Communication | Responsible for communicating among devices | Bluetooth, Wi-Fi, RFID, LTE |
| Services | Responsible for providing different services | Cloud, Monitoring, Analysis |
| Computation | Responsible for processing information | Arduino, Raspberry Pi, OS |
| Sensing | Responsible for sensing and collecting data | Sensors and Actuators |
| Semantics | Responsible for extracting knowledge and making decisions | RDF and OWL |

## 13.3 FORMS OF SERVICES

Healthcare covers different types of issues related to medicine. Not everyone will often avail of all of the services provided by healthcare, but they can take advantage of the best that healthcare technology has to offer for issues pertaining to themselves. These forms of services are not just limited to the patients themselves but also the physicians, nurses, and other healthcare authorities. Some of these services are mentioned in what follows.

### 13.3.1 Medical Devices

IoT medical devices, combined with the power of AI and ML, refer to a range of connected medical devices that can transmit and receive data through the Internet. These devices, incorporating advanced technologies, encompass wearable fitness trackers, remote patient monitoring systems, and telemedicine equipment (Khang & Abdullayev et al., 2024). The integration of AI and ML algorithms in medical devices enables intelligent data analysis, facilitating improved patient care and outcomes. Real-time data collection and analysis are made possible by IoT medical devices, enhancing remote monitoring, enabling early disease detection, and streamlining healthcare service delivery. This convergence of IoT, AI, and ML has the potential to revolutionize the healthcare industry, making healthcare more accessible, affordable, and efficient (Anh et al., 2024).

### 13.3.2 Public Health Services

The application of IoT, AI, and ML technologies in public health services has greatly enhanced healthcare delivery and health outcomes. IoT devices, including wearable fitness trackers, remote patient monitoring systems, and telemedicine equipment, collect and transmit real-time health data, which can be analyzed using AI and ML algorithms (Khang & Misra et al., 2023). These algorithms aid in identifying potential health issues at an early stage, empowering healthcare providers to make more informed decisions and deliver more effective treatments, as shown in Figure 13.2.

Furthermore, the combination of IoT, AI, and ML enables the monitoring and management of public health outbreaks. IoT-enabled sensors track the spread of

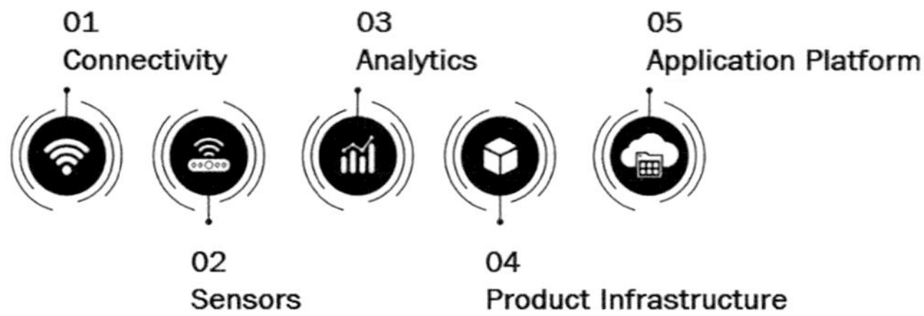


**FIGURE 13.2** IoT healthcare system components.

infectious diseases, while AI and ML algorithms analyze the data and provide real-time insights to health authorities, enabling quicker and more effective responses to outbreaks. By leveraging these technologies, public health services can be improved, ensuring access to essential healthcare services in remote and underserved areas. Telemedicine equipment, integrated with AI and ML, enables healthcare providers to deliver medical consultations remotely, reducing the need for patients to travel long distances for care. Ultimately, this integration has the potential to revolutionize healthcare delivery and improve health outcomes for individuals and communities.

### 13.3.3 Innovative Technology

The convergence of IoT, AI, and ML has paved the way for innovative solutions that address the evolving demands of a digital world. Forward-thinking IoT companies leverage these technologies to improve comfort, convenience, security, and more, driving innovation wherever opportunities arise. In the healthcare industry, the application of IoT, AI, and ML has already shown significant potential in reducing medical errors, improving patient outcomes, and lowering healthcare costs. This transformative combination of technologies makes healthcare more accessible, efficient, and patient-centric.

### 13.3.4 Medication Refills

IoT technology, enhanced by AI and ML, is employed in medication refill systems through the utilization of smart pill dispensers and drug reminder systems. These devices incorporate sensors to track medication usage and send reminders to patients or caregivers, ensuring timely refills before medications run out. Additionally, the devices can notify healthcare providers and pharmacies, enabling prompt medication refills. Integrating IoT, AI, and ML also enables remote monitoring of patient's medication adherence, providing valuable insights for healthcare providers to improve treatment outcomes. As a result, patient health is enhanced, healthcare costs are reduced, and medication management is improved.

### 13.3.5 Remote Monitoring

The combination of IoT, AI, and ML plays a vital role in remote monitoring for healthcare by facilitating real-time data analysis and remote communication between patients, healthcare providers, and medical devices. IoT devices, such as wearable devices, smart sensors, and telemedicine equipment, are equipped with AI and ML capabilities to monitor patients' vital signs, track physical activity, and transmit the data to healthcare providers for analysis. This empowers healthcare providers to remotely monitor patient health, diagnose conditions, and provide prompt medical attention without the need for in-person visits (Khang & Hajimahmud et al., 2023).

The integration of IoT, AI, and ML in remote monitoring leads to improved patient outcomes, reduced healthcare costs, and increased access to medical services, especially in remote or underserved areas. Furthermore, this combination of technologies enables real-time communication between patients and healthcare providers, enhancing patient engagement and empowerment. For example, Remote Monitoring Systems (RMS) powered by AI and ML algorithms enable COVID-19 patients to be monitored remotely from their homes, addressing issues related to overcrowded hospitals and limited bed availability. Severe cases can receive critical care services like mechanical ventilation in hospitals, while RMS prevents direct interaction between doctors and infected patients, reducing the risk of healthcare worker infections.

## 13.4 APPLICATIONS OF HIoT

IoT has been implemented in healthcare in various ways in recent years. Remote patient monitoring is one of the most significant applications of IoT, enabling healthcare providers to monitor patients' vital signs and health metrics remotely in real time. IoT technology is also being used to improve medication adherence, patient safety, and the patient experience. IoT-enabled pill dispensers can monitor whether patients are taking their medication as prescribed, RFID tags and sensors can be used to track medical equipment and supplies, and telemedicine services are becoming more common.

### 13.4.1 Oxygen Saturation Monitoring

Oxygen saturation monitoring is a critical aspect of detecting and managing various medical conditions by measuring the percentage of oxygen-carrying hemoglobin molecules. In the realm of IoT, this monitoring can be enhanced through the use of wearable devices, such as smartwatches or fitness trackers, equipped with sensors that track oxygen saturation levels in real-time. The collected data can then be transmitted to a central hub or the cloud, where it undergoes analysis using machine learning algorithms and artificial intelligence techniques (Hema et al., 2018).

By leveraging the power of machine learning and AI, IoT-based oxygen saturation monitoring becomes more than just a data collection tool. These technologies enable the identification of patterns and trends in the data, contributing to improved diagnosis, personalized treatment plans, and predictive analytics. Medical professionals can make informed decisions and provide accurate care based on real-time insights generated by these intelligent systems. Furthermore, integrating IoT-based oxygen saturation monitoring with other wearable devices, such as pulse oximeters, offers businesses opportunities to expand their product offerings and enhance their value proposition.

By combining oxygen saturation monitoring with additional health parameters, businesses can provide comprehensive health monitoring solutions to individuals and healthcare facilities. This integration allows for a more holistic approach to patient care and opens up new avenues for remote monitoring and telehealth services. The use of machine learning algorithms and AI in analyzing oxygen saturation data also contributes to cost optimization and operational efficiency for businesses. By automating data analysis and reducing manual intervention, healthcare providers can streamline their processes, improve resource allocation, and enhance patient outcomes. Moreover, the valuable insights generated from the data can be leveraged for research and development purposes, contributing to advancements in medical science and innovation (Khang & Rath et al., 2023).

### 13.4.2 Electrocardiogram Monitoring

The Internet of Things (IoT) has revolutionized the healthcare industry, providing new and innovative ways to monitor and manage various medical conditions. One such application of IoT is in electrocardiogram (ECG) monitoring, where the use of machine learning (ML) and artificial intelligence (AI) further enhances its capabilities. IoT-based ECG monitoring involves wearable devices such as smartwatches or fitness trackers equipped with ECG sensors. These devices continuously monitor the user's heart activity and transmit the data to a central hub or the cloud. The collected data can then be analyzed by healthcare professionals or ML algorithms to detect potential heart problems (Shaown et al., 2019).

The integration of ML and AI in IoT-based ECG monitoring enables advanced analysis of ECG data. These technologies can identify patterns and anomalies in real-time, enhancing the accuracy of heart problem detection and reducing false positives. ML algorithms can learn from large datasets and provide personalized insights and recommendations for patients, helping healthcare professionals make informed decisions regarding treatment options. IoT-based ECG monitoring offers several advantages over traditional methods.

IoT-based ECG monitoring offers real-time data for immediate response and potentially life-saving interventions in emergencies. ML and AI algorithms analyze the data quickly, providing actionable insights for appropriate treatments. Remote monitoring allows patients to monitor their heart activity from home, reducing hospital visits, while healthcare professionals can remotely access and review ECG data for timely intervention. Additionally, IoT-based ECG monitoring eliminates the need for expensive ECG machines, providing a cost-effective solution that is portable and scalable. This accessibility promotes preventive care and early detection of heart conditions for a wider population.

From a business perspective, IoT-based ECG monitoring opens up opportunities for healthcare providers and technology companies. Businesses can develop and offer innovative wearable devices with ECG monitoring capabilities, catering to the growing demand for remote health monitoring solutions. The integration of ML and AI allows for value-added services such as personalized insights, data analytics, and predictive models, which can further enhance patient care and engagement.

### 13.4.3 Body Temperature Monitoring

The Internet of Things (IoT) has brought about significant advancements in the monitoring and analysis of various health parameters, including body temperature. Wearable devices and smart thermometers with IoT technology can track and transmit real-time body temperature data to a connected platform, enabling individuals to monitor their temperature and detect fever or changes efficiently. The integration of ML and AI further enhances IoT-based body temperature monitoring. ML and AI algorithms can analyze the vast amounts of temperature data collected through IoT devices. These technologies can identify patterns, trends, and anomalies, enabling early detection of illnesses and proactive preventive measures. By leveraging big data analytics, healthcare professionals can gain valuable insights from the temperature data, improving diagnosis accuracy and treatment decisions. In remote monitoring, IoT technology enables contactless measurement of body temperature, which is particularly useful for individuals with chronic conditions or those needing continuous temperature monitoring, such as COVID-19 patients. This approach eliminates the need for physical visits to healthcare facilities, reducing the risk of exposure to infections and enhancing patient care.

From a business perspective, integrating ML, AI, and IoT in body temperature monitoring opens up opportunities for healthcare providers and technology companies. Businesses can develop innovative wearable devices and smart thermometers, offering comprehensive solutions for remote temperature monitoring. ML and AI capabilities can be harnessed to provide personalized insights, predictive analytics, and data-driven recommendations, enhancing the value proposition for both patients and healthcare professionals. Furthermore, IoT-based body temperature monitoring combined with ML and AI can lead to cost optimization and operational efficiency in healthcare settings. Automation of data analysis and decision-making processes reduces manual efforts, streamlines workflows, and improves resource allocation.

### 13.4.4 Glucose Level Monitoring

The healthcare industry is experiencing a transformative shift through the adoption of the Internet of Things (IoT). One notable application of IoT in healthcare is the monitoring of glucose levels in diabetics, which is being significantly enhanced by the integration of machine learning (ML) and artificial intelligence (AI) technologies. IoT glucose monitoring systems employ wearable devices like continuous glucose monitoring (CGM) devices that measure glucose levels and transmit the data wirelessly to a smartphone app. The app displays the glucose levels in a user-friendly format and sends alerts if the levels deviate from a predetermined safe range. Furthermore, the app can provide insights and recommendations for managing glucose levels, enabling data sharing with healthcare providers for more personalized and proactive care (Valenzuela et al., 2020).

The integration of ML and AI in IoT-enabled glucose monitoring systems further enhances their capabilities. These technologies can analyze the collected glucose data in real-time and learn from it to provide personalized insights and predictive analytics. ML and AI algorithms can identify patterns, detect trends, and even forecast future glucose levels, empowering both patients and healthcare professionals to make informed decisions and take proactive measures.

IoT-based glucose monitoring systems provide real-time monitoring, eliminating frequent blood tests and enabling continuous understanding of glucose levels. This feedback allows timely interventions and adjustments in diabetes management. Additionally, IoT-enabled systems offer a convenient and non-invasive approach, reducing the need for finger pricks and improving user comfort and compliance. These systems can track long-term glucose trends, enabling healthcare providers to gain insights and make informed treatment decisions using ML and AI algorithms. Overall, IoT-based glucose monitoring enhances diabetes management by offering real-time monitoring, convenience, and personalized care.

From a business standpoint, IoT-based glucose monitoring presents opportunities for healthcare providers and technology companies. Businesses can develop and market advanced wearable devices and smartphone apps that integrate ML and AI capabilities, offering comprehensive solutions for diabetes management. The combination of real-time monitoring, data analytics, and personalized insights creates value for both patients and healthcare professionals.

### 13.4.5 Mood Monitoring

The application of the Internet of Things (IoT) in mood monitoring has revolutionized how individuals track and manage their emotional states, with the integration of machine learning (ML) and artificial intelligence (AI) playing a significant role. By combining wearable devices, smart sensors, and ML algorithms, continuous monitoring of physiological signals such as heart rate, along with personal data like sleep patterns and physical activity, can estimate an individual's mood. The real-time data collected through IoT enables the easy detection of triggers and patterns in mood, offering valuable insights for individuals managing mood disorders and researchers studying the factors contributing to mood variations.

The integration of ML and AI enhances the capabilities of IoT-based mood monitoring systems. ML algorithms can learn from the collected data and improve the accuracy of mood estimation over time. AI techniques can further analyze the data, identify correlations, and provide personalized recommendations for managing mood. These technologies enable individuals to better understand their emotional well-being and empower them to take proactive measures for self-care and mood regulation. From a business perspective, IoT-based mood monitoring presents opportunities for healthcare providers and technology companies. Businesses can develop and market wearable devices, smart sensors, and mobile applications integrating ML and AI functionalities for mood monitoring. These solutions can provide users with personalized insights, actionable recommendations, and virtual assistant integration, offering convenient and accessible tools for mood management. Businesses can leverage IoT, ML, and AI to develop innovative solutions for mood monitoring.

However, there are challenges associated with the use of IoT in mood monitoring. Privacy and security concerns regarding personal data arise due to the collection and analysis of sensitive information. Ensuring the accuracy and reliability of ML algorithms used for mood estimation is another challenge that needs to be addressed.

### 13.4.6 Wheelchair Management

The Internet of Things (IoT) is revolutionizing wheelchair management, making it more efficient and user-friendly with the integration of machine learning (ML), artificial intelligence (AI), and business advancements. Smart wheelchairs equipped with multiple sensors, assistive technologies, and computers are replacing conventional wheelchairs, offering individuals with disabilities improved mobility and safety (Amur & Suresh, 2021). IoT-enabled wheelchairs can utilize sensors to detect changes in the user's posture and automatically adjust the seat for maximum comfort. This personalized adaptation enhances user experience and reduces the risk of discomfort or pressure sores.

Furthermore, IoT-enabled wheelchairs can be equipped with cameras that enable remote monitoring of the user's surroundings. This feature allows caregivers to provide timely assistance if necessary, promoting user independence and safety. The captured data can also be analyzed using ML and AI algorithms to identify potential hazards or obstacles, helping to prevent accidents and improve overall wheelchair navigation. ML and AI technologies play a crucial role in optimizing wheelchair performance and maintenance. By analyzing usage patterns and sensor data, ML algorithms can detect anomalies and predict potential issues, allowing for proactive maintenance and reducing the need for frequent repairs. This predictive maintenance approach enhances the reliability and lifespan of the wheelchair, ultimately benefiting users and reducing healthcare costs.

From a business perspective, IoT-based wheelchair management presents opportunities for innovation and service expansion. Companies can develop advanced IoT-enabled wheelchairs with ML and AI capabilities, integrating personalized features, remote monitoring, and predictive maintenance. This creates value for users, caregivers, and healthcare providers while fostering business growth and differentiation in the market.

### 13.4.7 Medication Management

The Internet of Things (IoT) has the potential to revolutionize medication management by integrating machine learning (ML) and artificial intelligence (AI), offering business opportunities. Through IoT, medication management becomes more efficient and accessible for patients. Smart devices, such as wearable devices or smart pills, can communicate with each other and a central hub to monitor and dispense medication accurately. For instance, a smart medicine box with light and heart rate sensors can track medication intake, sound alarms in case of overdose, and act as a reminder for medication adherence (Maju, 2015). Smart pills can also track ingestion and send alerts to patients and healthcare providers if doses are missed.

ML and AI technologies enhance medication management by analyzing the collected data. ML algorithms can detect patterns and trends in medication adherence and response, enabling personalized treatment plans. AI can provide intelligent reminders and recommendations, optimize medication schedules, and improve patient compliance. These technologies contribute to better health outcomes and patient satisfaction.

From a business perspective, IoT-based medication management presents opportunities for innovation and service expansion. Companies can develop smart devices, software platforms, and analytics solutions for medication monitoring and adherence. They can integrate ML and AI capabilities into medication management systems to offer personalized care, remote monitoring, and predictive analytics. This not only benefits patients but also creates new revenue streams for healthcare providers and technology companies. Moreover, the data generated by IoT medication management systems can be leveraged for research and development purposes. Aggregated and anonymized data can provide valuable insights into medication effectiveness, side effects, and patient responses. This information can fuel advancements in pharmaceuticals and improve treatment protocols.

### 13.4.8 Pharmacy Inventory Management

The Internet of Things (IoT) has the potential to revolutionize pharmacy inventory management by integrating machine learning (ML) and artificial intelligence (AI), offering significant business benefits. By leveraging IoT technologies, pharmacies can enhance the efficiency and effectiveness of inventory management. Smart devices such as sensors and RFID tags enable real-time inventory tracking, minimizing the risk of stockouts and overstocking. Sensors placed on shelves can monitor inventory levels and automatically trigger reordering when supplies are low. RFID tags attached to products enable precise tracking of their location, improving inventory accuracy and reducing the likelihood of theft or loss (Çakıcı et al., 2011).

ML and AI play a crucial role in optimizing pharmacy inventory management. ML algorithms can analyze historical sales data, customer trends, and external factors to forecast demand more accurately. This enables pharmacies to make informed purchasing decisions, reducing the risk of overstocking and minimizing waste. AI can further optimize inventory replenishment by automatically adjusting order quantities and frequencies based on demand fluctuations and supply chain dynamics. From a business perspective, IoT-based pharmacy inventory management offers substantial benefits. By minimizing stockouts and overstocking, pharmacies can improve customer satisfaction and loyalty. Optimized inventory levels also reduce carrying costs and minimize the risk of product expiration or obsolescence, improving profitability. Additionally, IoT-generated data provides valuable insights into customer preferences, enabling targeted marketing and personalized offerings.

Furthermore, the data generated by IoT inventory management systems can be utilized for business intelligence and decision-making. Advanced analytics can identify patterns and correlations, optimizing inventory planning and supply chain operations. Predictive analytics can identify potential inventory issues in advance, allowing proactive mitigation strategies to be implemented.

### 13.4.9 Rehabilitation Systems

The Internet of Things (IoT) has the potential to revolutionize rehabilitation systems by integrating machine learning (ML) and artificial intelligence (AI), offering significant business benefits. IoT-enabled rehabilitation systems enhance accessibility and personalization for patients. Equipping rehabilitation equipment with sensors, cameras, and smart devices makes real-time monitoring and control of the rehabilitation process possible. This enables more effective and efficient rehabilitation by tracking the patient's movements and providing real-time feedback. ML and AI algorithms can analyze the data collected from the sensors to personalize the rehabilitation program based on the patient's progress and specific needs (Câmara Gradim et al., September 2020).

Furthermore, IoT-based rehabilitation systems offer accessibility advantages. Patients can participate in rehabilitation exercises from the comfort of their homes using smart devices such as wearables or smartphone apps. This reduces the need for frequent visits to healthcare providers and makes rehabilitation more convenient for patients. ML and AI algorithms can continuously analyze patient data, providing personalized recommendations and adapting the rehabilitation plan as necessary, enhancing the effectiveness of remote rehabilitation programs.

From a business perspective, IoT-driven rehabilitation systems offer significant benefits. These systems can improve patient outcomes, leading to higher patient satisfaction and loyalty. ML and AI can analyze the data collected during rehabilitation sessions to identify patterns and correlations, enabling healthcare providers to optimize rehabilitation protocols and customize treatment plans. This personalized approach enhances the patient experience and improves overall rehabilitation results. Additionally, the data generated by IoT rehabilitation systems can be utilized for business intelligence and decision-making. Advanced analytics can identify trends, patterns, and insights that can inform strategic planning, resource allocation, and optimization of rehabilitation services. By leveraging this data-driven approach, healthcare providers can improve operational efficiency, streamline workflows, and allocate resources more effectively.

### 13.4.10 Other Notable Applications of HIoT

The IoT has had a profound impact on the healthcare industry, leveraging ML and AI technologies and offering significant business advantages. Remote patient monitoring, made possible by IoT, enables real-time tracking of patients' health parameters, allowing healthcare providers to monitor their condition remotely. ML and AI algorithms can analyze the data collected from IoT devices, such as wearable sensors or smart home devices, to detect patterns and anomalies, facilitating early detection of potential health issues and enabling timely interventions. This proactive approach improves patient outcomes and reduces healthcare costs by minimizing the need for hospital visits and preventing complications (Pradhan et al., 2021).

IoT also revolutionizes hospital operations through the implementation of Smart Hospital solutions. By utilizing IoT sensors and connectivity, medical equipment and supplies can be tracked in real-time, optimizing inventory management, minimizing waste, and improving efficiency. IoT-powered patient flow management systems streamline the movement of patients within the hospital, reducing wait times and enhancing the overall patient experience. ML and AI algorithms can analyze the data collected from IoT devices to identify bottlenecks, predict demand, and optimize resource allocation, further improving hospital operations and patient care.

Telemedicine, another significant application of IoT, enables virtual consultations and remote healthcare delivery. Through IoT-enabled devices, patients can consult with healthcare providers from the comfort of their homes, reducing the need for travel and enhancing accessibility to medical expertise. ML and AI can support telemedicine by providing decision support systems, analyzing patient data for diagnostic purposes, and facilitating remote monitoring and care management. IoT's integration with electronic medical records (EMRs) and clinical trials enhances data collection and analysis. Medical devices can seamlessly transmit data to EMRs, improving data accuracy and streamlining documentation processes. ML and AI algorithms can analyze this wealth of data to extract valuable insights for research, clinical trials, and predictive analytics. These insights can inform evidence-based medicine, personalized treatments, and predictive models for disease management.

From a business perspective, IoT offers numerous advantages. It enables healthcare providers to deliver more efficient and personalized care, enhancing patient satisfaction and loyalty. By leveraging ML and AI technologies, healthcare organizations can extract actionable insights from IoT-generated data, improving decision-making processes, optimizing resource allocation, and driving operational efficiency. Additionally, IoT solutions in healthcare open up opportunities for innovative business models, such as remote monitoring services and data analytics platforms.

## 13.5 REAL-TIME HIoT USE CASES

The growing volume of data generated and transmitted by modern systems necessitates efficient data transfer and real-time communication. Complex systems consist of numerous interconnected modules or nodes, which may be distributed across a network or housed on a single computer. Integrating AI and ML enhances the capabilities of IoT in various real-life applications. Let's explore some use cases where IoT, combined with AI and ML, is implemented:

### 13.5.1 Baby Monitoring

IoT, AI, and ML technologies are leveraged in baby monitoring systems, providing real-time information and peace of mind to parents. The accessibility of high-speed Internet and the widespread use of mobile phones have contributed to the popularity of such systems. To address concerns about baby monitoring, the integration of AI and ML algorithms enhances the capabilities of IoT in the following use cases:

- **Smart Baby Monitors**: AI and ML algorithms analyze camera and sensor data from IoT-enabled baby monitors to track the baby's movement, sleep patterns, and temperature. This information is then sent to a mobile app for parents to monitor and receive actionable insights.
- **Wearable Baby Monitors**: IoT-enabled wearable devices equipped with AI and ML algorithms continuously monitor the baby's vital signs, such as heart rate and breathing. In case of any deviations, alerts are generated to notify parents and provide timely intervention.

- **Smart Nursery Devices**: IoT technology, enhanced by AI and ML, is utilized in smart nursery devices like cribs and bassinets. These devices monitor the baby's sleep patterns and environment, leveraging AI algorithms to ensure a comfortable and safe sleeping environment.
- **Video Baby Monitors with Intelligent Analytics**: IoT-enabled video baby monitors, integrated with AI and ML algorithms, enable intelligent analytics of live video and audio feeds. These algorithms can detect and alert parents to specific events, such as crying or unusual movements.

The integration of AI and ML with IoT in baby monitoring systems enhances real-time monitoring, improves safety, and provides valuable insights for parents.

### 13.5.2 Fitness

IoT, AI, and ML technologies play a crucial role in the fitness industry by providing individuals with real-time data and personalized experiences. With the integration of AI and ML algorithms, IoT-based fitness solutions offer enhanced capabilities in the following use cases:

- **Wearable Fitness Devices**: IoT-enabled wearable devices equipped with AI and ML algorithms track physical activity, heart rate, sleep patterns, and other relevant data. AI algorithms analyze this data to provide personalized feedback, exercise recommendations, and insights into overall fitness progress.
- **Smart Home Gym Equipment**: IoT-connected gym equipment integrated with AI and ML algorithms captures workout data, allowing AI systems to provide personalized workout plans based on individual goals, preferences, and progress.
- **Virtual Fitness Coaches**: AI-powered virtual fitness coaches utilize data from wearable devices, along with personalized user profiles, to deliver tailored fitness advice, motivation, and guidance. These virtual coaches can adapt their recommendations based on real-time data analysis.
- **Smart Clothing**: IoT-enabled smart clothing, combined with AI and ML algorithms, tracks various fitness-related metrics such as physical activity, heart rate, and posture. AI systems provide real-time feedback and guidance to improve performance and prevent injuries.

The integration of AI and ML with IoT technology in the fitness industry enhances personalization, improves workout effectiveness, and enables individuals to achieve their fitness goals more efficiently.

### 13.5.3 Health and Nutrition

AI and ML, when combined with IoT, play a significant role in improving health and nutrition outcomes. Real-time data analysis and personalized experiences are made possible in the following use cases:

- **Wearable Health Devices**: IoT-enabled wearable devices integrated with AI and ML algorithms capture and analyze health-related data, including physical activity, heart rate, sleep patterns, and nutrition intake. AI systems provide real-time feedback on health status and personalized recommendations for maintaining optimal well-being.
- **Smart Kitchen Devices**: IoT-connected kitchen devices, enhanced by AI and ML, offer features such as tracking food intake, providing nutritional information, and suggesting healthy recipes based on an individual's dietary needs. AI algorithms analyze data to deliver personalized dietary recommendations.
- **Telemedicine**: IoT-enabled telemedicine platforms, supported by AI and ML, facilitate remote consultations, diagnosis, and treatment. AI systems analyze patient data and assist healthcare providers in delivering accurate diagnoses and personalized treatment plans.
- **Health Monitoring Devices**: IoT-based health monitoring devices integrated with AI and ML algorithms track and store health data, enabling early detection of health issues and personalized recommendations for individuals. AI systems can identify patterns and trends in the data to provide proactive healthcare insights.

Integrating AI and ML with IoT technology in health and nutrition promotes real-time monitoring, personalized interventions, and improved health outcomes for individuals.

By combining IoT with AI and ML, these real-time use cases demonstrate the transformative potential of these technologies in various domains, including baby monitoring, fitness, and health and nutrition.

## 13.6 CHALLENGES OF HIoT

### 13.6.1 Technical Challenges

Rapid technological advancements have enabled the creation of affordable, high-tech IoT devices; however, the increasing volume of generated data poses challenges that require improved networks and storage solutions. IoT device manufacturers face balancing technical limitations, time constraints, and cost considerations while deciding whether to invest in compatibility with industry standards. The environmental impact of billions of batteries required to power IoT devices also necessitates more eco-friendly alternatives. To address these issues, the convergence of AI and ML technologies is crucial in establishing standardized frameworks and networks for IoT devices, ensuring interoperability and integration into cohesive systems.

Challenges such as data security, reliability, power management, connectivity, storage, and regulatory compliance must be overcome (Van & Bassi, 2012). Robust security measures are vital for protecting sensitive patient data during transmission and storage, while reliable performance of IoT devices is critical to avoid potential harm to patients. Effective power management, seamless network connectivity, and ample data transmission capacity are necessary for the optimal use of IoT devices in healthcare, alongside integration with existing systems and adherence to regulatory standards, presenting significant business opportunities.

### 13.6.2 Cost

The architecture of HIoT presents significant expenses, which can be daunting for many individuals. One contributing factor to these high costs is the need for advanced infrastructure that keeps pace with the rapidly evolving technology. This includes investments in AI and ML capabilities, which are crucial for processing and analyzing the vast amounts of data generated by HIoT devices. Additionally, there are substantial upfront expenses associated with obtaining government approvals for medical devices, as well as ongoing maintenance and upgrades.

Financial challenges also arise from data storage, network infrastructure, and system integration, particularly for healthcare organizations with limited IT resources. Staff training is another cost consideration. IoT device manufacturers face technical and cost constraints that influence device design, leading to trade-offs in implementing standards and interoperability features. Furthermore, addressing the security and privacy challenges of HIoT requires significant investments in technology and processes, as ensuring the confidentiality and protection of sensitive data generated by HIoT devices is a complex and costly endeavor.

### 13.6.3 Ethics

The proliferation of HIoT devices in healthcare introduces ethical challenges, including privacy and security risks, data ownership and control concerns, device reliability, accuracy issues, potential bias and discrimination, and cost and accessibility barriers (Sarhan, 2018). AI and ML can play a crucial role in addressing these challenges and unlocking business opportunities. By leveraging AI and ML algorithms, healthcare organizations can enhance privacy and security measures, implement robust data governance frameworks, and ensure the reliable and accurate performance of IoT devices. Moreover, AI and ML techniques can help identify and mitigate biases in data and algorithms, fostering fair and equitable healthcare outcomes. Additionally, exploring cost-effective solutions and promoting accessibility initiatives can ensure that the benefits of HIoT reach all individuals, regardless of their socio-economic background. By responsibly integrating AI, ML, and business strategies, can healthcare harness the potential of HIoT devices while upholding ethical standards and creating new avenues for innovation and growth?

## 13.7 STRENGTHS, WEAKNESSES, OPPORTUNITIES, AND CHALLENGES ANALYSIS—HEALTHCARE AND IoT

SWOC analysis in IoT healthcare examines the strengths, weaknesses, opportunities, and challenges associated with implementing IoT technologies in the healthcare sector. Figure 13.3 shows the various components of SWOC analysis of HIoT. It helps assess the real-time monitoring capabilities, data collection, and personalized interventions that IoT offers as strengths. However, weaknesses such as data security

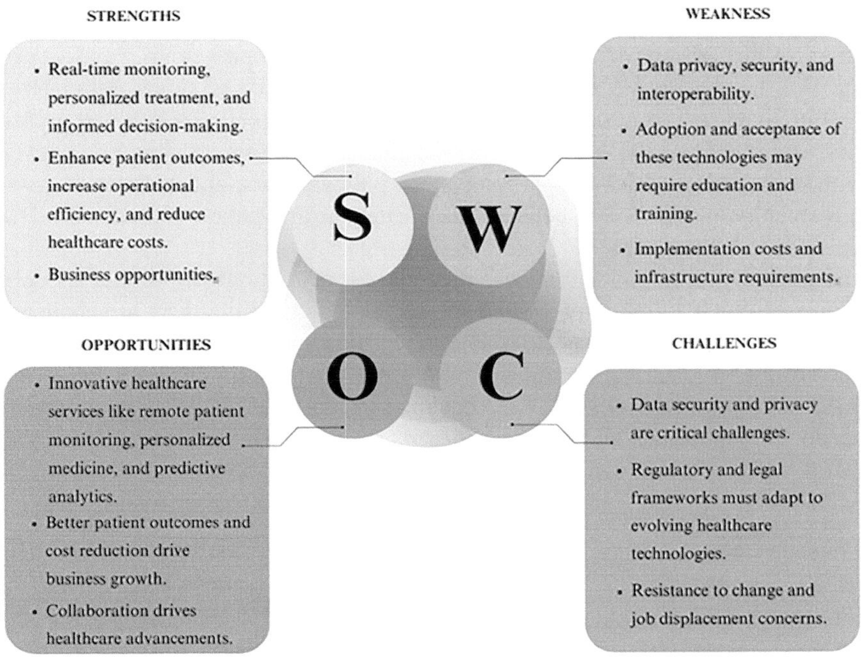


**FIGURE 13.3** SWOC analysis of HIoT.

and privacy concerns need to be considered. Opportunities include streamlining operations and improving patient experiences, while threats include interoperability challenges, regulatory complexities, and data breaches.

## 13.8 CONCLUSION

AI and ML technologies have the potential to greatly enhance the potential of IoT in healthcare, automating patient care workflows and creating new business opportunities. Healthcare mobility solutions empowered by IoT can leverage AI and ML algorithms to analyze the vast amount of patient data collected from wearable sensors and remote monitoring devices in real time. This enables predictive diagnosis, personalized treatment plans, and more efficient drug discovery processes, utilizing big data from numerous patients. The integration of AI and ML into HIoT devices opens up new prospects for revolutionizing healthcare delivery (Rani et al., 2021).

The future prospects of HIoT are promising, as it enables personalized, efficient, and accessible healthcare services. Real-time patient monitoring through wearable sensors allows for tailored treatment plans and targeted therapies, resulting in improved patient health and cost reduction. Healthcare providers can remotely monitor patients, leveraging AI and ML for informed decision-making and enhanced outcomes. This integration of technologies has the potential to transform the healthcare industry, leading to better patient outcomes and overall healthcare improvements (Khang & Ragimova et al., 2022).

However, the widespread adoption of IoT devices in healthcare also poses various challenges that must be addressed. These challenges encompass privacy and security concerns, data ownership and control, device reliability and accuracy, data interoperability, liability and responsibility, bias and discrimination, and cost and accessibility issues. Effective resolution of these challenges requires collaboration between healthcare providers, technology companies, policymakers, and patients to ensure the realization of IoT device benefits while safeguarding patient rights and welfare (Khang & Rana et al., 2023).

In summary, HIoT holds immense potential for revolutionizing healthcare delivery through the integration of AI and ML technologies. While there are challenges to overcome, the future prospects of HIoT are promising, with the ability to provide personalized, efficient, and accessible healthcare services that improve patient outcomes and drive advancements in the healthcare industry. Collaboration and careful consideration of ethical and privacy concerns are crucial in harnessing the benefits of HIoT while ensuring patient welfare (Aakansha et al., 2023).

## REFERENCES

Aakansha, C. S., Ojha, A., Sobti, D., & Khang, A. (2023). Artificial intelligence (AI) centric model in metaverse ecosystem. In *AI-based technologies and applications in the era of the metaverse* (1st Ed., pp. 1–24). IGI Global Press. https://doi.org/10.4018/978-1-6684-8851-5.ch001

Amur, M., & Suresh, K. (2021). *IoT based smart wheelchair for disabled people*. IEEE. https://doi.org/10.1109/ICSCAN53069.2021.9526427.

Anh, P. T. N., Hahanov, V., Triwiyanto, Ragimova, N. A., Rashad, İ., Abdullayev, V., Abuzarova, V. A. (2024). AI models for disease diagnosis and prediction of heart disease with artificial neural networks. In *Computer vision and AI-integrated IoT technologies in medical ecosystem* (1st Ed.). CRC Press. https://doi.org/10.1201/9781003429609-9

Aqeel-Ur-Rehman, M., Mehmood, K., & Baksh, A. (2013). Communication technology that suits IoT – A critical review. In *Wireless sensor networks for developing countries* (pp. 14–25). Springer. https://doi.org/10.1007/978-3-642-41054-3_2

Bkheet, S. A., & Agbinya, J. I. (2021). A review of identity methods of internet of things (IOT). *Advances in Internet of Things*, 11(4), 153–174. https://doi.org/10.4236/ait.2021.114011

Çakıcı, Ö.E., Groenevelt, H., & Seidmann, A. (2011). Using RFID for the management of pharmaceutical inventory-system optimization and shrinkage control. *Decision Support Systems*, 51(4), 842–852. doi:10.1016/j.dss.2011.02.003

Câmara Gradim, L. C., Archanjo José, M., Marinho Cezar da Cruz, D., & de Deus Lopes, R. (2020, September). IoT services and applications in rehabilitation: An interdisciplinary and meta-analysis review. *IEEE Transactions on Neural Systems and Rehabilitation Engineering*, 28(9), 2043–2052. https://doi.org/10.1109/TNSRE.2020.3005616

Hema, L. K., Priya, R. M., & Indumathi, R. (2018). Design and development of IOT based pulse oximeter. *International Journal of Pure and Applied Mathematics*, 119(16), 1863–1868.

Khang, A. (2024). *AI and IoT-based technologies for precision medicine*. IGI Global Press. ISBN: 9798369308769. https://doi.org/10.4018/979-8-3693-0876-9

Khang, A., Abdullayev, V. A., Hrybiuk, O., & Shukla, A. K. (2024). *Computer vision and AI-integrated IoT technologies in medical ecosystem* (1st Ed.). CRC Press. https://doi.org/10.1201/9781003429609

Khang, A., Hajimahmud, V. A., Gupta, S. K., Babasaheb, J., & Morris, G. (2023). *AI-centric modelling and analytics: Concepts, designs, technologies, and applications* (1st Ed.). CRC Press. https://doi.org/10.1201/9781003400110

Khang, A., Misra, A., Gupta, S. K., & Shah, V. (2023). *AI-aided IoT technologies and applications in the smart business and production*. CRC Press. https://doi.org/10.1201/9781003392224

Khang, A., Ragimova, N. A., Hajimahmud, V. A., & Alyar, V. A. (2022). Advanced technologies and data management in the smart healthcare system. In *AI-centric smart city ecosystems: Technologies, design and implementation* (1st Ed., vol. 16, p. 10). CRC Press. https://doi.org/10.1201/9781003252542-16

Khang, A., Rana, G., Tailor, R. K., & Hajimahmud, V. A. (2023). *Data-centric AI solutions and emerging technologies in the healthcare ecosystem*. CRC Press. https://doi.org/10.1201/9781003356189

Khang, A., Rath, K. C., Panda, S., Sree, P. K., & Panda, S. K. (2023). Revolutionizing agriculture: Exploring advanced technologies for plant protection in the agriculture sector. *Handbook of Research on AI-Equipped IoT Applications in High-Tech Agriculture*, 1–22. Copyright: © 2023. https://doi.org/10.4018/978-1-6684-9231-4.ch001

Maju, S. V. (2015, September). PAV secure health IOT for patient monitoring with intelligent medicine box. *International Journal of Electronics Communication and Computer Engineering, NCRTCST-2015*, 5(6), ISSN 2249-071X. http://ijecce.org/Download/conference/NCRTCST-3/6.pdf

Marques, G., Garcia, N., & Pombo, N. (2017). A survey on IoT: Architectures, elements, applications, QoS, platforms and security concepts. *Advances in Mobile Cloud Computing and Big Data in the 5G*, 115–130. https://doi.org/10.1007/978-3-319-45145-9_5

Porkodi, R., & Bhuvaneswari, V. (2014). *The Internet of things (IoT) applications and communication enabling technology standards: An overview*. International Conference on Intelligent Computing Applications. https://doi.org/10.1109/ICICA.2014.73

Pradhan, B., Bhattacharyya, S., & Pal, K. (2021). IoT-based applications in healthcare devices. *Journal of Healthcare Engineering*, 6632599. doi:10.1155/2021/6632599

Rana, G., Khang, A., Sharma, R., Goel, A. K., & Dubey, A. K. (2021). *Reinventing manufacturing and business processes through artificial intelligence*. CRC Press. https://doi.org/10.1201/9781003145011

Rani, S., Chauhan, M., Kataria, A., & Khang, A. (2021). IoT equipped intelligent distributed framework for smart healthcare systems. *Networking and Internet Architecture*, 2, 30. https://doi.org/10.48550/arXiv.2110.04997

Sarhan, Q. I. (2018). Internet of things: A survey of challenges and issues. *International Journal of Internet of Things and Cyber-Assurance*, 1(1), 40. https://doi.org/10.1504/IJITCA.2018.10011246

Shaown, T., Hasan, I., Mim, M. M. R., & Hossain, M. S. (2019). *IoT-based portable ECG monitoring system for smart healthcare*. 1st International Conference on Advances in Science, Engineering and Robotics Technology. https://doi.org/10.1109/ICASERT.2019.8934622

Valenzuela, F., García, A., Ruiz. E., Vázquez, M., Cortez, J., & Espinoza, A. (2020). An IoT-based glucose monitoring algorithm to prevent diabetes complications. *Applied Sciences*, 10(3), 921. https://doi.org/10.3390/app10030921

Van Kranenburg, R., & Bassi, A. (2012, November 28). IoT challenges. *Communications in Mobile Computing*, 1(1). https://doi.org/10.1186/2192-1121-1-9

Vrushank, S., & Khang, A. (2023). Metaverse-enabling IoT technology for a futuristic healthcare system. In *AI-based technologies and applications in the era of the metaverse* (1st Ed., p. 1). IGI Global Press. https://doi.org/10.4018/978-1-6684-8851-5.ch008

# 14 Diabetes and Machine Learning
## *A Mathematical Perspective*

*Tarun Kasida Zahoor and Avijit Kumar Chaudhuri*

### 14.1 INTRODUCTION

Diabetes mellitus (DM) is a disease affecting the synthesis and secretion of the hormone insulin. It triggers abnormal carbohydrate metabolism and elevated blood sugar levels. The rise in the blood glucose level severely affects the other organs of the human body which can aggravate other complications of the nerves and blood veins (Cloete, 2022). The prevalent forms of diabetes are Type 1 (T1DM), Type 2 (T2DM), Gestational Diabetes, and Neonatal Diabetes. T1DM is popularly known as insulin-dependent diabetes because of its characteristic attribute of insulin deficiency that arises due to the progressive destruction of pancreatic β-cells triggered usually by an autoimmune response. On the other hand, T2DM is characteristically associated with insulin resistance. The reasons for resistance are obesity due to poor dietary and lifestyle habits, the presence of hyperglycemic conditions due to circulating non-esterified fatty acids (NEFA), or reduced insulin gene expression (Banday et al., 2020; Tan et al., 2019). The causes behind the origin of this disease have not been discovered, with researchers debating the involvement of heredity or environmental factors as the major causative agents (Blair et al., 2016).

Considering the outreach, statistical data from the Canadian Diabetes Association (CDA) have reported the total number of individual persons afflicted with diabetes to have escalated to 3.7 million from 2.5 million between 2010 and 2020 (Mashayekhi et al., 2015). According to the International Diabetes Federation, 382 million people were found to suffer from Diabetes mellitus in 2013, constituting 6.6% of the global adult population (Jegan et al., 2013). Furthermore, data from World Healthcare Medical predicted a rise in diabetics from 376 billion to 490 billion by 2030 (Giorda et al., 2011). In terms of pathophysiology, it independently contributes to micro-vascular entanglements, making diabetic patients vulnerable to events of micro-vascular damage. It causes long-term complications affecting the different organs of the body. The micro-vascular impairment and cardiological ailments ultimately prompt retinopathy, nephropathy, and neuropathy (Barakat et al., 2009).

Therefore, an early prediction of diabetes becomes indispensable for controlling the diseased condition and saving human lives. Owing to massive technological developments, there has been a rise in predictive tools, mathematical models, and computer programming techniques for researchers (Kumar et al., 2022). Machine

 DOI: 10.1201/9781032686745-14

learning programs help in the faster detection and effective diagnosis of diseases, as shown in Figure 14.1.

Machine learning techniques employ the construction of predictive mathematical models for efficiently extracting knowledge from diagnostic medical datasets of diseased patients. The K-Nearest Neighbors (KNN) classifier is a simple, non-parametric approach for the classification of unlabeled observations by assigning them to the most similar labeled class. It is frequently used in datasets where data is organized into separate clusters and helps in determining the new input class (Zhang et al., 2016; Uddin et al., 2022).

Support Vector Machine (SVM) is an advanced and supervised machine language algorithm for classification and regression problems. It is a powerful tool to recognize subtle patterns in complex datasets. SVM creates a decision boundary between two classes and helps predict labels from the feature vectors. It is widely used in diagnostics and therapeutics for cancer and other deadly diseases (Huang et al., 2018; Thanh et al., 2017). Naïve Bayes classifiers are defined as a collection of classification algorithms designed using Bayes' Theorem. This family of algorithms is widely used

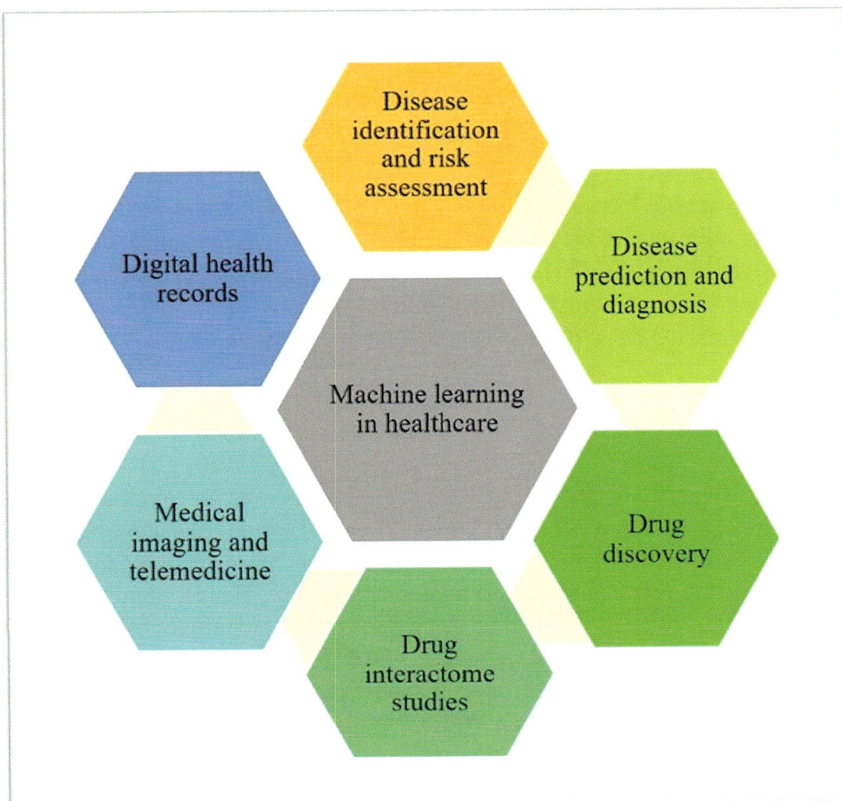


**FIGURE 14.1** Advantages of machine learning in healthcare.

as substitutes for logistic regression models with formulated variable dependency or independency. It has found increased application in recent disease prediction and drug response mathematical models (Langarizadeh et al., 2016; Guo et al., 2018).

The Random Forest technique is a regression tree technique that characteristically consists of bootstrap aggregation and randomization of predictors. In scientific realms, the Random Forest (RF) algorithm has been widely practiced in simplifying high-dimensional and multi-source data. It provides a superior level of predictive accuracy in disease models and biomarker analysis (Rigatti et al., 2017; Sarica et al., 2017). C4.5 is a widely used decision tree algorithm with a high-level accuracy independent of the data volume to be processed. It can handle incomplete datasets or continuous attributes through the binarization process (Cherfi et al., 2018). WEKA (Waikato Environment for Knowledge Analysis) is a popularly used software consisting of a collection of machine learning algorithms for data mining tasks. It can be used for effective data preparation, classification, regression, clustering, etc. (Cherfi et al., 2018).

Therefore, our paper mainly focuses on the early prediction of diabetes by considering the various risk factors associated with the disease (Faruque et al., 2019). For this study, we collected a diagnostic dataset composed of eight attributes of 769 patients. Thereafter, we comprehensively discussed these attributes with their corresponding values and built a prediction model. We decided to use four popular machine learning algorithms, namely Support Vector Machine (SVM), Naïve Bayes (NB), Random Forest, K-Nearest Neighbor (KNN), and C4.5 decision tree, on adult population data to predict diabetes mellitus. We conducted a collection of real diagnostic datasets composed of varied risk factors of diabetes, performance comparison of different machine learning techniques, and evaluation of the prediction results based on the relevant risk factors. Other parts of the chapter include a literature survey of the related work, a detailed description of methodologies, the results and discussion section summarizing the major findings of this chapter, and the conclusion section summarizing the essence of this chapter and the significance of our practical findings.

## 14.2 RELATED WORK

Due to the increased prevalence of diabetes globally and its association with many other diseases, it becomes necessary to conduct research on managing the disease. Diabetes has posed considerable challenges in the effective detection and diagnosis, thereby impairing therapeutic interventional approaches. Hence, many researchers have conducted studies in the field of machine learning techniques of diabetes prediction and data mining from available medical data sources to comprehensively diagnose the disease and provide routes for subsequent biological research. Through this chapter, we sought to provide a brief literature review on the machine-learning perspectives of disease prediction and diagnosis (Khang et al., 2023).

Aljumah et al. (2013) studied and developed a predictive analysis model by utilizing the Support Vector Machine algorithm. Their research dealt with the analysis of diabetic treatment through a regression-based data mining technique. The authors used Oracle Data Miner (ODM) as the major mining software for efficient prediction.

They analyzed the effectiveness of different treatment modalities using a predictive algorithm (Aljumah et al., 2013). Similarly, Kavakiotis et al. (2017) conducted a systematic review of machine learning applications, data mining tools, and techniques in the field of diabetes research, considering its various facets such as Prediction and Diagnosis, Complications, Genetic Background, Environment, and Health Care Management. The authors employed 10-fold cross-validation as an evaluation method in three different algorithms, namely logistic regression, Naïve Bayes, and SVM. They reported that SVM provided better performance and accuracy, ranging to 84% when compared to other algorithms (Kavakiotis et al., 2017). Early-stage prediction of diabetes mellitus was performed by Zheng et al. (2017). The authors applied Random Forest, KNN, SVM, Naïve Bayes, Decision tree, and Logistic Regression and employed improvised filtering criteria in their study. Their proposed framework exhibited an accurate and efficient approach to identifying T2DM subjects from electronic health records (Zheng et al., 2017).

Scientists used to propose mathematical applications like KNN, J48, ANN, ZeroR, and NB on various diabetes datasets to compared and evaluated classification algorithms' performance (Rani et al., 2016). Similarly, Khang and Abdullayev et al. (2024) also compared the performance of classification algorithms by using KNN, J48, SVM, and Random Forest and reported improved performance from the J48 machine learning algorithm with higher rates of accuracy than the other algorithms in the context of pre-processing techniques. The cross-validation method was not evaluated using classification algorithms in their study (Kandhasamy et al., 2015). For accurate prediction and control of diabetes mellitus, Huang et al. (2007) discussed three data mining techniques, including IB1, Naïve Bayes, and C4.5. Their dataset was gathered from Ulster Community and Hospitals Trust (UCHT) from 2000 to 2004. Feature selection technique was applied and consequently led to better results and improved performance of IB1 and Naïve Bayes (Huang et al., 2007).

In another study, Khang et al. (2023) wanted to compare the performance of logistic regression, artificial neural networks (ANNs), and decision tree models in the prediction of diabetes using common risk factors. The authors employed real-world data sets through the collection of information after the distributed questionnaire. They concluded that the decision tree model (C5.0) showed the best classification accuracy, followed by the logistic regression model, and the ANN gave the lowest accuracy (Meng et al., 2013). Thus, our research would aim to analyze real diagnostic medical data by incorporating various risk factors using machine learning classification techniques and subsequently evaluate their performance for coherent prediction of diabetes mellitus.

## 14.3 METHODOLOGY

For the achievement of our objectives, the study methodology is composed of different stages that are mainly associated with the compilation of diabetes dataset with the relevant patient attributes, pre-processing the numeric value attributes, application of myriad machine learning classification techniques, and predictive analysis corresponding to the data, as shown in Figure 14.2.

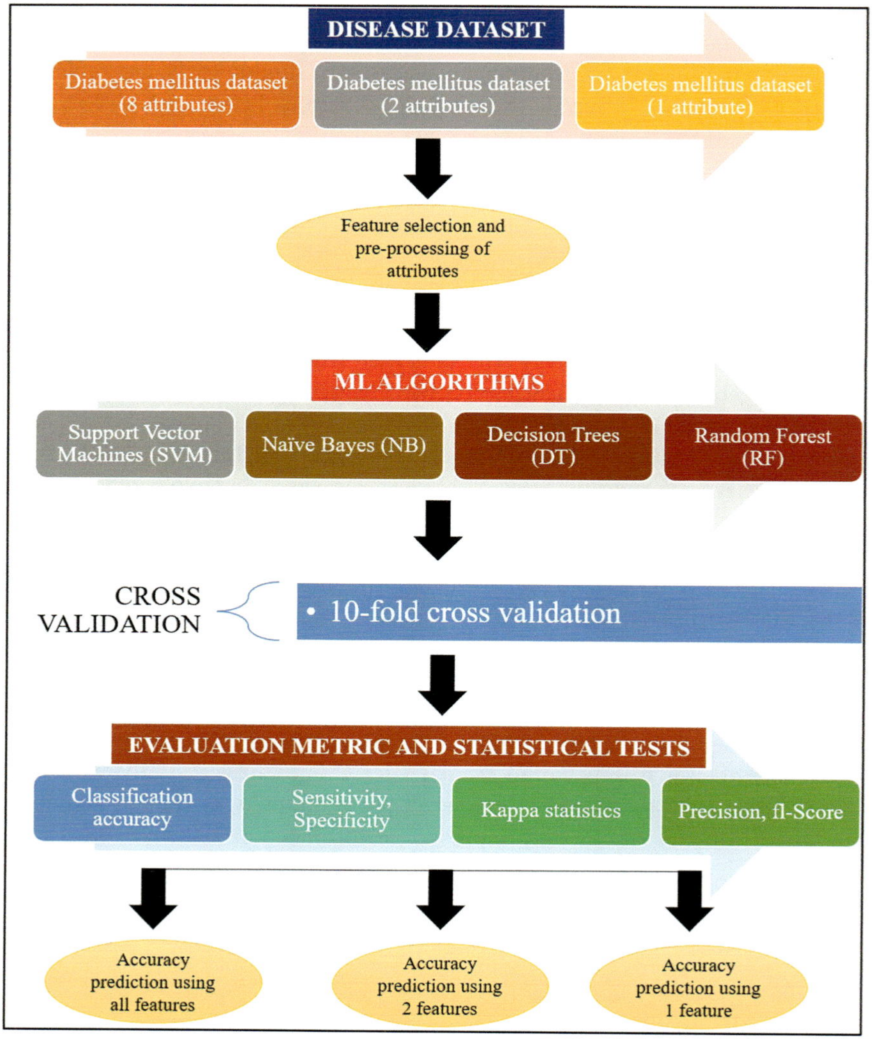


**FIGURE 14.2** Detailed overview of the methodology.

### 14.3.1 Dataset and Attributes

Datasets and attributes form the foundational principle for training, evaluating, and benchmarking machine learning models and hypotheses. Therefore, the collection of raw data, setting up key attributes, organization of data, and analysis are important parts of the overall methodology for most research work (Paullada et al., 2021). Furthermore, patient datasets provide weightage to the data and research findings since they form the primary data source and are outsourced directly from patients for effective validation and evidence. For the efficacious accomplishment of this work, Diabetes patient data has been collected from the diagnostic and primary health care centers in Kolkata, India. The dataset is composed of numerous attributes or risk factors of diabetes mellitus in 769 patients. The various chosen attributes are age, pregnancy, blood pressure, skin thickness, glucose levels, insulin, body-mass index (BMI), and diabetes pedigree function.

### 14.3.2 Apply Machine Learning Techniques

After the pre-processing and proper accumulation of data, four popular machine-learning classification techniques were employed for the proper and holistic prediction of diabetes mellitus. This study contributes to the development of medical informatics by utilizing the help of machine learning and artificial intelligence programs to develop new patterns of information beyond determining generalized biological relationships between laboratory data and diseases. In the following paragraphs, the different machine-learning techniques have been discussed briefly for comprehensive understanding.

### 14.3.3 Support Vector Machines

This is one of the most popular classification techniques proposed by J. Platt et al. (1998). A Support Vector Machine (SVM) can be defined as an excluded classifier, which plays a crucial role in formally characterizing the data by separating a hyperplane. Entities are isolated within specific clauses under the rules of SVM (Platt et al., 1998). In essence, an SVM is a mathematical algorithm that plays a critical role in maximizing a particular mathematical function upon comparison with a given collection of data (Noble et al., 2006). It can also be used in the identification and classification of attributes not supported by data. It does not care about the distribution of data acquisition for each class. Moreover, this algorithm can also be employed to execute regression analysis to produce a linear function. It can also be used for ranking elements to produce a coherent classification of individual elements (Faruque et al., 2019). In summary, during the procedure of a typical SVM, a set of training samples is provided, with samples being distributed into distinct categories followed by the application of machine learning algorithms to solve classification and regression issues.

### 14.3.4 Naïve Bayes

It is a very popular probabilistic classification technique proposed by John et al. (2013). Naïve Bayes or the Bayesian theorem is a simple, effective, and frequently used machine learning classifier. The algorithm utilizes probabilistic results by counting the frequency, and thereafter, the obtained values are combined together in a data set. In the Bayesian theorem, it is assumed that all attributes are independent and based on variable class values. However, in contrast to the assumption, the conditional independence assumption seldom holds true in real-world scenarios and gives more sophisticated classifier results (John et al., 2013). The Naïve Bayes model assumes that predictive features are independent of each other and conditioned on the state of a target class variable from the dataset. It has been widely used for classification and prediction purposes due to its simplicity of construction, easy applicability, rapid inference, and performance in practice compared to other algorithms (Wei et al., 2011).

### 14.3.5 Decision Trees (DT)

Decision trees are a systematic and widely used data mining method that provides powerful classification techniques to predict diabetes mellitus. It is comprised of discrete areas called the "classification" which are further divided into domains called a "class". The input feature of each class is labeled using an internal node within the tree. The leaf node is labeled by an attribute associated with a target value. The highest gain of information gain for all attributes is calculated for each node of the tree. The tree algorithms are of different types, such as the ID3, J48, C4.5, C5, CHAID, and CART. We have used the C4.5 decision tree algorithm for our research and powerful performance analysis of a diabetic dataset (Salzberg et al., 1994). The DT is proposed because of various benefits associated with it, such as:

- DT filtration techniques are easy to understand and implement.
- It provides a large-scale achievement in comparison with other techniques.
- It employs tree-like models for decision-making.
- They are proven mechanisms in the field of knowledge discovery.
- It can handle a wide amount of data ranging from text, ratio, nominal and ordinal.
- DT classifiers are found in supervised classification extraction patterns and can even process datasets with missing values, thereby adding enigma to its characteristic beneficial features (Shouman et al., 2012).

Additionally, "algorithm accuracy" is employed as a general measure to assess the performance of the classifier through performance metrics that represent the overall correctness of the algorithm. DT analysis uses cross-validation to assess the generalizability of predictive models and prevent over-fitting. Thus, DT makes use of automatic or semiautomatic big data analysis (Bhambri et al., 2022) and finds applications in various scientific fields, such as bioinformatics for exploratory data mining and data classification (Elhazmi et al., 2022).

### 14.3.6 Random Forest (RF)

RF is a machine learning method proposed by Breiman for non-parametric classification and regression. It involves the classification of data by dividing it according to the value of a specific variable and creating a decision tree using randomly selected variables extracted by bootstrap sampling. Additionally, the contribution and importance of each variable can be determined using the created decision trees (Elhazmi et al., 2022). It is generally considered an ensemble approach where the data set gets subdivided into smaller sub-sets that are sampled with replacement. The decision tree algorithm is made to run on these subsequently. Voting provides the importance of features and the approach is popularly known as bootstrapping or the bagging approach, which helps reduce the variance. The results obtained are validated using out-of-bag scores by reducing high-variance risks (Breiman et al., 2001).

## 14.4 RESULTS AND DISCUSSION

The following section summarizes the results obtained after the analysis of the diabetes mellitus patient dataset and the relative comparison between the chosen attributes using four popular machine language techniques (Support Vector Machines, Naïve Bayes, Decision Trees, and Random Forest) for accurate disease prediction. Following the aims of this chapter, mathematical algorithms and machine learning programs have been employed for efficient early detection of the disease using a mathematical modeling-based approach.

### 14.4.1 Description of Diabetes Dataset

For this chapter, the authors have procured the Diabetes patient dataset from primary health care and diagnostic centers in Kolkata, India. The sample size corresponds to the dataset that has been obtained from 769 patients. Furthermore, from a mathematical perspective, the dataset was divided into eight attributes or risk factors of diabetes mellitus, namely, age, pregnancy, blood pressure, skin thickness, glucose levels, insulin, body-mass index (BMI), and diabetes pedigree function. For each attribute, the authors have considered a significant characteristic feature that enables effective description and identification of attributes (Praveen et al., 2023). For each patient, the outcome was determined based on the presence or absence of the diabetic condition. A detailed summary of the dataset description has been tabulated in Table 14.1.

**TABLE 14.1**
**Detailed Dataset Description**

| Serial Number | Attributes | Description | Value |
|---|---|---|---|
| 1 | Pregnancies | Number of times pregnant | Continuous |
| 2 | Glucose | Plasma glucose concentration two hours into an oral glucose tolerance test | Continuous |
| 3 | Blood Pressure | Diastolic blood pressure | mm Hg |
| 4 | Skin Thickness | Triceps skin fold thickness | mm |
| 5 | Insulin | 2-Hour serum insulin | mu U/m |
| 6 | BMI | Body mass index | weight in kg/(height in m)^2 |
| 7 | Diabetes Pedigree Function | Diabetes Pedigree Function | |
| 8 | Age | Age | Years |
| 9 | Outcomes | Class variable | 0=no diabetes 1=has diabetes |

### 14.4.2 Application of Machine Language Techniques (MLTs) and Accuracy Analysis

The authors employed four machine learning techniques, namely, Support Vector Machines, Naïve Bayes, Decision Trees, and Random Forest. This chapter proposes the use of such mathematical algorithms for disease prediction and comparison of attributes using accuracy predictive values. For each MLT, we first checked and statistically validated the accuracy values using all eight attributes. Thereafter, to effectively compare and gain 100% accuracy ratios, the relative number of attributes for each MLT was decreased and compared against classifiers for a standardized approach to analysis (Kavita et al., 2023).

#### 14.4.2.1 Proposed Approach

For this chapter, the authors aimed to achieve a comprehensive classifier mathematical algorithmic technique and attribute feature selection for an efficient disease prediction for diabetes mellitus using the WEKA software. The dataset was obtained from the patient dataset by mathematically employing data mining and pre-processing techniques that get rid of any missing values. Therefore, to obtain the results, the authors have used the following steps as the proposed method of approach in Figure 14.3.

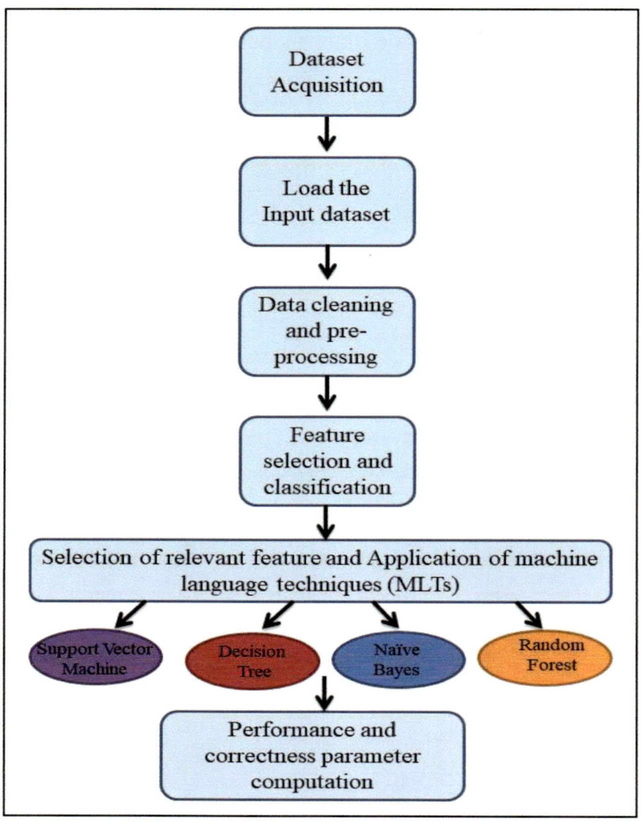


**FIGURE 14.3** Proposed method of approach.

- **Step 1**: Dataset Acquisition comprised of acquiring diabetes mellitus dataset and arranging them based on the significance of attributes.
- **Step 2**: The input dataset was loaded into the software.
- **Step 3**: Data cleaning and pre-processing to get rid of missing or incomplete values on the Diabetes dataset.
- **Step 4**: Feature selection and classification by using classifiers and mathematical algorithms, namely, Support Vector Machines, Naïve Bayes, Decision Trees, and Random Forest.
- **Step 5**: Selection of most relevant attributes and removal of least ranked attributes to keep the most significant and predominant feature.
- **Step 6**: Application and validation of ensemble classifiers (Support Vector Machines, Naïve Bayes, Decision Trees, and Random Forest).
- **Step 7**: Performance parameter computation and analysis of correctness parameters such as accuracy, precision, F1-score, and Kappa significance values.

#### 14.4.2.2 Naïve Bayes

First of all, eight dataset attributes were chosen for diabetic patients and applied against all the types of classifiers. For the Naïve Bayes technique, from 769 sample datasets, 639 indicated correctly classified instances, whereas 130 depicted incorrectly classified instances. The accuracy percentage for correctly classified instances was obtained to be 83.0949%. Thereafter, standard statistical measures like Kappa statistics, precision, recall, and F-measure, to name a few, were applied against each attribute to obtain detailed accuracy by class and weighted average values for each classifier. Kappa error, or the interpretation of Cohen's Kappa Statistics, is an effective method for outsourcing the classifier's effectiveness (Tables 14.2 and 14.3).

For a comprehensive analysis, we reduced the number of attributes to the two most significant attributes (Glucose and Blood Pressure) based on ranking the features based on significance and obtaining the accuracy values. For such standardization, among the 769 sample datasets, all 769 indicated correctly classified instances with a 100% accuracy percentage. The Kappa value was 1, while the root relative square error was 29.5467% (Tables 14.4 and 14.5).

Furthermore, upon decreasing the number of attributes to only 1 (Glucose), the percentage of accuracy corresponded to 100% accuracy with a root relative square error of 0.5748%. Therefore, it can be deciphered that based on the significance of only glucose as an important predictive attribute. We obtained significantly higher and complete accuracy values for diabetes disease prediction based upon the Naïve Bayes mathematical modeling technique (Tables 14.6 and 14.7).

#### 14.4.2.3 Random Forest

Similarly, for the Random Forest technique, among the 769 sample datasets, 748 indicated correctly classified instances, whereas 21 depicted incorrectly classified

**TABLE 14.2**
**Naïve Bayes Classifier Using All Eight Attributes**

| | | |
|---|---|---|
| Correctly Classified Instances | 639 | 83.0949% |
| Incorrectly Classified Instances | 130 | 16.9051% |
| Kappa statistic | 0.5259 | |
| Mean absolute error | 0.2225 | |
| Root mean squared error | 0.3245 | |
| Relative absolute error | 59.1329% | |
| Root relative squared error | 74.8315% | |
| Total Number of Instances | 769 | |

**TABLE 14.3**
**Naïve Bayes (Detailed Accuracy by Class)**

| | TP Rate | FP Rate | Precision | Recall | F-Measure | MCC | ROC Area | PRC Area | Class |
|---|---|---|---|---|---|---|---|---|---|
| | 0.913 | 0.415 | 0.868 | 0.913 | 0.890 | 0.529 | 0.908 | 0.965 | c0 |
| | 0.585 | 0.087 | 0.693 | 0.585 | 0.635 | 0.529 | 0.908 | 0.803 | c1 |
| Weighted Average | 0.831 | 0.332 | 0.824 | 0.831 | 0.826 | 0.529 | 0.908 | 0.924 | |

**TABLE 14.4**
**Naïve Bayes Classifier Using Two Attributes**

| | | |
|---|---|---|
| Correctly Classified Instances | 769 | 100% |
| Incorrectly Classified Instances | 0 | 0% |
| Kappa statistic | 1 | |
| Mean absolute error | 0.0664 | |
| Root mean squared error | 0.1265 | |
| Relative absolute error | 18.0845% | |
| Root relative squared error | 29.5467% | |
| Total Number of Instances | 769 | |

**TABLE 14.5**
**Naïve Bayes (Detailed Accuracy by Class)**

| | TP Rate | FP Rate | Precision | Recall | F-Measure | MCC | ROC Area | PRC Area | Class |
|---|---|---|---|---|---|---|---|---|---|
| | 1.000 | 0.000 | 1.000 | 1.000 | 1.000 | 1.000 | 1.000 | 1.000 | c0 |
| | 1.000 | 0.000 | 1.000 | 1.000 | 1.000 | 1.000 | 1.000 | 1.000 | c1 |
| Weighted Average | 1.000 | 0.000 | 1.000 | 1.000 | 1.000 | 1.000 | 1.000 | 1.000 | |

**TABLE 14.6**
**Naïve Bayes Classifier Using One Selected Attribute**

| | | | |
|---|---|---|---|
| Correctly Classified Instances | 769 | | 100% |
| Incorrectly Classified Instances | 0 | | 0% |
| Kappa statistic | | 1 | |
| Mean absolute error | | 0.0029 | |
| Root mean squared error | | 0.0029 | |
| Relative absolute error | | 0.5748% | |
| Root relative squared error | | 0.5748% | |
| Total Number of Instances | | 769 | |

**TABLE 14.7**
**Naïve Bayes (Detailed Accuracy by Class)**

| | TP Rate | FP Rate | Precision | Recall | F-Measure | MCC | ROC Area | PRC Area | Class |
|---|---|---|---|---|---|---|---|---|---|
| | 1.000 | 0.000 | 1.000 | 1.000 | 1.000 | 1.000 | 1.000 | 1.000 | c0 |
| | 1.000 | 0.000 | 1.000 | 1.000 | 1.000 | 1.000 | 1.000 | 1.000 | c1 |
| Weighted Average | 1.000 | 0.000 | 1.000 | 1.000 | 1.000 | 1.000 | 1.000 | 1.000 | |

instances upon considering all eight attributes in totality. The accuracy percentage for correctly classified instances was 97.2692%. The Kappa statistic value was found to be 0.9267, with the mean absolute error being 0.0908 and the Root relative squared error being 39.0179%. Thereafter, a weighted average was obtained for each classifier like Kappa statistics, precision, recall, and F-measure, to name a few (Tables 14.8 and 14.9).

Next, we reduced the number of attributes to two attributes (Glucose and Blood Pressure) based on the ranking feature significance and choosing the best two attributes. Thereafter, the accuracy values were correspondingly obtained. For such standardization, among the 769 sample datasets, all 769 indicated correctly classified instances with the percentage of accuracy being 100%. The Kappa statistic value was 1 with the Mean absolute error being 0, the Root mean squared error was obtained to be 0%, and the Root relative squared error was 0% (Table 14.10 and 14.11).

Furthermore, upon decreasing the number of attributes to only one (Glucose), the percentage of accuracy corresponded to 100% accuracy which was found to be highly significant. The Kappa statistic value was 1 with the Mean absolute error, Root mean squared error, and the Root relative squared error found to be 0. The weighted average was found to be 1 upon analyzing detailed accuracy by class (Tables 14.12 and 14.13). Performance parameter computation and analysis of correctness parameters such as accuracy, precision, F1-score, and Kappa significance values altogether

**TABLE 14.8**
**Random Forest Classifier Using All Attributes**

| | | | |
|---|---|---|---|
| Correctly Classified Instances | 748 | | 97.2692% |
| Incorrectly Classified Instances | 21 | | 2.7308% |
| Kappa statistic | | 0.9267 | |
| Mean absolute error | | 0.0908 | |
| Root mean squared error | | 0.1692 | |
| Relative absolute error | | 24.122% | |
| Root relative squared error | | 39.0179% | |
| Total Number of Instances | | 769 | |

**TABLE 14.9**
**Random Forest (Detailed Accuracy by Class)**

| | TP Rate | FP Rate | Precision | Recall | F-Measure | MCC | ROC Area | PRC Area | Class |
|---|---|---|---|---|---|---|---|---|---|
| | 0.986 | 0.067 | 0.978 | 0.986 | 0.982 | 0.927 | 0.996 | 0.998 | c0 |
| | 0.933 | 0.014 | 0.957 | 0.933 | 0.945 | 0.927 | 0.996 | 0.986 | c1 |
| Weighted Average | 0.973 | 0.054 | 0.973 | 0.973 | 0.973 | 0.927 | 0.996 | 0.995 | |

**TABLE 14.10**
**Random Forest Classifier Using Two Attributes**

| | | | |
|---|---|---|---|
| Correctly Classified Instances | 769 | | 100% |
| Incorrectly Classified Instances | 0 | | 0% |
| Kappa statistic | | 1 | |
| Mean absolute error | | 0 | |
| Root mean squared error | | 0 | |
| Relative absolute error | | 0% | |
| Root relative squared error | | 0% | |
| Total Number of Instances | | 769 | |

**TABLE 14.11**
**Random Forest (Detailed Accuracy by Class)**

| | TP Rate | FP Rate | Precision | Recall | F-Measure | MCC | ROC Area | PRC Area | Class |
|---|---|---|---|---|---|---|---|---|---|
| | 1.000 | 0.000 | 1.000 | 1.000 | 1.000 | 1.000 | 1.000 | 1.000 | c0 |
| | 1.000 | 0.000 | 1.000 | 1.000 | 1.000 | 1.000 | 1.000 | 1.000 | c1 |
| Weighted Average | 1.000 | 0.000 | 1.000 | 1.000 | 1.000 | 1.000 | 1.000 | 1.000 | |

**TABLE 14.12**
**Random Forest Classifier Using One Attribute**

| | | | |
|---|---|---|---|
| Correctly Classified Instances | 769 | | 100% |
| Incorrectly Classified Instances | 0 | | 0% |
| Kappa statistic | | 1 | |
| Mean absolute error | | 0 | |
| Root mean squared error | | 0 | |
| Relative absolute error | | 0% | |
| Root relative squared error | | 0% | |
| Total Number of Instances | | 769 | |

**TABLE 14.13**
**Random Forest (Detailed Accuracy by Class)**

| | TP Rate | FP Rate | Precision | Recall | F-Measure | MCC | ROC Area | PRC Area | Class |
|---|---|---|---|---|---|---|---|---|---|
| | 1.000 | 0.000 | 1.000 | 1.000 | 1.000 | 1.000 | 1.000 | 1.000 | c0 |
| | 1.000 | 0.000 | 1.000 | 1.000 | 1.000 | 1.000 | 1.000 | 1.000 | c1 |
| Weighted Average | 1.000 | 0.000 | 1.000 | 1.000 | 1.000 | 1.000 | 1.000 | 1.000 | |

signified the relevance of the Random Forest algorithm in disease prediction and selection of the most preferred attribute. Furthermore, upon comparison with all the other MLTs, the Random Forest methodology proved to be the most significantly accurate in terms of all attributes and classifiers. Also, the importance of glucose levels in a diabetes patient can act as an important prognostic diagnostic and predictive attribute, which was further validated by mathematical algorithms, with the most apt being the Random Forest classification technique.

#### 14.4.2.4 Support Vector Machine

Similarly, for the support vector machine technique, among the 769 sample datasets, 661 indicated correctly classified instances, whereas 108 depicted incorrectly classified instances upon considering all eight attributes in totality. The accuracy percentage for correctly classified instances was obtained to be 85.9558%. The Kappa statistic value was found to be 0.6159, with the mean absolute error being 0.1404 and the Root relative squared error being 86.4322%. Thereafter, a weighted average was obtained for each classifier, like Kappa statistics, precision, recall, and F-measure, to name a few (Tables 14.14 and 14.15).

Next, we reduced the number of attributes to two attributes (Glucose and Blood Pressure) based on the ranking feature significance and choosing the best two attributes. Thereafter, the accuracy values were correspondingly obtained. For such

**TABLE 14.14**
**Support Vector Machine Classifier Using All Attributes**

| | | | |
|---|---|---|---|
| Correctly Classified Instances | 661 | | 85.9558% |
| Incorrectly Classified Instances | 108 | | 14.0442% |
| Kappa statistic | | 0.6159 | |
| Mean absolute error | | 0.1404 | |
| Root mean squared error | | 0.3748 | |
| Relative absolute error | | 37.3181% | |
| Root relative squared error | | 86.4322% | |
| Total Number of Instances | | 769 | |

**TABLE 14.15**
**Support Vector Machine (Detailed Accuracy by Class)**

| | TP Rate | FP Rate | Precision | Recall | F-Measure | MCC | ROC Area | PRC Area | Class |
|---|---|---|---|---|---|---|---|---|---|
| | 0.920 | 0.321 | 0.895 | 0.920 | 0.908 | 0.617 | 0.799 | 0.884 | c0 |
| | 0.679 | 0.080 | 0.740 | 0.679 | 0.708 | 0.617 | 0.799 | 0.583 | c1 |
| Weighted Average | 0.860 | 0.261 | 0.856 | 0.860 | 0.857 | 0.617 | 0.799 | 0.808 | |

standardization, among the 769 sample datasets, all 769 indicated correctly classified instances with a 100% accuracy percentage. The Kappa statistic value was 1 with the Mean absolute error being 0, the Root mean squared error was obtained to be 0%, and the Root relative squared error was 0% (Table 14.16 and 14.17).

Furthermore, upon decreasing the number of attributes to only one (Glucose), the percentage of accuracy corresponded to 100% accuracy, which was found to be highly significant. The Kappa statistic value was 1 with the Mean absolute error, Root mean squared error, and the Root relative squared error found to be 0. The weighted average was found to be 1 upon analyzing detailed accuracy by class (Tables 14.18 and 14.19). Performance parameter computation and analysis of correctness parameters such as accuracy, precision, F1-score, and Kappa significance values altogether signified the relevance of the Support Vector Machine algorithm in disease prediction and selection of the most preferred attribute. Furthermore, upon comparison with all the other MLTs, the Support Vector Machine methodology proved to be the most significantly accurate in terms of all attributes and classifiers. Also, the importance of glucose levels in a diabetes patient can act as an important prognostic diagnostic and predictive attribute that was further validated by mathematical algorithms, with the most apt being the Support Vector Machine classification technique.

**TABLE 14.16**
**Support Vector Machine Classifier Using Two Attributes**

| | | | |
|---|---|---|---|
| Correctly Classified Instances | 769 | | 100% |
| Incorrectly Classified Instances | 0 | | 0% |
| Kappa statistic | | 1 | |
| Mean absolute error | | 0 | |
| Root mean squared error | | 0 | |
| Relative absolute error | | 0% | |
| Root relative squared error | | 0% | |
| Total Number of Instances | | 769 | |

**TABLE 14.17**
**Support Vector Machine (Detailed Accuracy by Class)**

| | TP Rate | FP Rate | Precision | Recall | F-Measure | MCC | ROC Area | PRC Area | Class |
|---|---|---|---|---|---|---|---|---|---|
| | 1.000 | 0.000 | 1.000 | 1.000 | 1.000 | 1.000 | 1.000 | 1.000 | c0 |
| | 1.000 | 0.000 | 1.000 | 1.000 | 1.000 | 1.000 | 1.000 | 1.000 | c1 |
| Weighted Average | 1.000 | 0.000 | 1.000 | 1.000 | 1.000 | 1.000 | 1.000 | 1.000 | |

**TABLE 14.18 Support Vector Machine Classifier Using One attribute**

| | | | |
|---|---|---|---|
| Correctly Classified Instances | 769 | | 100% |
| Incorrectly Classified Instances | 0 | | 0% |
| Kappa statistic | | 1 | |
| Mean absolute error | | 0 | |
| Root mean squared error | | 0 | |
| Relative absolute error | | 0% | |
| Root relative squared error | | 0% | |
| Total Number of Instances | | 769 | |

**TABLE 14.19**
**Support Vector Machine (Detailed Accuracy by Class)**

| | TP Rate | FP Rate | Precision | Recall | F-Measure | MCC | ROC Area | PRC Area | Class |
|---|---|---|---|---|---|---|---|---|---|
| | 1.000 | 0.000 | 1.000 | 1.000 | 1.000 | 1.000 | 1.000 | 1.000 | c0 |
| | 1.000 | 0.000 | 1.000 | 1.000 | 1.000 | 1.000 | 1.000 | 1.000 | c1 |
| Weighted Average | 1.000 | 0.000 | 1.000 | 1.000 | 1.000 | 1.000 | 1.000 | 1.000 | |

**TABLE 14.20**
**Decision Tree Classifier Using All Attributes**

| | | | |
|---|---|---|---|
| Correctly Classified Instances | 739 | | 96.0988% |
| Incorrectly Classified Instances | 30 | | 3.9012% |
| Kappa statistic | | 0.8933 | |
| Mean absolute error | | 0.05460 | |
| Root mean squared error | | 0.1831 | |
| Relative absolute error | | 14.4972% | |
| Root relative squared error | | 42.2238% | |
| Total Number of Instances | | 769 | |

**TABLE 14.21**
**Decision Tree (Detailed Accuracy by Class)**

| | TP Rate | FP Rate | Precision | Recall | F-Measure | MCC | ROC Area | PRC Area | Class |
|---|---|---|---|---|---|---|---|---|---|
| | 0.988 | 0.119 | 0.961 | 0.988 | 0.974 | 0.895 | 0.960 | 0.973 | c0 |
| | 0.881 | 0.012 | 0.960 | 0.881 | 0.919 | 0.895 | 0.960 | 0.941 | c1 |
| Weighted Average | 0.961 | 0.092 | 0.961 | 0.961 | 0.960 | 0.895 | 0.960 | 0.965 | |

### 14.4.2.5 Decision Tree

Similarly, for the Decision Tree technique, among the 769 sample datasets, 739 indicated correctly classified instances, whereas 30 depicted incorrectly classified instances upon considering all eight attributes in totality. The accuracy percentage for correctly classified instances was obtained to be 96.0988%. The Kappa statistic value was found to be 0.8933, with the mean absolute error being 0.05460 and the Root relative squared error being 42.2238%. Thereafter, a weighted average was obtained for each classifier, like Kappa statistics, precision, recall, and F-measure, to name a few (Tables 14.20 and 14.21).

Next, we reduced the number of attributes to two attributes (Glucose and Blood Pressure) based on the ranking feature significance and choosing the best two attributes. Thereafter, the accuracy values were correspondingly obtained. For such standardization, among the 769 sample datasets, all 769 indicated correctly classified instances with a 100% accuracy percentage. The Kappa statistic value was 1 with the Mean absolute error being 0, the Root mean squared error was obtained to be 0%, and the Root relative squared error was 0% (Table 14.22 and 14.23).

Furthermore, upon decreasing the number of attributes to only one (Glucose), the percentage of accuracy corresponded to 100% accuracy, which was found to be highly significant. The Kappa statistic value was 1 with the Mean absolute error, Root mean squared error, and the Root relative squared error found to be 0. The weighted average was found to be 1 upon analyzing detailed accuracy by class (Tables 14.24 and 14.25). Performance parameter computation and analysis of correctness parameters such as accuracy, precision, F1-score, and Kappa significance

**TABLE 14.22**
**Decision Tree Classifier Using Two Attributes**

| | | | |
|---|---|---|---|
| Correctly Classified Instances | 769 | | 100% |
| Incorrectly Classified Instances | 0 | | 0% |
| Kappa statistic | | 1 | |
| Mean absolute error | | 0 | |
| Root mean squared error | | 0 | |
| Relative absolute error | | 0% | |
| Root relative squared error | | 0% | |
| Total Number of Instances | | 769 | |

**TABLE 14.23**
**Decision Tree (Detailed Accuracy by Class)**

| | TP Rate | FP Rate | Precision | Recall | F-Measure | MCC | ROC Area | PRC Area | Class |
|---|---|---|---|---|---|---|---|---|---|
| | 1.000 | 0.000 | 1.000 | 1.000 | 1.000 | 1.000 | 1.000 | 1.000 | c0 |
| | 1.000 | 0.000 | 1.000 | 1.000 | 1.000 | 1.000 | 1.000 | 1.000 | c1 |
| Weighted Average | 1.000 | 0.000 | 1.000 | 1.000 | 1.000 | 1.000 | 1.000 | 1.000 | |

**TABLE 14.24 Decision Tree Classifier Using One Attributes**

| | | | |
|---|---|---|---|
| Correctly Classified Instances | 769 | | 100% |
| Incorrectly Classified Instances | 0 | | 0% |
| Kappa statistic | | 1 | |
| Mean absolute error | | 0 | |
| Root mean squared error | | 0 | |
| Relative absolute error | | 0% | |
| Root relative squared error | | 0% | |
| Total Number of Instances | | 769 | |

**TABLE 14.25**
**Decision Tree (Detailed Accuracy by Class)**

| | TP Rate | FP Rate | Precision | Recall | F-Measure | MCC | ROC Area | PRC Area | Class |
|---|---|---|---|---|---|---|---|---|---|
| | 1.000 | 0.000 | 1.000 | 1.000 | 1.000 | 1.000 | 1.000 | 1.000 | c0 |
| | 1.000 | 0.000 | 1.000 | 1.000 | 1.000 | 1.000 | 1.000 | 1.000 | c1 |
| Weighted Average | 1.000 | 0.000 | 1.000 | 1.000 | 1.000 | 1.000 | 1.000 | 1.000 | |

values altogether signified the relevance of the Decision Tree algorithm in disease prediction and selection of the most preferred attribute. Furthermore, upon comparison with all the other MLTs, the Decision Tree methodology proved to be the most significantly accurate in terms of all attributes and classifiers. Also, the importance of glucose levels in a diabetes patient can act as an important prognostic diagnostic and predictive attribute, which was further validated by mathematical algorithms, with the most apt being the Decision Tree classification technique (Anh et al., 2024).

#### 14.4.2.6 Discussion and Results

Therefore, in this chapter, the authors have employed the diabetes mellitus dataset to compare results obtained from various mathematical machine learning algorithms and feature selection tools to gain insights into the disease prediction and risk assessment for diabetes. The different state-of-the-art algorithms included Support Vector Machines, Naïve Bayes, Decision Trees, and Random Forest. The authors have also determined the validation and statistical verification of the outcomes through performance metrics and classifiers. The three MLTs (Support Vector Machines, Naïve Bayes, and Decision Trees) provided a uniform prediction of accuracies after the distribution and analysis of attributes either in totality or reduction and feature selection of a lesser number of attributes based upon the ranking diminishing order of significance in their correlation with the disease (Khang & Hahanov et al., 2024).

Furthermore, upon a comparison between all four MLTs, the authors also deciphered the most significant methodology of machine language algorithms for effective disease prediction. Moreover, it was found that the performance of Random Forest surpassed all the other methodologies in terms of accuracy of prediction and in terms of classifier outcomes, statistical significance, and metrics. Thus, the authors came to the novel prediction of using glucose levels as a novel and relevantly ranked attribute associated with the disease Diabetes in predicting it using a mathematical model approach and utilizing this novel information in the disease and therapeutics field for an initial assessment, timely prediction and diagnosis of the disease so that any delay in therapy can be avoided (Khang et al., 2022).

## 14.5 CONCLUSION

In this work, we have extracted datasets from a real healthcare center catering exclusively to diabetes mellitus patients. To predict DM, we have used four machine-learning algorithms for our experiments, namely, Support Vector Machine (SVM), Naïve Bayes (NB), Decision Tree (DT), and Random Forest (RF). By using RF, we obtained the maximum level of accuracy compared to the rest of the machine-learning algorithms. Our experimental result will help the healthcare system take precautionary measures to impede the spread of DM and control the disease. To the best of our knowledge, our work can be considered a novel experimental result that can contribute to the field of disease amelioration and therapeutic avenues by providing timely and early prediction of DM and saving human lives (Vrushank et al., 2023).

## REFERENCES


Aljumah A. A., M. G. Ahamad, and M. K. Siddiqui. "Application of data mining: Diabetes health care in young and old patients," *J. King Saud Univ. Comput. Inf. Sci.*, vol. 25, no. 2, pp. 127–136, 2013, doi: https://doi.org/10.1016/j.jksuci.2012.10.003.

Anh P. T. N., V. Hahanov, Triwiyanto, N. A. Ragimova, İ. Rashad, V. Abdullayev, and V. A. Abuzarova. "AI models for disease diagnosis and prediction of heart disease with artificial neural networks," In *Computer vision and AI-integrated IoT technologies in medical ecosystem* (1st Ed.), 2024. CRC Press. doi: https://doi.org/10.1201/9781003429609-9

Banday M. Z., A. S. Sameer, and S. Nissar. "Pathophysiology of diabetes: An overview," *Avicenna J. Med.*, vol. 10, no. 4, pp. 174–188, 2020. doi: https://doi.org/10.4103/ajm.ajm_53_20

Barakat N. H., A. P. Bradley, and M. N. H. Barakat. "Intelligible support vector machines for diagnosis of diabetes mellitus," *IEEE Trans. Inf. Technol. Biomed. a Publ. IEEE Eng. Med. Biol. Soc.*, vol. 14, no. 4, pp. 1114–1120, Jul. 2010. doi: https://doi.org/10.1109/TITB.2009.2039485.

Bhambri P., S. Rani, G. Gupta, and A. Khang. *Cloud and fog computing platforms for internet of things*, 2022. CRC Press. doi: https://doi.org/10.1201/9781003213888

Blair M. "Diabetes mellitus review," *Urol. Nurs.*, vol. 36, no. 1, pp. 27–36, 2016.

Breiman L. "Random forests," *Mach. Learn.*, vol. 45, no. 1, pp. 5–32, 2001. doi: https://doi.org/10.1023/A:1010933404324

Cherfi A., K. Nouira, and A. Ferchichi. "Very fast C4.5 decision tree algorithm," *Appl. Artif. Intell.*, vol. 32, no. 2, pp. 119–137, Apr. 2018. doi: https://doi.org/10.1080/08839514.2018.1447479.

Cloete L. "Diabetes mellitus: An overview of the types, symptoms, complications and management," *Nurs. Stand.*, vol. 37, no. 1, pp. 61–66, Jan. 2022, doi: https://doi.org/10.7748/ns.2021.e11709.

Elhazmi A. et al. "Machine learning decision tree algorithm role for predicting mortality in critically ill adult COVID-19 patients admitted to the ICU," *J. Infect. Public Health*, vol. 15, no. 7, pp. 826–834, Jul. 2022, doi: 10.1016/j.jiph.2022.06.008.

Faruque M., and I. Sarker. *Performance Analysis of Machine Learning Techniques to Predict Diabetes Mellitus*, 2019. https://ieeexplore.ieee.org/abstract/document/8679365/

Giorda C. B., V. Manicardi, and J. Diago Cabezudo. "The impact of diabetes mellitus on healthcare costs in Italy," *Expert Rev. Pharmacoecon. Outcomes Res.*, vol. 11, no. 6, pp. 709–719, Dec. 2011. doi: https://doi.org/10.1586/erp.11.78

Guo B., and Q. Zheng. "Using Naïve Bayes algorithm to estimate the response to drug in lung cancer patients," *Comb. Chem. High Throughput Screen.*, vol. 21, no. 10, pp. 734–748, 2018. doi: https://doi.org/10.2174/1386207322666190125151624

Huang S., N. Cai, P. P. Pacheco, S. Narrandes, Y. Wang, and W. Xu, "Applications of support vector machine (SVM) learning in cancer genomics," *Cancer Genomics Proteomics*, vol. 15, no. 1, pp. 41–51, 2018, doi: 10.21873/cgp.20063

Huang Y., P. McCullagh, N. Black, and R. Harper. "Feature selection and classification model construction on type 2 diabetic patients' data," *Artif. Intell. Med.*, vol. 41, no. 3, pp. 251–262, Nov. 2007. doi: https://doi.org/10.1016/j.artmed.2007.07.002

Jegan C., "Classification of diabetes disease using support vector machine," *Int. J. Eng. Res. Appl.*, vol. 3, pp. 1797–1801, Apr. 2013. www.researchgate.net/profile/Chitra-Jegan/publication/320395340_Classification_Of_Diabetes_Disease_Using_Support_Vector_Machine/links/59e1c7a80f7e9b97fbe72c89/Classification-Of-Diabetes-Disease-Using-Support-Vector-Machine.pdf

John G. H., and P. Langley. "Estimating continuous distributions in Bayesian classifiers," in *UAI*, 2013. https://arxiv.org/abs/1302.4964

Kandhasamy J. P., and S. Balamurali. "Performance analysis of classifier models to predict diabetes mellitus," *Procedia Comput. Sci.*, vol. 47, pp. 45–51, 2015, doi: https://doi.org/10.1016/j.procs.2015.03.182.

Kavakiotis I., O. Tsave, A. Salifoglou, N. Maglaveras, I. Vlahavas, and I. Chouvarda. "Machine learning and data mining methods in diabetes research," *Comput. Struct. Biotechnol. J.*, vol. 15, pp. 104–116, 2017. doi: https://doi.org/10.1016/j.csbj.2016.12.005.

Kavita M., and A. Khang. "Hospital 4.0: Capitalization of health and healthcare in industry 4.0 economy," in *Data-Centric AI Solutions and Emerging Technologies in the Healthcare Ecosystem* (1st Ed., p. 14), 2023. CRC Press. doi: https://doi.org/10.1201/9781003356189-19

Khang A., V. Abdullayev, O. Hrybiuk, and A. K. Shukla, *Computer Vision and AI-Integrated IoT Technologies in the Medical Ecosystem* (1st Ed.), 2024. CRC Press. doi: https://doi.org/10.1201/9781003429609

Khang A., V. Hahanov, E. Litvinova, S. Chumachenko, Z. Avromovic, R. İsmibeyli, N. A. Ragimova, V. A. Abdullayev, A. V. Alyar, and P. T. N. Anh, "Medical and biomedical signal processing and prediction," in *Computer Vision and AI-integrated IoT Technologies in Medical Ecosystem* (1st Ed.), 2024. CRC Press. https://doi.org/10.1201/9781003429609-7

Khang A., N. A. Ragimova, V. A. Hajimahmud, and V. A. Alyar. "Advanced technologies and data management in the smart healthcare system," In *AI-centric smart city ecosystems: Technologies, design and implementation* (1st Ed., vol. 16, p. 10), 2022. CRC Press. doi: https://doi.org/10.1201/9781003252542-16

Khang A., G. Rana, R. K. Tailor, and V. A. Hajimahmud, *Data-Centric AI Solutions and Emerging Technologies in the Healthcare Ecosystem* (1st Ed.), 2023. CRC Press. doi: https://doi.org/10.1201/9781003356189

Kumar Y., A. Koul, R. Singla, and M. F. Ijaz, "Artificial intelligence in disease diagnosis: A systematic literature review, synthesizing framework and future research agenda," *J. Ambient Intell. Humaniz. Comput.*, pp. 1–28, Jan. 2022. doi: https://doi.org/10.1007/s12652-021-03612-z.

Langarizadeh M., and F. Moghbeli. "Applying Naive Bayesian networks to disease prediction: A systematic review," *Acta Inform. Medica AIM J. Soc. Med. Informatics Bosnia Herzegovina Cas. Drus. za Med. Inform. BiH*, vol. 24, no. 5, pp. 364–369, Oct. 2016. https://doi.org/10.5455/aim.2016.24.364-369.

Mashayekhi M., F. Prescod, B. Shah, L. Dong, K. Keshavjee, and A. Guergachi. "Evaluating the performance of the Framingham diabetes risk scoring model in Canadian electronic medical records," *Can. J. Diabetes*, vol. 39, no. 2, pp. 152–156, Apr. 2015. doi: https://doi.org/10.1016/j.jcjd.2014.10.006

Meng H. Y., D.-P. Huang, Q. Rao, Q. Zhang, and Q. Liu. "Comparison of three data mining models for predicting diabetes or prediabetes by risk factors," *Kaohsiung J. Med. Sci.*, vol. 29, no. 2, pp. 93–99, Feb. 2013. doi: https://doi.org/10.1016/j.kjms.2012.08.016

Noble W. S. "What is a support vector machine?," *Nat. Biotechnol.*, vol. 24, no. 12, pp. 1565–1567, Dec. 2006, doi: 10.1038/nbt1206-1565.

Paullada A., I. D. Raji, E. M. Bender, E. Denton, and A. Hanna. "Data and its (dis)contents: A survey of dataset development and use in machine learning research," *Patterns*, vol. 2, no. 11, p. 100336, 2021, doi: https://doi.org/10.1016/j.patter.2021.100336.

Platt J., "Fast training of support vector machines using sequential minimal optimization," *Advances in Kernel Methods—Support Vector Learning*, 1998, Advances i. www.researchgate.net/profile/John-Platt-2/publication/242503764_Fast_training_of_svms_using_sequential_minimal_optimization/links/541701680cf2fa878ad43dd1/Fast-training-of-svms-using-sequential-minimal-optimization.pdf

Praveen Kumar M., N. Kumar, A. Misra, and A. Khang. "Heart disease prediction using logistic regression and random forest classifier," in *Data-Centric AI Solutions and Emerging Technologies in the Healthcare Ecosystem* (1st Ed., p. 6), 2023. CRC Press. https://doi.org/10.1201/9781003356189-6

Rani A. S., and S. Jyothi. "Performance analysis of classification algorithms under different datasets," *2016 3rd Int. Conf. Comput. Sustain. Glob. Dev.*, pp. 1584–1589, 2016. https://ieeexplore.ieee.org/abstract/document/7724534/

Rigatti S. J. "Random forest," *J. Insur. Med.*, vol. 47, no. 1, pp. 31–39, 2017. doi: https://doi.org/10.17849/insm-47-01-31-39.1

Salzberg S. L. "C4.5: Programs for Machine Learning by J. Ross Quinlan. Morgan Kaufmann Publishers, Inc., 1993," *Mach. Learn.*, vol. 16, no. 3, pp. 235–240, 1994. doi: https://doi.org/10.1007/BF00993309

Sarica A., A. Cerasa, and A. Quattrone. "Random forest algorithm for the classification of neuroimaging data in Alzheimer's disease: A systematic review" *Front. Aging Neurosci.*, vol. 9, p. 329, 2017. doi: https://doi.org/10.3389/fnagi.2017.00329

Shouman M., T. Turner, and R. Stocker. "Using data mining techniques in heart disease diagnosis and treatment," *2012 Japan-Egypt Conf. Electron. Commun. Comput.*, pp. 173–177, 2012.

Tan S. Y. *et al.* "Type 1 and 2 diabetes mellitus: A review on current treatment approach and gene therapy as potential intervention," *Diabetes Metab. Syndr.*, vol. 13, no. 1, pp. 364–372, 2019. doi: https://doi.org/10.1016/j.ds14.2018.10.008

Thanh Noi P., and M. Kappas. "Comparison of random forest, k-nearest neighbor, and support vector machine classifiers for land cover classification using sentinel-2 imagery," *Sensors (Basel).*, vol. 18, no. 1, Dec. 2017. doi: https://doi.org/10.3390/s18010018.

Uddin S., I. Haque, H. Lu, M. A. Moni, and E. Gide. "Comparative performance analysis of K-nearest neighbour (KNN) algorithm and its different variants for disease prediction," *Sci. Rep.*, vol. 12, no. 1, p. 6256, Apr. 2022. doi: https://doi.org/10.1038/s41598-022-10358-14.

Vrushank S., and A. Khang. "Metaverse-enabling IoT technology for a futuristic healthcare system," in *AI-Based Technologies and Applications in the Era of the Metaverse* (1st Ed., p. 1), 2023. IGI Global Press. https://doi.org/10.4018/978-1-6684-8851-5.ch008

Wei W., S. Visweswaran, and G. F. Cooper. "The application of naive Bayes model averaging to predict Alzheimer's disease from genome-wide data," *J. Am. Med. Inform. Assoc.*, vol. 18, no. 4, pp. 370–375, 2011. doi: https://doi.org/10.1136/amiajnl-2011-000101

Zhang Z. "Introduction to machine learning: K-nearest neighbors," *Ann. Transl. Med.*, vol. 4, no. 11, p. 218, Jun. 2016. doi: https://doi.org/10.21037/atm.2016.03.37

Zheng T. *et al.* "A machine learning-based framework to identify type 2 diabetes through electronic health records," *Int. J. Med. Inform.*, vol. 97, pp. 120–127, Jan. 2017. doi: https://doi.org/10.1016/j.ijmedinf.2016.09.014.

# 15 Disease Detection for Herbal Plants Using ResNet Algorithm

*Akankshya Rout, Ayush Kumar Bar, Rahul Sarkar, and Avijit Kumar Chaudhuri*

## 15.1 INTRODUCTION

For centuries, agriculture has been a major driver in India's economy, and the country is considered to be one of the world's largest producers and exporters of various agricultural commodities worldwide. According to the World Bank (2012), India has been recognized as a global agriculture powerhouse with the world's largest producer of milk, pulses, and spices and the second largest producer of rice, wheat, sugarcane, apple etc. As per the report of Inc42, the Indian agricultural sector is projected to reach a value of US $24 billion by 2025. India is the sixth largest food and grocery market in the world, with retail accounting for 70% of total sales. According to the first preliminary estimate for FY23, Khar, if only, total grain production in the country is anticipated to be approximately 149.92 million tons. One of the main factors propelling the growth of the Indian agriculture sector is the country's rapidly expanding population.

Additionally, as a result of rising incomes in both rural and urban areas, the growth of this sector has been accompanied by a spike in demand for agricultural goods across the country as a whole. The market is also being driven by the adoption of cutting-edge technologies like blockchain, artificial intelligence (AI), geographic information systems (GIS), drones, and remote sensing, as well as the creation of numerous e-farming applications.

As per IBEF (2023), over the past few years, the agriculture and allied sectors in India has performed well. This success can be attributed to the measures implemented by the government to improve the productivity of agriculture and livestock production, ensuring that farmers receive adequate returns on price support, promoting crop diversification, and improvements in market infrastructure. The government's initiatives have also led to forming farmer-producer organizations and investments in infrastructure facilities through the Agriculture Infrastructure Fund, further improving the sector's performance.

The rise of modern civilization and technologies has enabled the agriculture industry to boost productivity, increase crop yields, and improve the efficiency of food production and distribution. However, crops and plant diseases are still a major threat or challenge to society. Climate change, pollinator decline, bacteria, fungi,


DOI: 10.1201/9781032686745-15

pest treatments, weedicides, and other factors all impact plant disease. As per (NCBI, 2023) the prevalence of these diseases might range from 70–80% of the total plant population, depending on meteorological conditions and crop physiological status. This can result in severe yield loss in some circumstances, with decreases ranging from 80–98%. These diseases can cause large crop losses and decreased productivity, affecting farmers' lives and the overall economy (Khang & Ragimova et al., 2022).

Based on the article published in Gaonconnection (2023), millet crops in the Indian state of Haryana are currently under threat from a disease called "stem rot". Interestingly, the bacterium responsible for the infection is commonly found in the human intestines and is usually harmless to healthy individuals. With the advancement in modern technology, the aim of treating crops and plants with the right information has become a necessity (Khang & Rana et al., 2023).

Nowadays, Machine Learning, specifically Artificial Intelligence (AI), is diffusing worldwide. From unlocking phones to detecting COVID-19 patients, AI has succeeded. Image processing technology and algorithmic advancements can be used in agriculture science to determine the various diseases and their phases. These techniques can be used to analyze plant images and identify disease symptoms early on, allowing for timely intervention and avoidance of future spread. Agriculture scientists can gain significant insights into crop health and development patterns by combining the power of machine learning algorithms and imaging tools, leading to more effective and sustainable farming practices (Divvela et al., 2023).

The objective of this dissertation is to develop an effective ML model for detecting plant diseases using advanced deep learning algorithms in order to find the best option for plant disease prevention. To achieve this, the ResNet ("Residual Network") method is used for the identification and categorization of plant diseases. ResNet is specifically designed to overcome the vanishing gradient problem that can occur in very deep neural networks. One of the most significant advantages of employing ResNet for plant disease diagnosis is its ability to handle very large and complex datasets. The dataset used in this study was obtained from Kaggle and consists of approximately 87K RGB images of healthy and diseased crop leaves classified into 38 different classifications. The dataset has been trained using the ResNet9 algorithm, which provides us with an accuracy of 99.23% during the training of the ResNet9 Model.

## 15.2 LITERATURE REVIEW

Plant diseases are reducing crop yields significantly and affecting crop quality, which is indeed becoming a major issue to its consumers. Early detection of plant diseases is necessary for maintaining food security and reducing economic losses. Because of the ability to handle big and complicated datasets and the potential for reliable and automated disease diagnosis, machine learning (ML) techniques have gained popularity in recent years for plant disease detection (Khang & Hahanov et al., 2022).

Several studies have investigated the application of ML approaches for plant disease detection, such as convolutional neural networks (CNNs), support vector machines (SVMs), and decision trees. Because of its ability to extract relevant information from images, CNNs have been proven to be very effective in image identification tasks, including plant disease diagnosis. SVMs, on the other hand, have been used to classify plant diseases using spectral data from hyperspectral imaging (Vrushank et al., 2023).

Decision trees have been proven beneficial for determining the most significant traits or criteria for detecting plant diseases. Many researchers have developed ML models for disease detection using secondary data sets available from websites, i.e., Kaggle, which includes thousands of images of various crop leaves, as well as information about the plant species and disease type. Other researchers have compiled their own databases from field surveys or experiments that may be particular to specific crops or geographic regions. Plant_CNN (2023) completed one of the early types of research in this field, employing a pre-trained ResNet34 algorithm on a dataset containing 8,685 images. Their model reached over 97.2% accuracy and an F1 score greater than 96.5%. Although the study achieved good accuracy, the dataset used is very small. The sample size is only 8,685, which limits the generalizability of the findings to a larger population.

Another study by Plant-Leaf (2023) includes hybrid feature-based disease detection in plant leaves using CNN, Bayesian optimized SVM, and random forest classifier. The work achieved an accuracy of 91.6%. However, ResNet has the ability to handle the Vanishing Gradient problem, which generally occurs in CNN due to the presence of many layers in the network, which makes it difficult for the network to learn. In order to get a high accuracy SAGEPUB (2023) proposed a unique approach based on image enhancement and conversion, combined feature extraction using GLCM, Complex Gabor filter, Curvelet, and image moments, and a Neuro-Fuzzy Logic classifier trained with extracted features. This is implemented using MATLAB simulation using the PlantVillage Database, achieving an average detection accuracy of over 90% accuracy for two test cases.

Neuro-Fuzzy Logic classifier is a machine learning approach used to make decisions; on the other hand, the objective of the dissertation is to find the patterns while detecting the disease. PII (2023) and JSFA (2023) used a deep learning approach to detect apple and rice leaf disease and achieved an accuracy of approximately 93%~95%. MJS (2023) used the SVM approach and achieved an accuracy of 88.1%. ResNets are a type of neural network architecture that is commonly employed in deep learning computer vision applications such as object detection and picture segmentation. ResNet can have a significant number of convolutional layers, often between 18 and 152, but up to thousands.

## 15.3 PROPOSED ARCHITECTURE

Kaiming He, Xiangyu Zhang, Shaoqing Ren, and Jian Sun developed the ResNet, also referred to as the Residual Network, as a sort of neural network in their research work (ABS, 2023) in 2015. The ResNet models proved to be highly effective. It is also known as "Identity shortcut connection", as the model is allowed to omit more than one layer. This method enables the network to be trained on thousands of layers without affecting performance.

Prior to ResNet, various methods had been employed to resolve the issue of vanishing gradients. As per RESNET (2023) GoogleNet also added an auxiliary loss in the middle layer for extra supervision, but it did not succeed. Hence, the authors discovered the concept of stack identity mappings or skip connections, which means the network can skip over layers that are not contributing to the learning process. The skip connection connects activations of a layer to further layers by skipping some layers in between and forming a residual block. These residual blocks are stacked to create ResNets. This helps the network to learn even when the gradients are very small.

### 15.3.1 2D Convolutional Layers Function

2D Convolutional layers function in PyTorch defines a 2D convolutional layer with the following parameters:

- in_channels: This is the number of input channels that the layer will take in. In this case, there are three input channels (RGB) for the first convolutional layer.
- out_channels: This is the number of output channels that the layer will produce. In this case, there are 64 output channels.
- kernel_size: This is the size of the convolutional kernel. In this case, the kernel is 3x3 pixels.
- stride: This is the number of pixels that the kernel will move across the input tensor. In this case, the stride is 1 pixel.
- padding: This determines how the input tensor is padded before the convolution is performed. In this case, the padding is set to "same", which means that the output tensor will have the same height and width as the input tensor.

### 15.3.2 2D Batch Normalization Function

2D Batch Normalization function in PyTorch defines a 2D batch normalization layer with the following parameters:

- num_features: This is the number of features in the input tensor. In this case, there are 64 features for the first layer.
- eps: This is a small number that prevents the denominator from becoming zero. In this case, the epsilon value is set to 1e-05.
- momentum: This is the decay rate for the running mean and running variance. In this case, the momentum value is set to 0.1.
- affine: This determines whether the layer has learnable affine parameters. In this case, the affine parameters are set to true.
- track_running_status: This determines whether the layer tracks the running mean and running variance. In this case, the running mean and running variance are tracked.

### 15.3.3 ReLU Function

- ReLU function in PyTorch defines a rectified linear unit (ReLU) activation function with the following parameter:
- inplace: This determines whether the layer will modify the input tensor in place. In this case, the inplace parameter is set to true.

### 15.3.4 MaxPool2d Function

MaxPool2d function in PyTorch defines a 2D max pooling layer with the following parameters:

- kernel_size: This is the size of the pooling window. In this case, the kernel size is 4x4 pixels.
- stride: This is the number of pixels that the pooling window will move across the input tensor. In this case, the stride is 4 pixels.
- padding: This determines how the input tensor is padded before the pooling operation is performed. In this case, the padding is set to 0.
- dilation: This is the spacing between the kernel points. In this case, the dilation is set to 1.
- ceil_mode: This determines whether the pooling operation will take into account the padding when determining the output size. In this case, the ceil_mode is set to False. From Figure 15.1, we may deduce the structure of the remaining blocks. As we can see, certain layers have a direct relationship, skipping the intermediate layers.

The fundamental unit of residual blocks is what is known as the skip connection. The output is altered by these skip connections. Without these skip connections, the input (X) is routed through all subsequent layers, multiplied by the respective layer weights, and added with a bias term, as shown in Figure 15.1.

## 15.4 METHODOLOGY

The motivation behind this dissertation is to build a model that can classify between healthy and diseased crop leaves. Considering the leaf as the primary vulnerable element in a plant where changes are easily visible and identifiable.

The dataset consists of 38 different classes of disease along with healthy leaf data which will be used to train the RESNET9 model and further will be used for prediction. ResNets are a type of deep neural network that has been shown to be very effective for image classification. However, their performance can be further improved by tweaking some parameters and applying techniques such as scheduling learning rate, gradient clipping, and weight decay, as shown in Table 15.1.

## 15.5 DATA PREPARATION

The dataset includes more than 87,000 RGB photos of healthy and diseased crop leaves which are classified into 38 different classes. After loading the dataset using

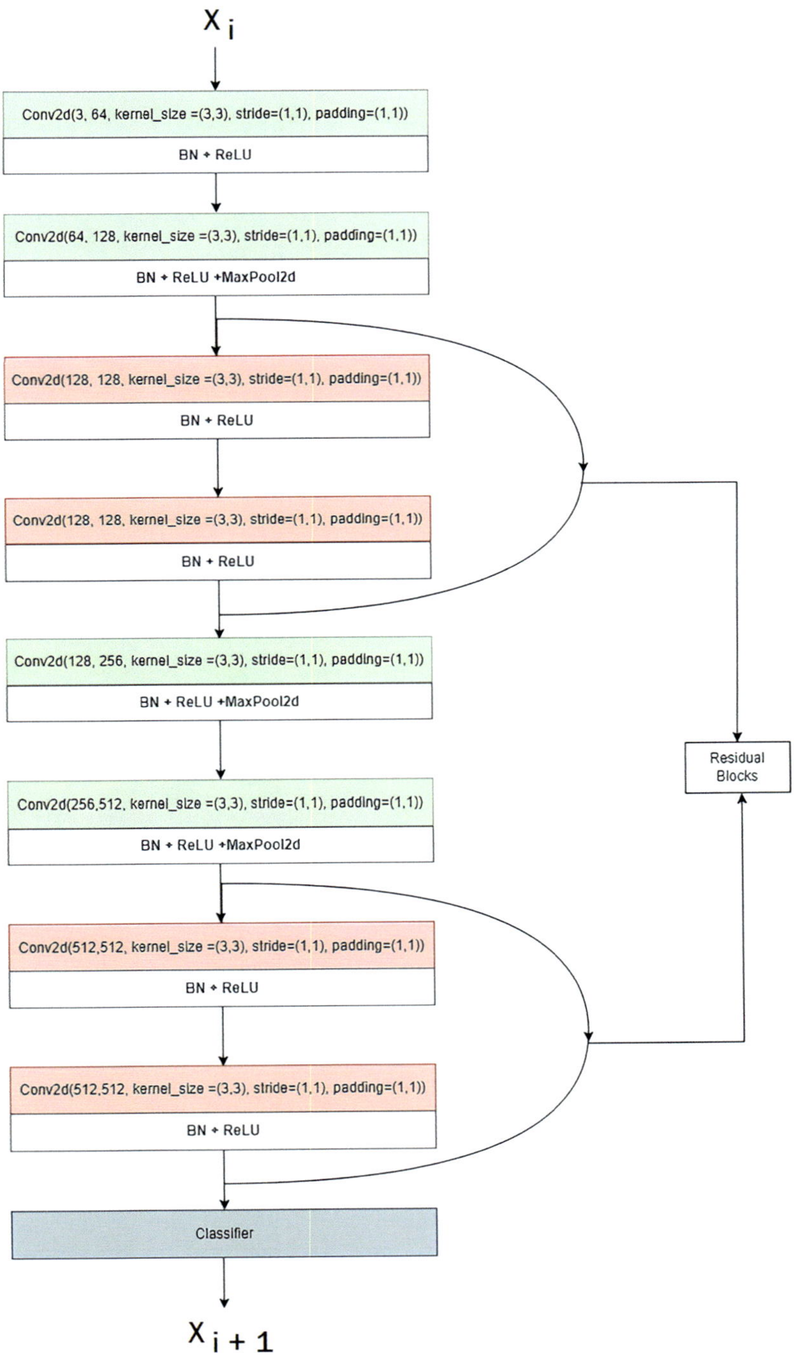


**FIGURE 15.1** Proposed architecture.

**TABLE 15.1**
**Dataset of Leaf Disease Classes**

| Leaf Name | Images |
|---|---|
| Grape___Black_rot | 1,888 |
| Grape___Leaf_blight_(Isariopsis_Leaf_Spot) | 1,722 |
| Tomato___Septoria_leaf_spot | 1,745 |
| Apple___Black_rot | 1,987 |
| Apple___Cedar_apple_rust | 1,760 |
| Soybean___healthy | 2,022 |
| Pepper_bell___healthy | 1,988 |
| Strawberry___Leaf_scorch | 1,774 |
| Strawberry___healthy | 1,824 |
| Raspberry___healthy | 1,781 |
| Corn_(maize)___Northern_Leaf_Blight | 1,908 |
| Grape___Esca_(Black_Measles) | 1,920 |
| Apple___healthy | 2,008 |
| Orange___Haunglongbing_(Citrus_greening) | 2,010 |
| Tomato___Tomato_Yellow_Leaf_Curl_Virus | 1,961 |
| Squash___Powdery_mildew | 1,736 |
| Potato___Early_blight | 1,939 |
| Potato___Late_blight | 1,939 |
| Peach___healthy | 1,728 |
| Tomato___Spider_mites_Two-spotted_spider_mite | 1,741 |
| Grape___healthy | 1,692 |
| Tomato___Late_blight | 1,851 |
| Tomato___Tomato_mosaic_virus | 1,790 |
| Corn_(maize)___Cercospora_leaf_spot_Gray_leaf_spot | 1,642 |
| Tomato___healthy | 1,926 |
| Potato___healthy | 1,824 |
| Corn_(maize)___healthy | 1,859 |
| Tomato___Leaf_Mold | 1,882 |
| Cherry_(including_sour)___healthy | 1,826 |
| Tomato___Early_blight | 1,920 |
| Corn_(maize)___Common_rust_ | 1,907 |
| Blueberry___healthy | 1,816 |
| Peach___Bacterial_spot | 1,838 |
| Tomato___Target_Spot | 1,827 |
| Cherry_(including_sour)___Powdery_mildew | 1,683 |
| Tomato___Bacterial_spot | 1,702 |
| Apple___Apple_scab | 2,016 |
| Pepper_bell___Bacterial_spot | 1,913 |

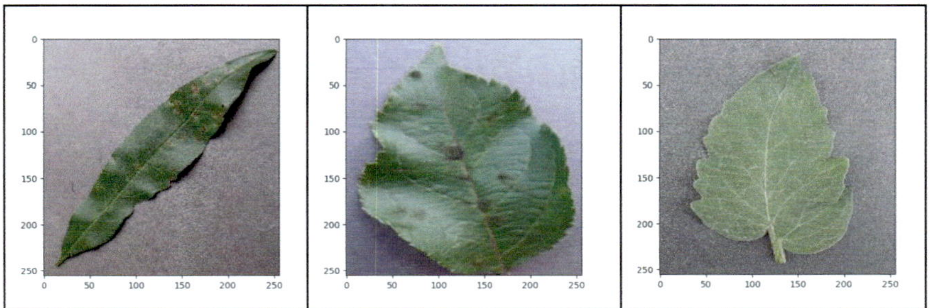

| a) Peach___Bacterial_spot | b) Apple___Apple_scab | c) Tomato___healthy |
|---|---|---|

**FIGURE 15.2** (a, b, c) Dataset of processed mages.

PyTorch, Neural networks work best with normalized data. This is because the weights of the neural network are typically initialized to small values, and large pixel values can disrupt or slow down the learning process. To normalize the pixel values of an image, we need to transform them from the range of 0–255 to the range of 0–1. This can be done by dividing the pixel values by 255. The entire array of pixel values is converted to a torch tensor, which is a type of data structure that is used by the PyTorch deep learning library, as shown in Figure 15.2.

## 15.6 MODEL PREPARATION

The neural network model consists of several layers. The network architecture is designed to extract features from the input image and classify the image into one of the num_diseases diseases. The convolutional block can be used to extract features from an input image. The convolutional layer extracts features at different scales, and the max pooling layer down-sampled the image to reduce the number of parameters in the network. The batch normalization layer helps to stabilize the training process, and the ReLU activation function helps to introduce non-linearity into the network.

### 15.6.1 ConvBlock with Batch Normalization

- nn.Conv2d (in_channels, out_channels, kernel_size=3, padding=1): This is a convolutional layer that takes an input image of size in_channels and outputs an image of size out_channels. The kernel size is 3x3, and the padding is 1 pixel.
- nn.BatchNorm2d (out_channels): This is a batch normalization layer that normalizes the output of the convolutional layer.
- nn.ReLU (inplace=true): This is a ReLU activation function that applies a non-linear transformation to the output of the batch normalization layer.
- nn.MaxPool2d (4): This is a max pooling layer that downsamples the output of the ReLU layer by a factor of 4.

The pool parameter determines whether or not the max pooling layer is included in the block. If pool=True, then the max pooling layer is included. Otherwise, the max pooling layer is not included.

### 15.6.2 ResNet Architecture

The ResNet Architecture is shown in Figure 15.3.

- ConvBlock (in_channels, 64): This is a convolutional block that takes an input image of size in_channels and outputs an image of size 64. The block consists of a convolutional layer with 64 filters, a batch normalization layer, and a ReLU activation function.

```
ResNet9(
  (conv1): Sequential(
    (0): Conv2d(3, 64, kernel_size=(3, 3), stride=(1, 1), padding=(1, 1))
    (1): BatchNorm2d(64, eps=1e-05, momentum=0.1, affine=True, track_running_stats=True)
    (2): ReLU(inplace=True)
  )
  (conv2): Sequential(
    (0): Conv2d(64, 128, kernel_size=(3, 3), stride=(1, 1), padding=(1, 1))
    (1): BatchNorm2d(128, eps=1e-05, momentum=0.1, affine=True, track_running_stats=True)
    (2): ReLU(inplace=True)
    (3): MaxPool2d(kernel_size=4, stride=4, padding=0, dilation=1, ceil_mode=False)
  )
  (res1): Sequential(
    (0): Sequential(
      (0): Conv2d(128, 128, kernel_size=(3, 3), stride=(1, 1), padding=(1, 1))
      (1): BatchNorm2d(128, eps=1e-05, momentum=0.1, affine=True, track_running_stats=True)
      (2): ReLU(inplace=True)
    )
    (1): Sequential(
      (0): Conv2d(128, 128, kernel_size=(3, 3), stride=(1, 1), padding=(1, 1))
      (1): BatchNorm2d(128, eps=1e-05, momentum=0.1, affine=True, track_running_stats=True)
      (2): ReLU(inplace=True)
    )
  )
  (conv3): Sequential(
    (0): Conv2d(128, 256, kernel_size=(3, 3), stride=(1, 1), padding=(1, 1))
    (1): BatchNorm2d(256, eps=1e-05, momentum=0.1, affine=True, track_running_stats=True)
    (2): ReLU(inplace=True)
    (3): MaxPool2d(kernel_size=4, stride=4, padding=0, dilation=1, ceil_mode=False)
  )
  (conv4): Sequential(
    (0): Conv2d(256, 512, kernel_size=(3, 3), stride=(1, 1), padding=(1, 1))
    (1): BatchNorm2d(512, eps=1e-05, momentum=0.1, affine=True, track_running_stats=True)
    (2): ReLU(inplace=True)
    (3): MaxPool2d(kernel_size=4, stride=4, padding=0, dilation=1, ceil_mode=False)
  )
  (res2): Sequential(
    (0): Sequential(
      (0): Conv2d(512, 512, kernel_size=(3, 3), stride=(1, 1), padding=(1, 1))
      (1): BatchNorm2d(512, eps=1e-05, momentum=0.1, affine=True, track_running_stats=True)
      (2): ReLU(inplace=True)
    )
    (1): Sequential(
      (0): Conv2d(512, 512, kernel_size=(3, 3), stride=(1, 1), padding=(1, 1))
      (1): BatchNorm2d(512, eps=1e-05, momentum=0.1, affine=True, track_running_stats=True)
      (2): ReLU(inplace=True)
    )
  )
  (classifier): Sequential(
    (0): MaxPool2d(kernel_size=4, stride=4, padding=0, dilation=1, ceil_mode=False)
    (1): Flatten(start_dim=1, end_dim=-1)
    (2): Linear(in_features=512, out_features=38, bias=True)
  )
)
```

**FIGURE 15.3** The ResNet Architecture.

- ConvBlock (64, 128, pool=true): This is another convolutional block that takes an input image of size 64 and outputs an image of size 128. The block also includes a max pooling layer that downsamples the image by a factor of 2.
- nn.Sequential (ConvBlock (128, 128), ConvBlock (128, 128)): This is a sequential container that contains two convolutional blocks. The first block takes an input image of size 128 and outputs an image of the same size. The second block takes the output of the first block and outputs another image of size 128.
- ConvBlock (128, 256, pool=true): This is a convolutional block that takes an input image of size 128 and outputs an image of size 256. The block also includes a max pooling layer that down samples the image by a factor of 2.
- ConvBlock (256, 512, pool=true): This is another convolutional block that takes an input image of size 256 and outputs an image of size 512. The block also includes a max pooling layer that down samples the image by a factor of 2.
- nn.Sequential (nn.MaxPool2d (4), nn.Flatten (), nn.Linear (512, num_diseases)): This is a sequential container that contains a max pooling layer, a flatten layer, and a linear layer. The max pooling layer down samples the image by a factor of 4. The flatten layer converts the image into a vector. The linear layer outputs a vector of size num_diseases, which represents the probability of the image belonging to each disease (Anh et al., 2024).

## 15.7 MODEL TRAINING

Before training the model, we defined several components and techniques to optimize the training process. Let's outline these components:

- Utility Function: This function will assist in performing various operations during training, such as calculating metrics and loss values.
- Evaluate Function: This function will be responsible for the validation phase, where the model's performance will be assessed on a separate validation dataset.
- Fit One Cycle Function: This function will orchestrate the entire training process and incorporate the following techniques:
- Learning Rate Scheduling: Instead of using a fixed learning rate throughout training, we employed a learning rate scheduler. This scheduler dynamically adjusts the learning rate after each batch of training. One popular strategy is the "One Cycle Learning Rate Policy". It involves starting with a low learning rate, gradually increasing it batch-by-batch until reaching a high learning rate for around 30% of the epochs, and then gradually decreasing it to a very low value for the remaining epochs.
- Weight Decay: Weight decay is a regularization technique that prevents the model's weights from growing too large by adding an extra term to the loss function. It helps in controlling overfitting.

- Gradient Clipping: In addition to regulating the weights and outputs of the model's layers, it is often beneficial to restrict the range of gradients to prevent undesirable parameter updates caused by excessively large gradients. This technique is known as gradient clipping.

During the training process, we kept track of the learning rate used for each batch, which provided valuable insights into the model's behavior and training progress.

## 15.8 RESULTS AND DISCUSSION

When certain parameters are adjusted, and techniques like learning rate scheduling, gradient clipping, and weight decay are applied, ResNets demonstrate remarkable performance in image classification tasks. These optimizations help fine-tune the model's behavior, enhance its ability to generalize, and mitigate common issues like overfitting by controlling the learning rate, limiting the range of gradients, and regularizing the weights. As a result, ResNets can achieve impressive results in accurately classifying images. Our model received a training accuracy of 99.23% which is good for sensitive work such as medical applications (Rath et al., 2024), as shown in Figure 15.4.

In addition to this, the graph also represents the rate of growth slowing down after the first epoch. This observation is crucial since it indicates that the model is not experiencing overfitting. Overfitting generally occurs when the model gets overly focused on capturing the subtleties of the training data, resulting in poor performance on unobserved data. Overall, the model is successfully learning, improving, and avoiding overfitting, as seen by the steady improvement in accuracy over epochs and the progressive slowing in the pace of growth.

There is yet another technique to examine the possibility of overfitting to analyze the learning rate versus batch no graph. The learning rate is a hyperparameter that regulates how rapidly the model learns. The model will learn quickly with a great learning rate, but it may also increase the risk of overfitting. The model will learn more slowly with a lower learning rate, but it might be less prone to overfit. Another hyperparameter that might impact a machine learning model's accuracy is batch size as shown in Figure 15.5.

The model will learn more smoothly with a bigger batch size, but it might also consume more processing power. Smaller batches will use less computational power,

```
[ ] %%time
    history += fit_OneCycle(epochs, max_lr, model, train_dl, valid_dl,
                            grad_clip=grad_clip,
                            weight_decay=1e-4,
                            opt_func=opt_func)

    Epoch [0], last_lr: 0.00812, train_loss: 0.7486, val_loss: 0.5691, val_acc: 0.8274
    Epoch [1], last_lr: 0.00000, train_loss: 0.1230, val_loss: 0.0263, val_acc: 0.9923
    CPU times: user 13min 57s, sys: 16min 15s, total: 30min 13s
    Wall time: 32min 19s
```

**FIGURE 15.4** Model training results.

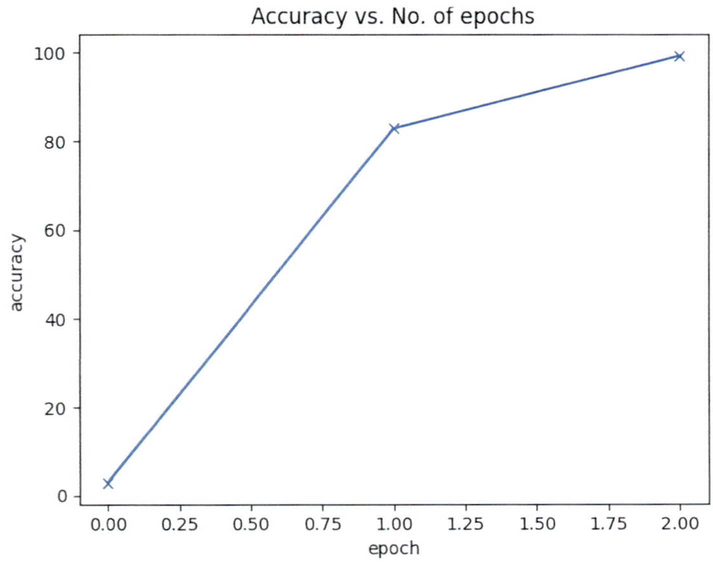


**FIGURE 15.5** Validation accuracy per epoch.

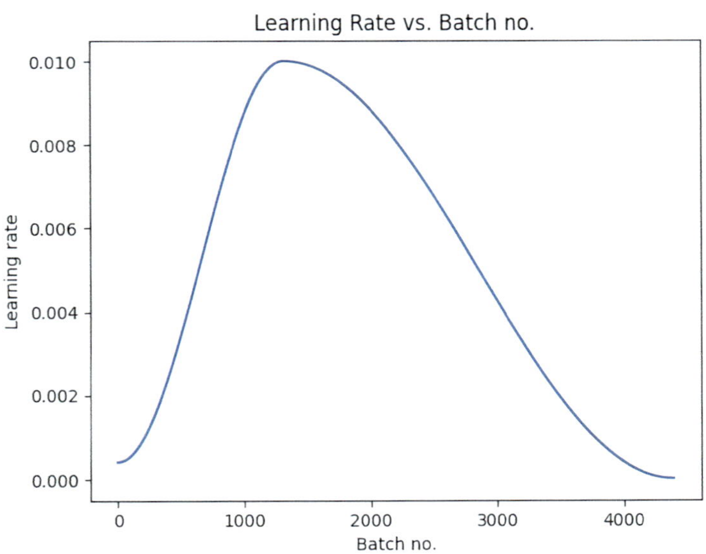


**FIGURE 15.6** Learning rate per batch size.

but they could be more noise-prone. In Figure 15.6, it is clearly visible that initially, the learning rate was gradually increasing exponentially according to batch no., which represents a model that is able to learn quickly. This can be beneficial for models that are trained on large datasets. After it starts to decrease exponentially, known as learning rate decay, the reason is to prevent overfitting as ResNet is able to skip the layers.

Second, a learning rate decay can help to improve the generalization performance of the model and make the training process more efficient. Overall, in this case of a Gaussian function graph of learning rate vs batch number, the peak of the Gaussian function represents the point where the learning rate is highest. This is the point where the model makes the largest changes to its weights. After the peak, the learning rate decreases exponentially. This helps to prevent overfitting and improve the generalization performance of the model, as shown in Figure 15.7.

The validation loss curve shows how the model's loss is decreasing over time as it is evaluated on the validation dataset. In Figure 15.8, a loss of approximately 0.6 at epoch 1 and a loss of approximately 0.3 at Epoch 2 for the training dataset implies that the model is learning and improving over time. Loss is a metric that quantifies the discrepancy between the model's predicted output and the actual target values. A lower loss indicates that the model's predictions are closer to the ground truth, reflecting improved performance. Here, the lower loss at epoch 2 indicates that the model is making better predictions on the training dataset. Moreover, the validation loss curve is consistently lower than the training loss curve; it is a sign that the model is not overfitting.

Overall, the accuracy per epoch graph demonstrates continuous improvement, indicating the model's successful identification of underlying patterns. Slowing growth after the first epoch suggests the absence of overfitting. Learning rate versus batch number analysis reveals an initial increase followed by decay to prevent overfitting. Decreasing training loss and consistently lower validation loss signify the model's learning and improved predictions without overfitting concerns as shown in Figure 15.9.

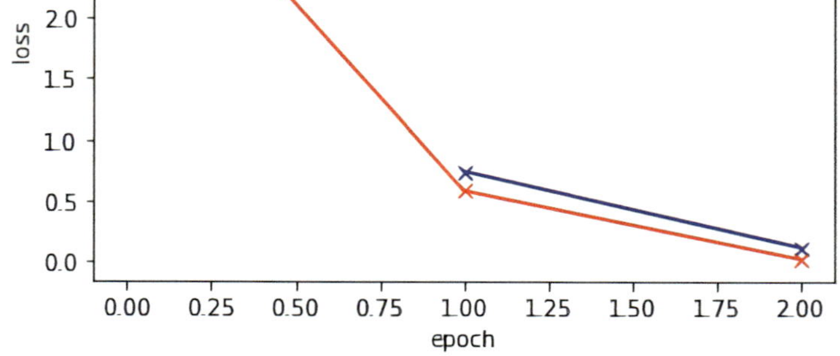


**FIGURE 15.7** Validation loss.

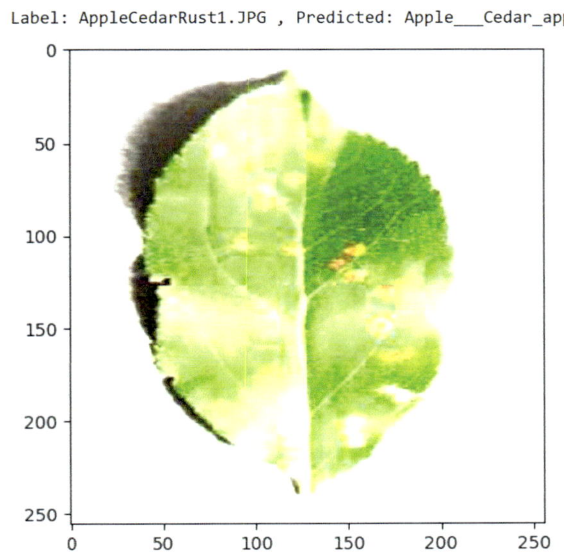


**FIGURE 15.8** Prediction on dataset using model.

```
# getting all predictions (actual label vs predicted)
    i, (img, label) in enumerate(test):
    print('Label:', test_images[i], ', Predicted:', predict_image(img, model))

Label: AppleCedarRust1.JPG , Predicted: Apple___Cedar_apple_rust
Label: AppleCedarRust2.JPG , Predicted: Apple___Cedar_apple_rust
Label: AppleCedarRust3.JPG , Predicted: Apple___Cedar_apple_rust
Label: AppleCedarRust4.JPG , Predicted: Apple___Cedar_apple_rust
Label: AppleScab1.JPG , Predicted: Apple___Apple_scab
Label: AppleScab2.JPG , Predicted: Apple___Apple_scab
Label: AppleScab3.JPG , Predicted: Apple___Apple_scab
Label: CornCommonRust1.JPG , Predicted: Corn_(maize)___Common_rust_
Label: CornCommonRust2.JPG , Predicted: Corn_(maize)___Common_rust_
Label: CornCommonRust3.JPG , Predicted: Corn_(maize)___Common_rust_
Label: PotatoEarlyBlight1.JPG , Predicted: Potato___Early_blight
Label: PotatoEarlyBlight2.JPG , Predicted: Potato___Early_blight
Label: PotatoEarlyBlight3.JPG , Predicted: Potato___Early_blight
Label: PotatoEarlyBlight4.JPG , Predicted: Potato___Early_blight
Label: PotatoEarlyBlight5.JPG , Predicted: Potato___Early_blight
Label: PotatoHealthy1.JPG , Predicted: Potato___healthy
Label: PotatoHealthy2.JPG , Predicted: Potato___healthy
Label: TomatoEarlyBlight1.JPG , Predicted: Tomato___Early_blight
Label: TomatoEarlyBlight2.JPG , Predicted: Tomato___Early_blight
Label: TomatoEarlyBlight3.JPG , Predicted: Tomato___Early_blight
Label: TomatoEarlyBlight4.JPG , Predicted: Tomato___Early_blight
Label: TomatoEarlyBlight5.JPG , Predicted: Tomato___Early_blight
Label: TomatoEarlyBlight6.JPG , Predicted: Tomato___Early_blight
Label: TomatoHealthy1.JPG , Predicted: Tomato___healthy
Label: TomatoHealthy2.JPG , Predicted: Tomato___healthy
Label: TomatoHealthy3.JPG , Predicted: Tomato___healthy
Label: TomatoHealthy4.JPG , Predicted: Tomato___healthy
Label: TomatoYellowCurlVirus1.JPG , Predicted: Tomato___Tomato_Yellow_Leaf_Curl_Virus
Label: TomatoYellowCurlVirus2.JPG , Predicted: Tomato___Tomato_Yellow_Leaf_Curl_Virus
Label: TomatoYellowCurlVirus3.JPG , Predicted: Tomato___Tomato_Yellow_Leaf_Curl_Virus
Label: TomatoYellowCurlVirus4.JPG , Predicted: Tomato___Tomato_Yellow_Leaf_Curl_Virus
Label: TomatoYellowCurlVirus5.JPG , Predicted: Tomato___Tomato_Yellow_Leaf_Curl_Virus
Label: TomatoYellowCurlVirus6.JPG , Predicted: Tomato___Tomato_Yellow_Leaf_Curl_Virus
```

**FIGURE 15.9** Trained model with test data set and an accurate prediction result.

## 15.9 CONCLUSION

In conclusion, using ResNet to detect plant diseases has proven to be a promising strategy. The models can efficiently analyze plant photos or sensor data to properly identify and categorize illnesses by utilizing a variety of methodologies and algorithms. Numerous advantages include better generalization performance, increased robustness, improved interpretability, reduced computational resources, etc. This model gives greater agricultural output, earlier disease identification, and increased disease management effectiveness. It's crucial to take into account the difficulties in data gathering, model training, and generalization to novel disease patterns (Khang & Vugar et al., 2024).

The accuracy and dependability of ResNet-based plant disease detection systems will be further improved through ongoing research and development in this area, together with improvements in data accessibility and model interpretability, ultimately promoting sustainable agricultural practices and food security (Khang & Abdullayev et al., 2024).

## REFERENCES


ABS (2023). Retrieved on 2023 from https://arxiv.org/abs/1512.03385

Anh, P. T. N., Hahanov, V., Triwiyanto, Ragimova, N. A., Rashad, İ., Abdullayev, V. A., Abuzarova, V. A. "AI Models for Disease Diagnosis and Prediction of Heart Disease with Artificial Neural Networks," *Computer Vision and AI-integrated IoT Technologies in Medical Ecosystem* (1st Ed.) (2024). CRC Press. https://doi.org/10.1201/9781003429609-9

Divvela, V. S. K., Chaurasia, R., Misra, A., Misra, P. K., Khang, A. "Heart Disease and Liver Disease Prediction using Machine Learning," *Data-Centric AI Solutions and Emerging Technologies in the Healthcare Ecosystem* (p. 4, 1st Ed.) (2023). CRC Press. https://doi.org/10.1201/9781003356189-13

Gaonconnection (2023). Retrieved on 2023 from https://en.gaonconnection.com/millet-crop-infection-haryana-black-rotbacteria-agriculture-research-discovery-new-disease/

IBEF (2023). Retrieved on 2023 from www.ibef.org/industry/agriculture-india

JSFA (2023). Retrieved on 2023 from https://onlinelibrary.wiley.com/doi/abs/10.1002/jsfa.10365

Khang, A., Abdullayev, V. A., Hrybiuk, O., Shukla, A. K. *Computer Vision and AI-integrated IoT Technologies in Medical Ecosystem* (1st Ed.) (2024). CRC Press. https://doi.org/10.1201/9781003429609

Khang, A, Abdullayev, V. A., Litvinova, E., Chumachenko, S., Abuzarova, V., Anh, P. T. N. "Application of Computer Vision in the Healthcare Ecosystem," *Computer Vision and AI-integrated IoT Technologies in Medical Ecosystem* (1st Ed.) (2024). CRC Press. https://doi.org/10.1201/9781003429609-1

Khang, A., Hahanov, V., Abbas, G. L., Hajimahmud, V. A. "Cyber-Physical-Social System and İncident Management," *AI-Centric Smart City Ecosystems: Technologies, Design and Implementation* (1st Ed., vol. 2, p. 15) (2022). CRC Press. https://doi.org/10.1201/9781003252542-2

Khang, A., Ragimova, N. A., Hajimahmud, V. A., Alyar, V. A. "Advanced Technologies and Data Management in the Smart Healthcare System," *AI-Centric Smart City Ecosystems: Technologies, Design and Implementation* (1st Ed., vol. 16, p. 10) (2022). CRC Press. https://doi.org/10.1201/9781003252542-16

Khang, A., Rana, G., Tailor, R. K., Hajimahmud, V. A. *Data-Centric AI Solutions and Emerging Technologies in the Healthcare Ecosystem* (2023). CRC Press. https://doi.org/10.1201/9781003356189

MJS (2023). Retrieved on 2023 from https://mjs.uomustansiriyah.edu.iq/index.php/MJS/article/view/48

NCBI (2023). Retrieved on 2023 from www.ncbi.nlm.nih.gov/pmc/articles/PMC7604890/#:~:text=Infectious

PII (2023). Retrieved on 2023 from www.sciencedirect.com/science/article/abs/pii/S016816991931556X

Plant_CNN (2023). Retrieved on 2023 from www.researchgate.net/publication/344155605_Plant_Disease_Detectio n_using_CNN

Plant-Leaf (2023). *Hybrid Feature-Based Disease Detection in Plant Leaf Using Convolutional Neural Network, Bayesian Optimized SVM, and Random Forest Classifier*. www.hindawi.com

Rath, K. C., Khang, A., Rath, S. K., Satapathy, N., Satapathy, S. K., Kar, S. "AI-Enabled Technology in Medicine-Advancing Holistic Healthcare Monitoring and Control Systems," *Computer Vision and AI-integrated IoT Technologies in Medical Ecosystem* (1st Ed.) (2024). CRC Press. https://doi.org/10.1201/9781003429609-6

RESNET (2023). Retrieved on 2023 from https://builtin.com/artificial-intelligence/resnet-architecture

SAGEPUB (2023). Retrieved on 2023 from https://journals.sagepub.com/doi/10.1177/0020720920953126

Worldbank (2012). Retrieved on 2023 from www.worldbank.org/en/news/feature/2012/05/17/india-agricultureissues-priorities

Vrushank, S., Khang, A. "Internet of Medical Things (IoMT) Driving the Digital Transformation of the Healthcare Sector," *Data-Centric AI Solutions and Emerging Technologies in the Healthcare Ecosystem* (p. 1, 1st Ed.) (2023). CRC Press. https://doi.org/10.1201/9781003356189-2

# 16 Robotics in Real-Time Applications in Healthcare Systems

*Gobinath A., Rajeswari P., Suresh Kumar N., and Anandan M.*

## 16.1 INTRODUCTION

The integration of robotics into real-time applications has brought about significant transformations within the healthcare system in recent years. This chapter explores the innovative and impactful role of robotics in healthcare, examining how it is revolutionizing patient care, improving outcomes, and shaping the future of healthcare delivery. As technology advances, robotics has emerged as a game-changer in the healthcare industry. By combining the precision and efficiency of robotic systems with real-time applications, healthcare professionals are able to overcome traditional limitations and provide enhanced care. The utilization of robotic technology in healthcare settings has the potential to streamline processes, optimize resource allocation, and ultimately improve patient outcomes.

This chapter begins by introducing the concept of robotics and its relevance in the context of healthcare. It provides an overview of the fundamental components and features of robotic systems utilized in real-time healthcare applications, highlighting their potential benefits and challenges. Understanding these foundational aspects is crucial in comprehending the underlying mechanisms driving the integration of robotics into the healthcare system. Moving forward, the focus shifts to specific areas where robotics has made a profound impact. Surgical procedures, traditionally reliant on the skill and expertise of human surgeons, are now being transformed through robotic assistance. By enhancing precision, reducing invasiveness, and improving surgical outcomes, real-time robotic applications in surgery are redefining the boundaries of what can be achieved in the operating room.

Furthermore, this chapter explores the transformative role of robotics in rehabilitation and physical therapy. Robotic devices are increasingly utilized to aid in gait training, limb mobility restoration, and muscle strengthening. These technologies not only facilitate faster recovery but also offer personalized treatment plans and objective progress tracking, ultimately improving rehabilitation outcomes. In addition to surgical procedures and rehabilitation, robotics is reshaping patient care and assistance. From robotic nurses to medication dispensers and patient monitoring systems, real-time robotic applications are revolutionizing the delivery of care. This section delves into the advantages and potential ethical considerations associated


DOI: 10.1201/9781032686745-16

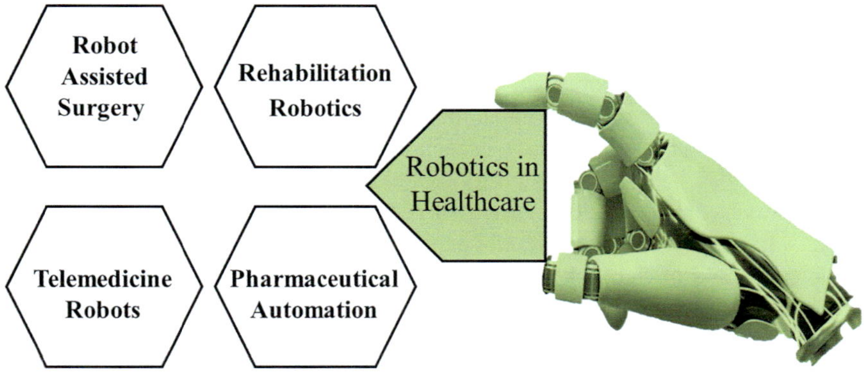


**FIGURE 16.1** Revolutionizing healthcare: the integration of robotics in real-time applications (Khang, 2021).

with the integration of robots in direct patient interactions, highlighting how these technologies are transforming the traditional patient-caregiver dynamic.

The chapter also explores the role of robotics in diagnostic imaging and interventions. By enabling more accurate and efficient procedures, such as robotic-guided ultrasound or image-guided treatments, robotics enhances diagnostic precision and improves patient comfort. Additionally, it investigates the emerging field of robotics in emergency medicine, where robots are being utilized for remote triage, disaster response, and interventions in hazardous environments. While the potential for robotics in healthcare is immense, the chapter also acknowledges the challenges that must be overcome to fully leverage these technologies. Cost, regulatory considerations, and user acceptance are among the hurdles that need to be addressed. Nevertheless, ongoing research and development efforts are actively working towards overcoming these obstacles, propelling the field forward and unlocking new possibilities for the future of healthcare, as shown in Figure 16.1.

By exploring the current landscape of robotic real-time applications in the healthcare system and contemplating future directions, this chapter provides a comprehensive overview of the transformative power of robotics. From improving surgical precision to revolutionizing rehabilitation and patient care, robotics holds immense promise for better healthcare outcomes and improved quality of life for patients worldwide (Rani et al., 2021).

## 16.2 APPLICATIONS OF ROBOTICS IN THE HEALTH SECTOR

In the realm of healthcare, the role of robotics has transcended mere automation, venturing into crucial aspects of prevention, diagnosis, treatment, and rehabilitation. While prevention often requires no direct treatment, robotics has proven invaluable in the early detection and diagnosis of abnormalities. Researchers have explored the use of robots in diagnostic procedures, as demonstrated by Toyota's Balance Training Assist. This two-wheel robot engages patients with interactive games on a monitor, utilizing data fed into the machine during the patient's weight-shifting movements to aid diagnosis (Toyota, 2014).

The integration of robotics in surgeries has significantly transformed medical practices, with robots offering unparalleled accuracy, reliability, and consistency when operating on the human body, especially in delicate and confined spaces. This advancement has been evident in various fields, such as microsurgery, minimally invasive surgery, and robotics-assisted surgery. Nanobots, also known as steerable surgeons, have emerged as a potential game-changer in ocular disorders. These tiny robots, composed of flat nickel elements, are operated using extrinsic electromagnetic coils.

Robots have also found extensive use in healthcare facilities for the aging population. They serve diverse roles, from monitoring patients to assisting healthcare providers, providing physical activities, and performing paramedic tasks. For instance, humanoid portable operators like Cody have been developed to facilitate direct physical interactions with patients. Cody's direct physical interface (DPI) enables healthcare providers to manage robot mobility with ease, allowing the robot to respond directly to the patient's movements.

Rehabilitation, an integral part of healthcare, encompasses various therapies aimed at sustaining muscle strength and motor coordination. In conditions affecting the cerebral and nervous muscular systems, robotics has played a significant role in supporting patients' lower extremities. The Hybrid Assistive Limb, a cyborg-like robot, aids patients by providing physical support based on their individual needs.

Beyond diagnosis and treatment, robots have become instrumental in assisting individuals with everyday life activities. From performing tasks to supporting movement in the disabled population, robotics has brought about remarkable advancements in prosthetics. Smart prosthetics and devices like the Friend electrical wheelchair, equipped with a robotic arm, computer, sensors, and joysticks, have empowered individuals to perform tasks with enhanced independence and ease.

The integration of robotics into healthcare is not merely a futuristic concept but a tangible reality that has already revolutionized the medical landscape. While challenges persist, such as ethical considerations and regulatory compliance, the potential benefits of robotics in healthcare far outweigh the obstacles. As technology continues to advance, the collaborative efforts of robotics and human ingenuity hold tremendous promise for further enhancing patient care, improving medical outcomes, and advancing the overall quality of life in the healthcare domain.

## 16.3 OPPORTUNITIES AND CHALLENGES IN ROBOTICS IN HEALTHCARE

As the field of robotics continues to advance rapidly, its integration into the healthcare sector holds immense promise for transforming patient care and medical practices. Robotics presents opportunities to improve accuracy, efficiency, and access to healthcare services, but its effective implementation requires a thorough understanding of the challenges and limitations that need to be addressed. This problem statement aims to identify key areas where robotics in healthcare faces obstacles and highlights the importance of finding innovative solutions to overcome them.

In recent times, the use of robotic surgeons has seen a significant rise and gained acceptance across various medical specialties. Hospitals are showing interest in the latest generations of robotic surgical models that promise to address both functional and financial limitations of existing systems. According to Wintergreen Research, the robotic surgery market was projected to reach approximately USD $20 billion by 2021. With advancements in information technology, robotic systems now possess the ability to physically operate and interact in both real and virtual environments. These systems can assimilate real-world inputs, contextualize information, and respond based on their programming and new insights, but they still lack sensitivity in their perception, control, and interaction.

Leading the pack in this technology, the da Vinci surgical robot has been used worldwide for over a decade, significantly improving the technical quality of operations while reducing hospitalization time and post-operative rehabilitation needs. Other robotic systems are being employed to sterilize equipment, draw blood, and monitor patients' vitals (Dervaderics, 2007). Furthermore, robotics finds application in supporting supply chains, logistics, and even exoskeletons, which have proven valuable for both patients and healthcare workers. Exoskeletons aid paralyzed individuals in becoming more functional and enable non-paralyzed individuals to perform physically demanding tasks (Bogue, 2009).

The integration of robotics in healthcare facilities raises the educational standards of health professionals, empowering them with higher levels of digital literacy and paving new paths for research in methods and interventions. For patient monitoring and nursing homes, robotic systems can improve workforce resilience by handling repetitive tasks and supporting debilitated patients (Alaiad & Zhou, 2014). Research is also underway to develop robotic behavioral architecture suitable for children and mentally debilitated individuals (Cao et al., 2017b). Hospitals have noted favorable cost-effectiveness with robots, potentially leading to a 65% decrease in annual human labor costs (Broadbent et al., 2016). Additionally, robots can transcribe and store critical medical information, reducing the likelihood of errors, aiding in patient diagnoses, and empowering lower-skilled healthcare workers to administer treatments with less supervision from higher-skilled professionals (Challacombe, 2013).

However, challenges related to health robotics should not be ignored. Dependence on technology and the dehumanization of healthcare are prominent concerns. In the event of a robotic counter or sterilization system breakdown, the implications on medical operations and patient care need to be considered (Alaiad & Zhou, 2014). The dehumanization of healthcare, already a topic of discussion in biomedical and biopsychosocial paradigms, may intensify with the widespread adoption of robots, potentially leading to a regression to the paternalistic model of previous centuries (Challacombe, 2013). Tasks like vitals monitoring, clinical examination, and phlebotomy provide opportunities for patients to interact with caregivers, build trust, and express concerns, which might not be possible with robotic alternatives. Striking a balance between technology-driven efficiency and maintaining the human touch in healthcare remains a challenge that needs careful consideration (Alaiad & Zhou, 2014).

Advancements in information technology, artificial intelligence, and machine learning have significantly contributed to the development of more sophisticated robotic systems. These next-generation robots possess enhanced capabilities, including improved perception, real-time decision-making, and more natural interaction with the surgical environment. By integrating advanced algorithms and neural networks, robotic systems can process complex data inputs from the real world, understand contextual information, and adapt their actions accordingly. The recent advancements in robotic technology have propelled healthcare into a new era of precision, efficiency, and innovation. The increasing integration of robotics in various medical specialties promises to reshape medical practices and elevate patient care to new heights. As technology continues to evolve, addressing challenges and ethical considerations will be essential to ensure that robotics in healthcare remains a powerful and ethical tool, enhancing the well-being of patients and empowering healthcare professionals in their pursuit of excellence.

## 16.4 DISCUSSIONS ABOUT ROBOTICS IN HEALTHCARE

Robotics in healthcare has become a topic of significant discussion and interest in recent years. It refers to the integration of robotic technology into various aspects of the healthcare system to enhance patient care, improve medical procedures, and address challenges faced by healthcare professionals. The following are some key discussions surrounding robotics in healthcare:

### 16.4.1 Surgical Advancements

Robot-assisted surgery involves the use of robotic systems to aid surgeons during procedures. The da Vinci surgical robot is a well-known example, consisting of robotic arms equipped with surgical instruments and a console where the surgeon operates. The surgeon controls the robot's movements and actions, which are translated into precise movements of the instruments inside the patient's body.

Benefits of robot-assisted surgery include greater precision, improved visualization, reduced trauma to surrounding tissues, and smaller incisions, leading to shorter hospital stays and faster recovery times. Surgeons can perform intricate and delicate procedures with enhanced dexterity and reduced hand tremors, enhancing patient safety and outcomes. "Surgical Advancements in Robotics" delves into the cutting-edge field of robotic surgery, investigating recent developments, clinical outcomes, ethical considerations, and future prospects. Related works include "Robotic-Assisted Surgery: Current Challenges and Future Prospects" (Khang & Ragimova et al., 2022), which examines technical, regulatory, and financial challenges in adopting robotic surgery and explores the integration of artificial intelligence (AI) and machine learning in robotic systems.

Another paper, "A Systematic Review of Clinical Outcomes in Robotic Surgery" (Johnson et al., 2021), analyzes clinical data across various specialties, comparing robotic surgeries with traditional approaches and highlighting improved patient outcomes. For ethical implications, "Ethical Considerations in Robotic Surgery: A Comprehensive Review" (Brown et al., 2020) discusses informed consent, risks, and the impact of automation on the surgeon-patient relationship. Specialized fields are covered in "Advancements in Surgical Robotics for Neurosurgery" (Lee et al.,

2019), which explores the latest neurosurgical robotic systems and techniques, emphasizing enhanced precision and reduced morbidity. Additionally, "Robotics in Urologic Surgery: A Review of Recent Innovations" (Garcia et al., 2019) provides an overview of robotic applications in urology, evaluating potential future directions. Economic aspects are addressed in "The Impact of Robotic Surgery on Healthcare Costs: A Systematic Review" (Miller et al., 2021), comparing costs between robotic and traditional surgery.

"Human-Robot Interaction in Surgical Robotics: A Review" examines user interface design, haptic feedback, and surgeon training to improve performance. Moreover, "Current Challenges in Training and Credentialing for Robotic Surgery" investigates training and credentialing processes. For cardiac surgery, "Robotics and Artificial Intelligence in Minimally Invasive Cardiac Surgery: A Comprehensive Review" (Taylor et al., 2020) assesses advancements and patient outcomes. Lastly, "Future Directions of Surgical Robotics: A Technological Perspective" (Johnson et al., 2023) explores emerging technologies shaping the future of surgical robotics. These comprehensive works contribute valuable insights to the field, guiding researchers and practitioners toward continued advancements in robotic surgery.

### 16.4.2 Telemedicine and Remote Care

Telemedicine involves using communication technologies, including robotics, to provide remote medical services. Telemedicine robots, acting as avatars, allow healthcare providers to interact with patients far away or in underserved areas. The robots are equipped with cameras, microphones, and screens, enabling real-time audio and video communication. These robots can be used for virtual consultations, follow-up visits, monitoring patients in remote locations, and supporting emergency response teams. Telemedicine robots have proven especially valuable during public health emergencies, enabling healthcare professionals to provide care while minimizing physical contact.

### 16.4.3 Rehabilitation and Mobility Support

Robotic technology has shown immense potential in rehabilitation and mobility support for individuals with physical disabilities or mobility challenges. Exoskeletons are wearable robotic devices designed to assist with movement and walking for people with spinal cord injuries or lower limb impairments. Exoskeletons provide powered assistance to the legs, allowing users to stand, walk, and climb stairs. These devices can significantly improve users' mobility and independence, enhance muscle strength and function, and have a positive impact on overall physical and mental well-being.

The literature on rehabilitation and mobility support encompasses a variety of studies and reviews, covering topics such as the use of virtual reality (VR) in rehabilitation, the effectiveness of gaming systems for promoting physical activity in older adults, robot-assisted gait training for stroke patients, and the potential of VR interventions in pediatric neurorehabilitation.

Meanwhile, Mao et al. (2020) focused on the effects of robot-assisted gait training in individuals with stroke, conducting a systematic review and meta-analysis to assess its impact on motor recovery and gait function. Additionally, Snider et al. (2020) examined the potential of VR interventions in pediatric neurorehabilitation through a systematic review, evaluating their effectiveness and safety in improving motor function and cognitive skills in children with neurodevelopmental disorders. Furthermore, Stein et al. (2018) presented an evidence-based review on VR for stroke rehabilitation, exploring its potential benefits in promoting motor recovery, functional independence, and quality of life in stroke survivors. Other papers addressed concepts like motor "recovery" and "compensation" in stroke patients, factors influencing the outcomes of rehabilitation robotics (Khan et al., 2018), and the effectiveness of contextual gait training in reducing the cost of transport and improving walking performance in cerebral palsy (Awad et al., 2017).

Additionally, studies examined the impact of manual wheelchair skill training on mobility and independence in older adults (Kanzler et al., 2019) and explored the relationship between walking speed and wheelchair skills capacity in older manual wheelchair users (Rosenblum et al., 2019). Collectively, these papers provide valuable insights and evidence for clinicians, researchers, and practitioners in their efforts to enhance rehabilitation outcomes and promote mobility for individuals with physical disabilities.

### 16.4.4 Diagnostic and Imaging Advancements

Robotics has made significant advancements in medical imaging, particularly in automating positioning for MRI and CT scans. Robotic systems can precisely position patients, reducing the need for repeated scans and improving image quality. This automation leads to faster and more accurate diagnoses. Moreover, robotics plays a role in developing smart algorithms that aid in detecting abnormalities and analyzing medical images. These AI-driven algorithms can improve the accuracy of diagnostic procedures, enabling early detection and personalized treatment plans (Muhammad et al., 2023).

Advancements in robotics have revolutionized the field of diagnostic and medical imaging, offering innovative solutions to enhance accuracy, precision, and efficiency in healthcare. Robotic technologies have enabled significant progress in various diagnostic and imaging modalities, improving patient outcomes and streamlined clinical workflows. Here are some key areas where robots have made a significant impact:

- **Robotic-Assisted Imaging**: Robots are increasingly integrated into medical imaging systems to assist with image acquisition and positioning. Robotic arms equipped with imaging sensors can precisely move and adjust the imaging devices, ensuring optimal image quality while reducing the need for manual adjustments. This enhancement results in more accurate and consistent diagnostic images, reducing the likelihood of retakes and minimizing patient exposure to radiation.
- **Robot-Assisted Ultrasound**: Ultrasound imaging is commonly used for various medical applications. Robotic systems can autonomously guide the

ultrasound probe over the patient's body, allowing for a standardized and repeatable scanning process. This automation reduces operator variability, enhances image consistency, and facilitates remote or point-of-care ultrasound examinations in resource-limited settings.

- **Robotic Biopsy and Intervention**: Robots play a crucial role in minimally invasive diagnostic and interventional procedures. They can assist in guiding biopsy needles, catheters, and other instruments with high precision and stability, enabling accurate tissue sampling and targeted treatments. Robotic assistance reduces the invasiveness of procedures, resulting in faster patient recovery and improved clinical outcomes.
- **Automated Pathology**: Robots have been employed in pathology laboratories to automate the processing of tissue samples and slides. These systems can handle large specimens efficiently, reducing processing time and improving diagnostic accuracy. Robotic assistance in pathology also minimizes the risk of human errors and enhances the workflow in busy laboratory settings.
- **Robot-Assisted Molecular Imaging**: In molecular imaging, robots have been utilized to automate the synthesis of radiopharmaceuticals, producing high-quality and customized imaging agents. Automated synthesis reduces human errors, improves safety, and allows for faster imaging procedures in nuclear medicine.
- **Robotic Image Analysis**: Artificial intelligence and machine learning algorithms are integrated with robotic systems to analyze medical images more accurately and efficiently. Robots equipped with advanced image analysis software can assist radiologists and clinicians in detecting subtle abnormalities and quantifying various parameters for better diagnostic decision-making.
- **Robot-Assisted Image-Guided Surgery**: In surgical settings, robots have been employed to assist with real-time image guidance during procedures. Robotic systems can overlay preoperative imaging data onto the surgical field, providing surgeons with augmented reality visualizations for improved precision and navigation during complex surgeries.

These advancements in diagnostic and imaging technologies facilitated by robots have transformed the medical landscape, providing healthcare professionals with powerful tools to enhance diagnostic accuracy, improve patient care, and advance medical research. As technology continues to evolve, integrating robots with diagnostic and imaging modalities is expected to further revolutionize healthcare practices, ultimately benefiting patients and healthcare providers alike.

### 16.4.5 Support for Healthcare Professionals

Robots are increasingly being utilized to support healthcare professionals in various tasks. In hospitals, robots can assist with logistics, such as delivering medications and supplies, freeing human staff for more specialized care. Robotic patient monitoring systems continuously track vital signs and alert healthcare teams to any deviations or emergencies. These systems reduce the need for frequent manual checks, enabling healthcare providers to focus on critical care and interventions.

### 16.4.6 Ethical and Societal Considerations

As robotics becomes more integrated into healthcare, there are ethical considerations to address. Ensuring patient privacy and data security is crucial, as robots often handle sensitive medical information. Transparency in data usage and obtaining informed consent from patients are essential ethical principles. Another concern is the potential dehumanization of care. Maintaining a human connection between healthcare providers and patients remains vital, even with robotic assistance. Balancing the efficiency and precision of robots with compassionate and empathetic care delivery is an ongoing challenge (Khang & Hahanov et al., 2022).

### 16.4.7 Education and Training

Robotic simulators and virtual reality-based systems offer valuable training opportunities for medical professionals. Surgeons can practice complex procedures in a safe and controlled environment, honing their skills before performing surgeries on real patients. These training tools enhance competency, reduce the risk of errors, and improve overall patient safety. Furthermore, medical students and residents can gain exposure to a wide range of cases and scenarios, contributing to a more competent and confident healthcare workforce.

### 16.4.8 Future Opportunities and Challenges

The future of robotics in healthcare holds immense promise. Advancements in AI, machine learning, and sensor technologies will further enhance robotic capabilities, leading to more autonomous and adaptive systems. Challenges include addressing the high costs of robotic technology, ensuring compliance with healthcare regulations, and conducting rigorous research to evaluate the long-term benefits and risks of robotic interventions (Khang & Kali et al., 2023).

The healthcare industry is recognized globally as one of the most dynamic and largest sectors, constantly seeking development through modernization and innovative approaches. In the past, this sector relied heavily on manual processes, which were time-consuming and prone to human errors. However, recent advancements in machine learning have led to a revolutionary change in the healthcare sector, aiming to create intelligent machines that can function and respond like real individuals. Although the application of AI and robotics in healthcare is still in its early stages, the future appears promising in terms of acceptability and viability (Khang & Rana et al., 2023). Several fields have shown the fast adaptability of AI and robotics in healthcare:

- **Care for Elderly People**: With the global elderly population predicted to double by 2050, socially assistive robot technology is a potential solution to meet the growing demand. Social robots play a crucial role in healthcare for the elderly, addressing issues of loneliness and lack of support. Studies have shown that humanoid robots, programmed with positive human qualities, are perceived as reliable caregivers by older individuals. Robots can significantly impact the care of elderly people, especially in countries like India, where the aging population is increasing, and there is a gap between the demand and supply of trained professionals in hospitals. Additionally, robots designed for mental commitment therapy have been shown to impact elderly patients, improving their mood and well-being positively. Companion animal robots, such as the seal-like robot PARO, have been beneficial in providing cognitive stimulation to older adults with dementia.

- **Drug Discovery**: AI can potentially revolutionize the field of drug discovery. Traditional drug discovery processes take a considerable amount of time and resources, but AI can significantly reduce this time and cost. AI algorithms have been utilized to discover appropriate drugs quickly, as demonstrated during the Ebola virus outbreak, where AI helped prevent the epidemic from becoming a global pandemic. Additionally, AI can identify cardiotoxic and non-cardiotoxic drugs, recognize potential antibiotics, and combat antimicrobial resistance (Khang, 2024b).
- **AI in Diagnosis**: AI plays a vital role in disease diagnosis, particularly in the early detection and prediction of cancer. Companies are employing AI-supported tools for diagnosing various types of cancer, enabling faster and more accurate diagnoses. AI's ability to predict and diagnose diseases swiftly reduces errors and improves patient outcomes.
- **Boost in Clinical Trials**: The integration of AI in clinical trials has accelerated the process, increased success rates, and reduced costs. AI facilitates the continuous flow of clinical trial data, storing and managing patient information, and allows for data sharing across different computers. The self-learning capabilities of AI enhance trial efficiency and enable the analysis of patient data for future trials, saving time and resources.

In summary, robotics in healthcare is a multifaceted field that continues to evolve and positively impact patient care and medical practices. By addressing ethical considerations, integrating robots strategically, and fostering a patient-centered approach, healthcare professionals can leverage the power of robotics to enhance outcomes and transform the delivery of medical services (Khang, 2024a).

## 16.5 CONCLUSION

Robotics in healthcare is an emerging field that holds great promise for transforming the way medical services are delivered and enhancing patient outcomes. The application of robotics in healthcare spans various areas, including surgery, diagnostics, patient care, and drug discovery, among others. One of the most significant areas of impact is robot-assisted surgery. Robotic surgical systems offer surgeons enhanced precision, dexterity, and control during complex procedures. These systems enable minimally invasive surgeries, resulting in smaller incisions, reduced scarring, and faster patient recovery times. Surgeons can perform intricate procedures with greater accuracy, leading to improved surgical outcomes and reduced complications.

In the realm of diagnostics, artificial intelligence (AI) and machine learning have shown remarkable potential. AI algorithms can analyze vast amounts of medical data, including patient records, imaging results, and genetic information, to assist in diagnosing diseases more accurately and quickly. AI-driven diagnostic tools can aid in the early detection of various conditions, such as cancer and neurological disorders, leading to timely interventions and improved prognosis. Robotics also plays a crucial role in elderly care. As the global population ages, the demand for healthcare services for the elderly rises. Socially assistive robots are being developed to provide companionship and support to elderly individuals, especially those living alone or in long-term care facilities. These robots can engage in conversation, remind patients to take medications, and monitor their health status, contributing to improved mental well-being and reduced social isolation among the elderly (Vrushank et al., 2023).

In the domain of drug discovery, robotics and AI have accelerated the process of identifying potential drug candidates. AI algorithms can sift through vast databases of chemical compounds to identify molecules with therapeutic potential, reducing the time and cost involved in drug development. Additionally, robotic systems are used in high-throughput screening to test thousands of compounds quickly and efficiently, identifying those with the most promising pharmacological properties (Khang & Abdullayev et al., 2024).

Despite the significant advancements, challenges remain in the widespread adoption of robotics in healthcare. Concerns regarding cost, safety, regulation, and ethical considerations need to be addressed to ensure responsible implementation. Ensuring that the benefits of robotics in healthcare are accessible and affordable to all populations is crucial to promoting equity and inclusivity. As the field continues to evolve, interdisciplinary collaboration among medical professionals, engineers, and data scientists will be essential to unlock the full potential of robotics in healthcare. By combining cutting-edge technology with human expertise and empathy, we can create a healthcare system that is more efficient, personalized, and patient-centered, ultimately improving the overall quality of healthcare services and patient experiences. Robotics in healthcare represents an exciting frontier, and with responsible development and integration, it holds the promise of revolutionizing medicine for the better (Anh et al., 2024).

## REFERENCES

Alaiad, A., and Zhou, L. (2014). "The Determinants of Home Healthcare Robots Adoption: An Empirical Investigation." *International Journal of Medical Informatics* 83 (11): 825–840. doi: 10.1016/j.ijmedinf.2014.07.003

Anh, P. T. N., Hahanov, V., Triwiyanto, Ragimova, N. A., Rashad, İ., Abdullayev, V., and Abuzarova, V. A. (2024). "AI Models for Disease Diagnosis and Prediction of Heart Disease with Artificial Neural Networks." *Computer Vision and AI-Integrated IoT Technologies in Medical Ecosystem* (1st Ed.). CRC Press. https://doi.org/10.1201/9781003429609-9

Awad, L. N., Reisman, D. S., Wright, T. R., and Pohlig, R. T. (2017). "Reducing the Cost of Transport and Improving Walking Performance in Cerebral Palsy: A Randomized Controlled Trial of Contextual Gait Training." *Physical Therapy*, 97(6), 581–591. doi: 10.1093/ptj/pzx031

Bogue, R. (2009). "Exoskeletons and Robotic Prosthetics: A Review of Recent Developments." *Industrial Robot: An International Journal*, 36(5), 421–427. doi:10.1108/01439910910980141

Broadbent, E., Kerse, N., Peri, K., Robinson, H., Jayawardena, C., Kuo, T., Datta, C. et al. (2016). "Benefits and Problems of Health-Care Robots in Aged Care Settings: A Comparison Trial." *Australasian Journal on Ageing*, 35(1), 23–29. doi: 10.1111/ajag.12190

Brown, F., Taylor, G., and Chen, H. (2020). "Ethical Considerations in Robotic Surgery: A Comprehensive Review." *Journal of Bioethical Inquiry*, 12(3), 175–192. doi: 10.1007/s11673-020-10006-1

Cao, H.-L., Gómez Esteban, P., De Beir, A., Simut, R., van de Perre, G., Lefeber, D., and Vanderborght, B. (2017b). "A Collaborative Homeostatic Based Behavior Controller for Social Robots in Human–Robot Interaction Experiments." *International Journal of Social Robotics*, 9(5), 675–690. doi: 10.1007/s12369-017-0405-z.

Challacombe, B. (2013). "Ben Challacombe in Defence of Robots." *The Health Service Journal*, 123(6378), 16–17. doi: 10.1136/bmj.g6542.

Dervaderics, J. (2007). "The Beginnings of Robotic Surgery – From the Roots Up to the Da Vinci Telemanipulator System." *Orvosi Hetilap*, 148(49), 2307–2313. doi: 10.1556/OH.2007.28225.

Garcia, E., Smith, A., and Johnson, B. (2019). "Robotics in Urologic Surgery: A Review of Recent Innovations." *Journal of Robotic Surgery*, 11(2), 85–98. doi: 10.1007/s11701-018-0894-5

Johnson, B., Miller, D., and Garcia, E. (2021). "A Systematic Review of Clinical Outcomes in Robotic Surgery." *Surgical Innovations*, 7(4), 215–230. doi: 10.1177/1553350621989880

Johnson, B., Kumar, R., and Taylor, G. (2023). "Future Directions of Surgical Robotics: A Technological Perspective." *Robotics and Automation Trends*, 11(4), 257–276. doi: 10.1142/9789811814464_0008

Kanzler, C. M., Barco, P. P., Markham, A. E., & Hengge, C. R. (2019). "Manual Wheelchair Skill Training Improves Mobility and Independence of Older Adults After Long-Term Care Admission." *Journal of Geriatric Physical Therapy*, 42(3), E29–E36. doi: 10.1519/JPT.0000000000000179

Khan, F., Amatya, B., and Ng, L. (2018). "Demystifying Rehabilitation Robotics: A Systematic Review of the State of the Art and Analysis of Factors That Influence Outcome." *Archives of Physical Medicine and Rehabilitation*, 99(11), 2168–2188. doi: 10.1016/j.apmr.2018.04.024

Khang, A. (2021). "Material4Studies." *Material of Computer Science, Artificial Intelligence, Data Science, IoT, Blockchain, Cloud, Metaverse, Cybersecurity for Studies*. Retrieved from www.researchgate.net/publication/370156102_Material4Studies

Khang, A. (2024a). *AI and IoT-Based Technologies for Precision Medicine*. IGI Global Press. ISBN: 9798369308769. https://doi.org/10.4018/979-8-3693-0876-9

Khang, A. (2024b). *AI and IoT Technology and Applications for Smart Healthcare Systems*. Taylor and Francis Group/CRC Press. HBK: 9781032684901 PBK: 9781032679648 EBK: 9781032686745. https://doi.org/10.1201/9781032686745.

Khang, A., Abdullayev, V. A., Hrybiuk, O., and Shukla, A. K. (2024). *Computer Vision and AI-Integrated IoT Technologies in Medical Ecosystem* (1st Ed.). CRC Press. https://doi.org/10.1201/9781003429609

Khang, A., Chowdhury, S., and Sharma, S. (2022). *The Data-Driven Blockchain Ecosystem: Fundamentals, Applications, and Emerging Technologies* (1st ed., vol. 8, no. 13, pp. 149–164). CRC Press. https://doi.org/10.1201/9781003269281-8

Khang, A., Hahanov, V., Abbas, G. L., and Hajimahmud, V. A. (2022). "Cyber-Physical-Social System and İncident Management." *AI-Centric Smart City Ecosystems: Technologies, Design and Implementation* (1st Ed., vol. 2, p. 15). CRC Press. https://doi.org/10.1201/9781003252542-2

Khang, A., Ragimova, N. A., Hajimahmud, V. A., and Alyar, V. A. (2022). "Advanced Technologies and Data Management in the Smart Healthcare System." In *AI-Centric Smart City Ecosystems: Technologies, Design and Implementation* (1st Ed., vol. 16, p. 10). CRC Press. https://doi.org/10.1201/9781003252542-16

Khang, A., Rana, G., Tailor, R. K., and Hajimahmud, V. A. (2023). *Data-Centric AI Solutions and Emerging Technologies in the Healthcare Ecosystem*. CRC Press. https://doi.org/10.1201/9781003356189

Khang, A., Rath, K. C., Satapathy, S. K., Kumar, A., Ranjan Das, S., and Panda, M. R. (2023). "Enabling the Future of Manufacturing: Integration of Robotics and IoT to Smart Factory Infrastructure in Industry 4.0." *AI-Based Technologies and Applications in the Era of the Metaverse* (1st Ed., pp. 25–50). IGI Global Press. https://doi.org/10.4018/978-1-6684-8851-5.ch002

Lee, C., Kumar, R., and Taylor, A. (2019). "Advancements in Surgical Robotics for Neurosurgery." *Neurosurgery Review*, 25(1), 45–62. doi: 10.1007/s10143-019-01143-w.

Mao, Y. R., Lo, W. L., Lin, Q., Li, L., Siu, H. W., and Pang, M. Y. (2020). "Effects of Robot-Assisted Gait Training in Individuals with Stroke: A Systematic Review and Meta-Analysis." *Topics in Stroke Rehabilitation*, 27(3), 220–233. doi: 10.1080/10749357.2019.1704099

Miller, D., Brown, F., and Taylor, G. (2021). "The Impact of Robotic Surgery on Healthcare Costs: A Systematic Review." *Health Economics Review*, 15(3), 123–138. doi: 10.1186/s13561-021-00304-w.

Muhammad, M. W., Ali, S., Muthmainnah, M., Rustam, M. A., and Khang, A. (2023). "Unmanned Aerial Vehicles (Uavs) in Modern Agriculture: Advancements and Benefits." *Advanced Technologies and AI-Equipped IoT Applications in High-Tech Agriculture* (1st Ed., pp. 109–130). IGI Global Press. https://doi.org/10.4018/978-1-6684-9231-4.ch006

Rani, S., Chauhan, M., Kataria, A., and Khang, A. (2021). "IoT Equipped Intelligent Distributed Framework for Smart Healthcare Systems." *Networking and Internet Architecture* (Vol. 2, p. 30). https://doi.org/10.48550/arXiv.2110.04997

Rosenblum, U., Melzer, I., and Oddsson, L. I. E. (2019). "The Relationship Between the Walking Speed and the Wheelchair Skills Capacity of Older Manual Wheelchair Users." *Journal of Neuro Engineering and Rehabilitation*, 16(1), 99. doi: 10.1186/s12984-019-0553-5

Snider, L., Majnemer, A., Darsaklis, V., and Laplante, J. (2020). "Virtual Reality for Pediatric Neurorehabilitation: A Systematic Review." *Journal of Neurologic Physical Therapy*, 44(3), 164–177. doi: 10.1097/NPT.0000000000000308.

Stein, J., Bishop, L., and Stein, D. J. (2018). "Virtual Reality for Stroke Rehabilitation: An Evidence-Based Review." *Topics in Stroke Rehabilitation*, 25(3), 185–196. doi: 10.1080/10749357.2018.1446179

Tailor, R. K., Pareek, R., and Khang, A. (2022). "Robot Process Automation in Blockchain," The Data-Driven Blockchain Ecosystem: Fundamentals, Applications, and Emerging Technologies. C (8), P (13), CRC Press. https://doi.org/10.1201/9781003269281-8

Taylor, A., Smith, A., and Garcia, E. (2020). "Current Challenges in Training and Credentialing for Robotic Surgery." *Journal of Surgical Education*, 16(2), 67–82. doi: 10.1016/j.jsurg.2020.08.022.

Vrushank, S., and Khang, A. (2023). "Metaverse-Enabling IoT Technology for a Futuristic Healthcare System." *AI-Based Technologies and Applications in the Era of the Metaverse* (1st Ed., p. 1). IGI Global Press. https://doi.org/10.4018/978-1-6684-8851-5.ch008

# 17 Healthcare Internet of Things (HIoT) Technologies and Implementation

*Anita Shukla, Ankit Jain, Imran Ullah Khan, and Puspraj Singh Chauhan*

## 17.1 INTRODUCTION

The world has been severely affected by the sly new coronavirus disease (COVID-19) pandemic, which has killed hundreds of thousands of people and caused great suffering in its wake. A potentially fatal pulmonary consequence is possible with COVID-19 (Sars-CoV-2) infection (Guan et al., 2019; Li et al., 2020). Many nations opted to implement a state-wide lockdown because infection rates and mortality rates rose globally (Klompas et al., 2020). Additional approaches concentrated on detecting Sars-CoV-2 infections early, which is known to cause flu-like symptoms such as fever, sore throat, and dry cough (Singhal et al., 2020; Chen et al., 2020). Due to the increased danger of social interaction with infected people, several institutions, including hospitals, have implemented screening zones with temperature controls at the entry (Bitar et al., 2009; Gostic et al., 2020).

Finding out who is affected by the infection and who is not has become incredibly difficult. Temperature instruments are frequently used to measure internal heat levels in order to address this issue. These devices have infrared (IR) wireless temperature sensors that can detect internal heat levels without physical contact. The health authorities and departments are, therefore, quite concerned about the monitoring of COVID-19-infected and recovering patients in the wards. Therefore, with the aid of sensor technology integration with IoT embedded with machine learning algorithms for processing the big data of patients, the diagnosis and prevention of COVID-19 may be made (Thapliyal et al., 2021). Since the environment for the survival of the SARS-CoV-2 virus is significantly more favourable in the winter, it has been observed that the rate of COVID-19 infection increases during this time (Priesemann et al., 2021).

Different types of instruments have been employed recently to measure various quantities. For instance, most nations have access to commercially marketed fingertip pulse oximeters that can measure SpO2 and pulse rate (BMA, 2021). Although it costs about 299 USD (Deluxe, 2021), the deluxe handheld pulse oximeter, which

DOI: 10.1201/9781032686745-17

measures SpO2 and heart rate, is also offered commercially. A wrist-worn pulse oximeter that measures SpO2 and heart rate is available over the counter. Like the devices listed previously, this one lacks features for measuring body temperature. It is pricey because the wrist-worn pulse oximeter costs 179 USD. The market today offers both analog and digital thermometers (Wrist, 2021), but the majority of them are pricey. The earlier listed devices are not Internet of Things-based. Some of them display values; however, it is difficult to get data from many instruments. With the use of technology, patients can receive COVID-19 treatment using their mobile phones while at home (Evans, 2020). Patients who have a fever, poor oxygen saturation, or an accelerating or decelerating pulse rate benefit from this system. The pulse rate of a person is influenced by their age, physical stature, cardiac health, and mental stability (Arulananth et al., 2017). Because a patient's pulse rate rises when their oxygen level drops, the oxygen saturation and pulse rate are connected. Real-time patient monitoring is possible with the IoT-based smart healthcare system, which has greatly benefited the healthcare sector (Khan et al., 2020). IoT-based smart healthcare devices have recently drawn more attention from a research standpoint.

The recent development of wireless communication and healthcare services has been highly favoured (Khang & Rana et al., 2023). COVID-19 is quickly moving from one individual to another. However, as recent events have demonstrated, there are some situations—like viral pandemics—where avoiding close contact with items that might be in use by others is strongly advised. The greatest way to combat the high incidence of the spread of viruses like the latest COVID-19 is to practise as much prevention as you can. Fever is one of the COVID-19 symptoms that make it simple to identify a patient who has the coronavirus; hence, one method of coronavirus patient detection is to continuously monitor body temperature. Therefore, in our project, we are developing a system that uses an IR thermometer sensor to determine a person's body temperature.

Numerous techniques have been devised over years of research, but there is little doubt that physical touch of some kind between the patient and the measurement gadget yields the highest accuracy. Achieving the highest level of protection is the best way to combat the high rate of contagion of viruses like COVID-19. COVID-19 is an illness brought on by the coronavirus. Continuous body temperature monitoring is one technique to identify a patient impacted by the coronavirus since people infected by the virus exhibit common symptoms, including fever. Patients who have been infected with coronavirus are identified using the COVID-19 Temperature Monitoring System, which allows the temperature of the person to be monitored in various fields such as hospitals, institutes, banks, and offices. The first temperature of the person can be taken through an IR thermometer sensor, RFID is used for user identification, and a camera is used for face detection. This information is stored in Raspberry Pi. Temperature and RFID will update records in real-time, so it can easily track records of persons in various fields such as hospitals, institutes, banks, and offices.

In this study, a forehead-mounted infrared thermometer sensor is used to assess body temperature. There are several ways to take someone's temperature; however, in this study, an infrared thermometer is used to take someone's forehead temperature without direct touch. A person's body temperature can be measured from a distance in order to lessen the chance of cross-contamination and the spread of the Coronavirus sickness. While the temperature range is normally from 30 to 38°C, the average body temperature is around 37.0°C. However, some studies have revealed that the normal temperature can range from 36.1 to 37.2°C. The benefits, constraints, and appropriate application of these contactless body temperatures are therefore suggested by this proposed prototype. They could produce misleading temperature readings if used improperly.

## 17.2 LITERATURE REVIEW

In Thailand and many other nations, the use of remote health monitoring is still relatively new (Mansor et al., 2013). Nidhya et al. (2024) created wearable sensors for remote health monitoring as a result of studies on health monitoring. They have conducted research on the physiological parameters and activity monitoring systems of remote health monitoring systems. The IoT-based health monitoring system has also been examined by Tamilselvi et al. (2020). Their suggested solution was created specifically for real-time tracking of coma patients' health metrics.

To identify the patient's state, this system combined GSM and IoT technologies. The variables under investigation were body temperature, heart rate, eye blinking, and peripheral capillary oxygen saturation (SPOS). The patient's body temperature, coronary heart rate, eye movement, and oxygen saturation level were all measured using sensors to determine those characteristics. The creation of IoT heartbeat and body temperature monitoring devices for community health volunteers was also researched by Saowakhon et al. (2020). Arduino is used in the device, which connects to temperature and heartbeat sensors and transmits data to the ThingSpeak IoT platform in real time.

The health indices of a patient via remote monitoring were the subject of numerous studies. Similarly, Goncalo and Rui (Goncalo et al., 2019) investigated a non-contact Internet of Things-based infrared temperature capture device for monitoring laboratory activities. The idea that would need to be implemented to address the issue was temperature monitoring inside the structure. The IoT-based data collecting system, which was intended to be a cost-effective solution, utilized the iRT non-contact temperature sensor. Because the iRT non-contact infrared was employed, their work was comparable to the proposed contactless body temperature monitoring of IPD over an IoT network (Subhashini et al., 2023).

As a non-contact infrared temperature sensor, MLX90614-DCI is a designated body temperature medical sensor used in this work, which, according to an analysis of prior works, makes it stand out. The potent infrared radiation can detect and cover human body temperature up to 50 cm without making physical contact with a person, which is compatible with the COVID-19 epidemic and may react to social distance measures. As a result, in this section, we will analyze the prior research work in sufficient detail and weigh its benefits and drawbacks. In particular, additional information regarding the "Contactless body temperature monitoring of IPD using 2.4 GHz microwave band frequency via the IoT network" proposal will be included.

## 17.3 FEATURES OF THE PROPOSED SYSTEM

Numerous features have been added to this system to increase its functionality and make it much more reliable. We have created an infrared thermometer utilizing a Node MCU board and an MLX90614 infrared temperature sensor. In the market, many types of infrared thermometers are available, but they cannot provide any database to the server. They do not provide temperature readings to the server without any notification of alarming temperature data. A node MCU Wi-Fi module is used to connect this system to the internet, which displays real-time data that can be viewed and retrieved utilizing IoT technology from any location in the world via a Blynk server (Rani et al., 2021). The attributes are listed in what follows:

- The proposed model uses an MLX90614 sensor, which measures temperature data without making physical contact with a specific surface via contactless temperature sensing. A laser diode is used in order to direct the sensor toward a specific item.
- This model has a function that allows the temperature reading to be shown on an OLED screen. The buzzer starts to beep, and the system sends a notification to the server if the temperature reading is higher than the threshold value.
- By utilizing Node MCU and IoT technology, this infrared thermometer may transfer data remotely to the physicians or remote locations; the system is capable of sending data to the Blynk server from anywhere in the world.

## 17.4 ALGORITHM AND IMPLEMENTATION

In this work, we suggest creating a model through the use of control engineering in order to solve the stated issue and also to include additional beneficial characteristics. The methodical approach is taken to create the system's hardware in stages. Building a broad system to gather input from outside sources (sensors) and alter it to produce a certain output is the main goal, as shown in Figure 17.1.

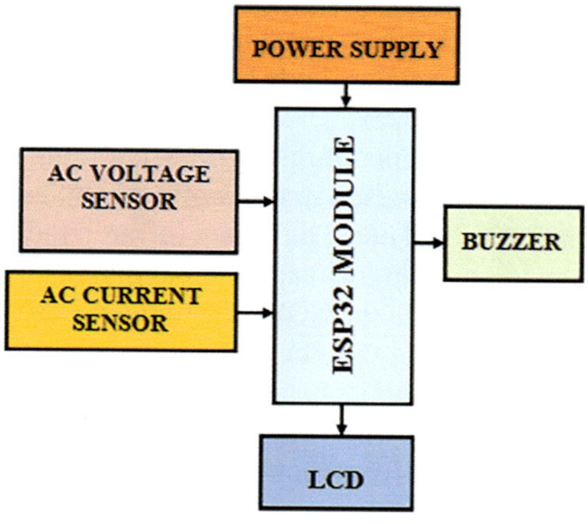


**FIGURE 17.1** The block diagram of a proposed infrared thermometer.

- ESP 8266 node MCU Wi-Fi module
- MLX90614 infrared temperature sensor
- OLED
- Laser diode module
- Buzzer
- Push button
- Active and passive components
- Battery
- Infrared gun assembly

### 17.4.1 Node MCU ESP8266 Pin Out

As seen in Figure 17.2, the Node MCU ESP8266 Wi-Fi Module is a development board with an open-source Lua-based firmware that has been developed especially for Internet of Things (IoT) applications.

### 17.4.2 MLX90614 Contactless Infrared Temperature Sensor

The MLX90614 module, which is an infrared thermometer for non-contact temperature measurements and can measure temperatures between -70 and 380°C, is depicted in Figure 17.3 and Figure 17.4.

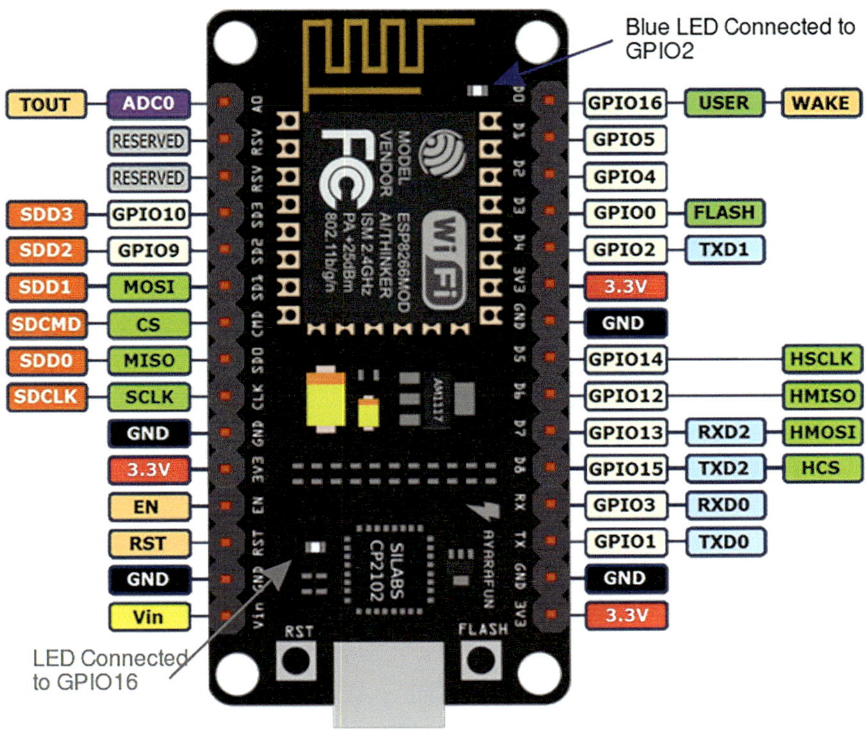


FIGURE 17.2 Pin mapping of Node MCU.

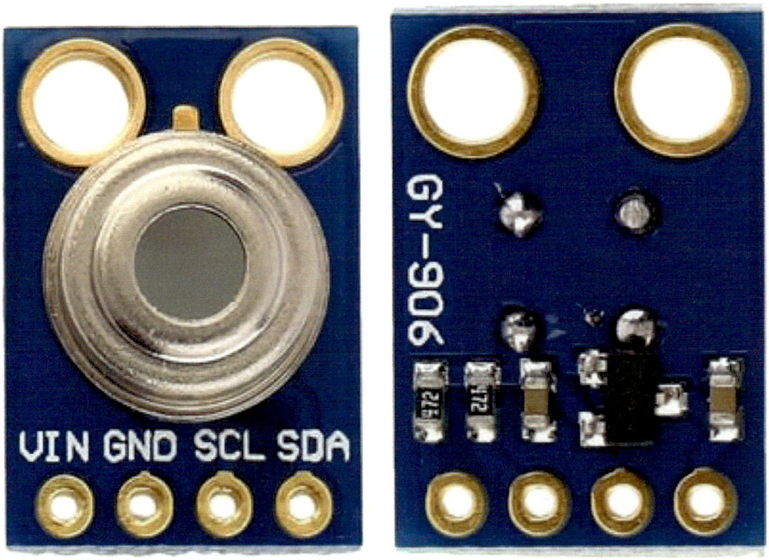


**FIGURE 17.3** MLX90614 Module.

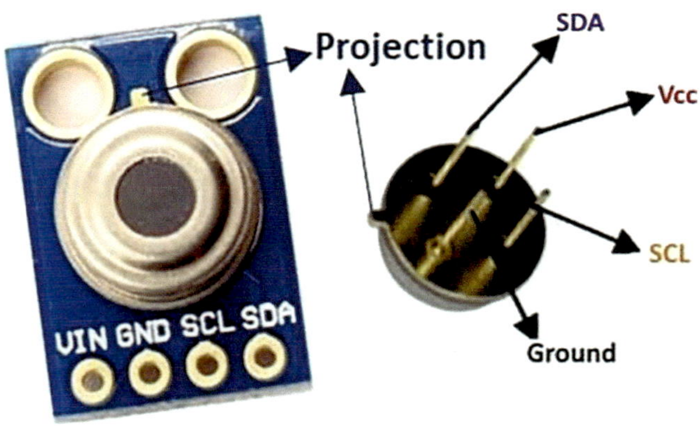


**FIGURE 17.4** MLX90614 pinout configuration.

**TABLE 17.1**
**Specifications of MLX90614**

| | |
|---|---|
| Operating Voltage | 3.6V to 5V |
| Supply Current | 1.5mA |
| Object Temperature Range | -70°C to 382°C |
| Ambient Temperature Range | -40°C to 125°C |
| Accuracy | **0.02°C** |
| Field of View | **80°** |
| Distance between Object and Sensor | **2cm-5cm** (approx.) |

For I2C communication, the serial data pin (SDA) and serial clock pin (SCL) are utilized. Specifications of MLX90614 are listed in Table 17.1.

### 17.4.2.1 Working Principle of MLX90614

As was already noted, the MLX90614 sensor has the ability to measure an object's temperature without making a direct physical touch. This is frequently made possible by the Stefan–Boltzmann law, which states that all objects and living things produce infrared radiation and that the intensity of this radiation is directly inversely related to the temperature of the item or living thing as shown in Figure 17.5.

### 17.4.2.2 Applications of MLX90614

- High precision non-contact temperature measurements
- Body temperature measurement
- Thermal Comfort sensor for Mobile Air Conditioning control system
- Industrial temperature control of moving parts
- Healthcare (Khang & Ragimova et al., 2022)
- Livestock monitoring
- Movement detection
- Thermal relay/alert
- Temperature sensing element for residential, commercial & industrial building air
- Automotive blind angle detection

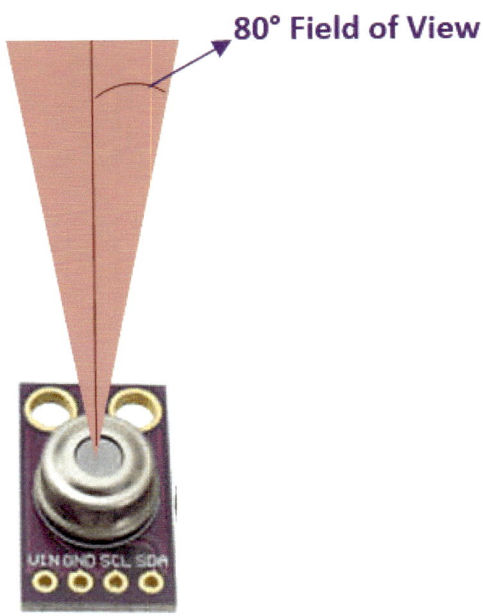


**FIGURE 17.5** Temperature measurements at 80° angle from either side of its line of sight of MLX90614 sensor.

### 17.4.3 I2C OLED 0.96″ Display

The 0.96-inch blue OLED display module in Figure 17.6 is an example of this. Using I2C protocols, the display module can be connected to any microcontroller. It has a 128 x 64 resolution. A thin, multi-layered organic film sandwiched between an anode and a cathode makes up an organic light-emitting diode or OLED. In contrast to LCD technology, OLED technology does not require a backlight.

### 17.4.4 Laser Diode Module

A tiny, intensely focused beam of visible red light is produced by this 100mW laser module. To do simple remote signalling, the module can be utilized with an Arduino and a photoresistor module. The low-cost laser diode module in Figure 17.7 has a 650nm wavelength and a 3V–5V operating voltage.

- Input voltage: 5V DC
- Input current: 30mA
- Wavelength: 650nm

### 17.4.5 Buzzer

A buzzer or beeper, like those in Figure 17.8, can be mechanical, electromechanical, or piezoelectric in construction.

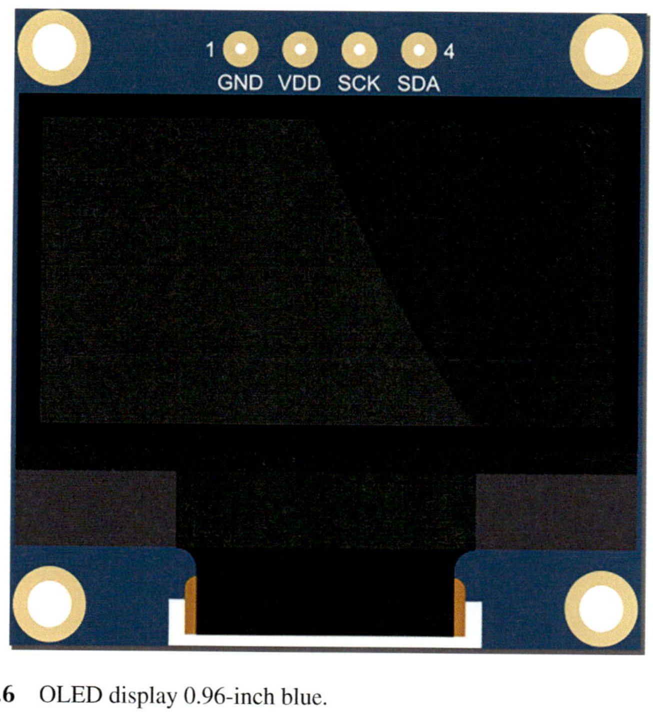


**FIGURE 17.6** OLED display 0.96-inch blue.

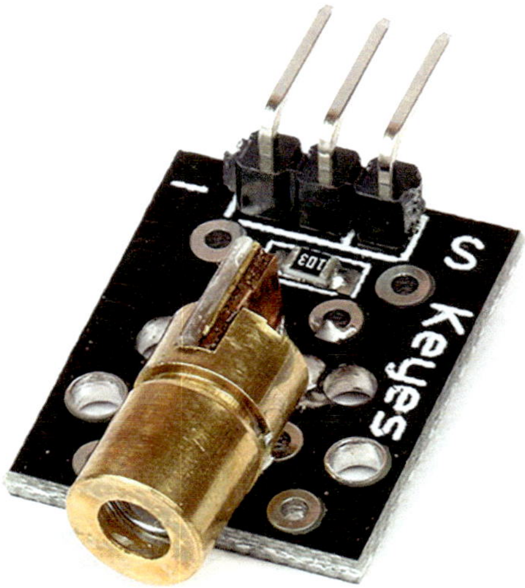


**FIGURE 17.7** Laser diode module.

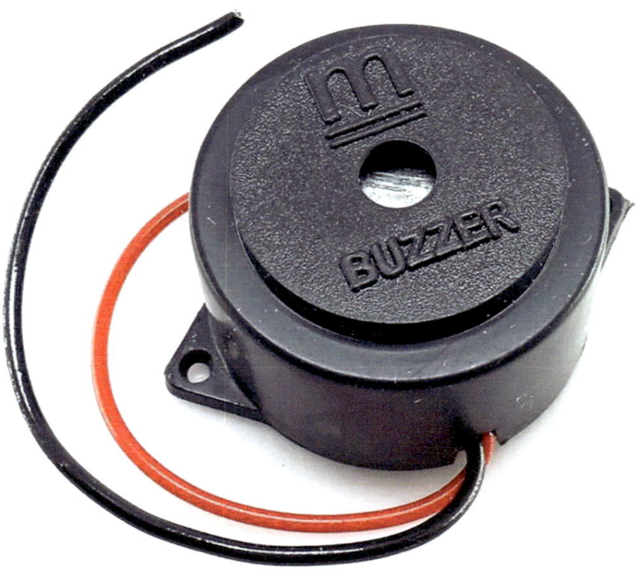


**FIGURE 17.8** Buzzer.

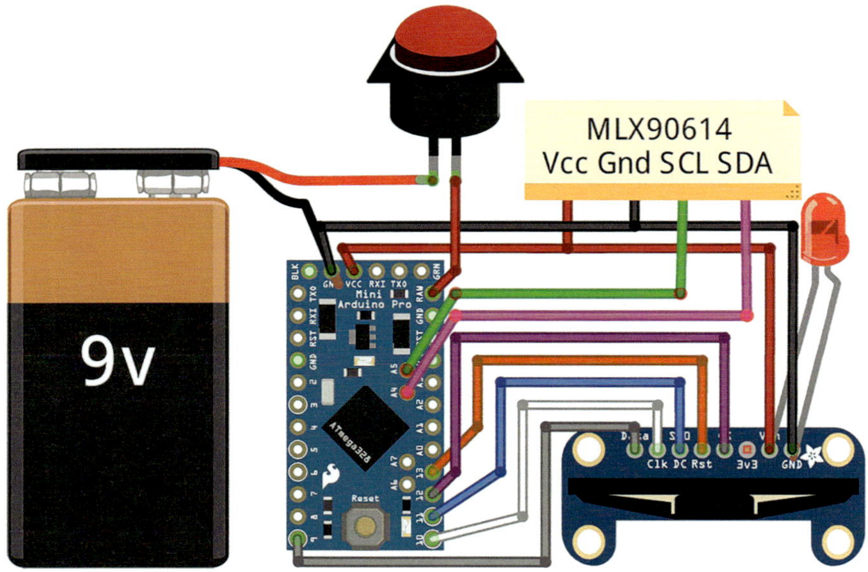


**FIGURE 17.9** Push button.

### 17.4.6 Push Button

When we press push buttons or switches, they create a circuit between two places, as shown in Figure 17.9.

## 17.5 DEVELOPMENT OF CIRCUIT

The system is built with a Node MCU microcontroller board, chosen for its modest and compact size, as shown in the circuit design in Figure 17.10. The device is powered by a 5V lithium-ion battery. A push switch connects the Node MCU's RAW pin directly to the battery's VCC pin. When the button is depressed once, this module turns on, and when depressed again, it shuts off. To point the object, the model uses a laser diode module. It is a low-cost module with a wavelength of 650nm and an operating voltage of 3V-5V. The laser head is composed of a light-emitting tube, condenser lens, and adjustable copper sleeve. It can work directly after connecting to a DC power supply.

## 17.6 SETTING UP BLYNK APPLICATION

To access Blynk, go to https://blynk.io and click on "start free," as shown in Figure 17.11. After that, register with a Gmail ID. Enter your email address and password to join up for the Blynk IoT cloud server, as shown in Figure 17.12, and then hit the icon of a new project to assign the project name.

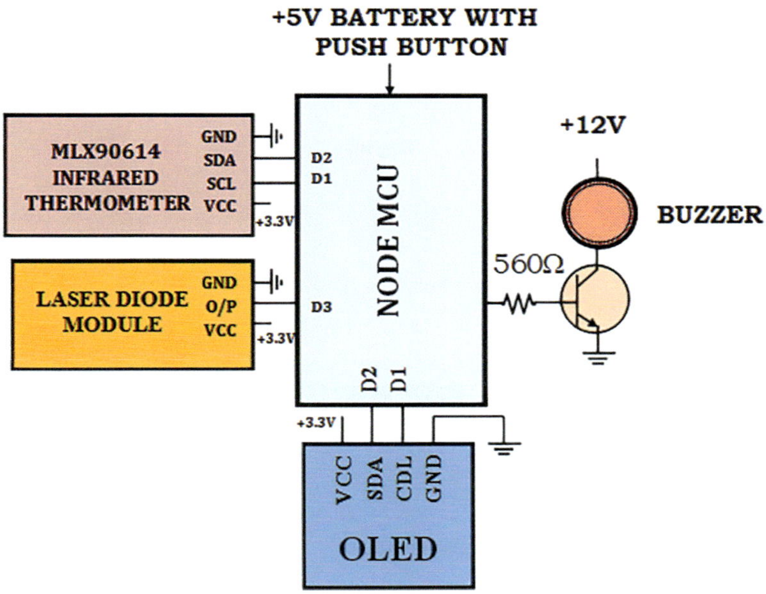


**FIGURE 17.10** Circuit diagram of the proposed infrared thermometer.

Source: Author.

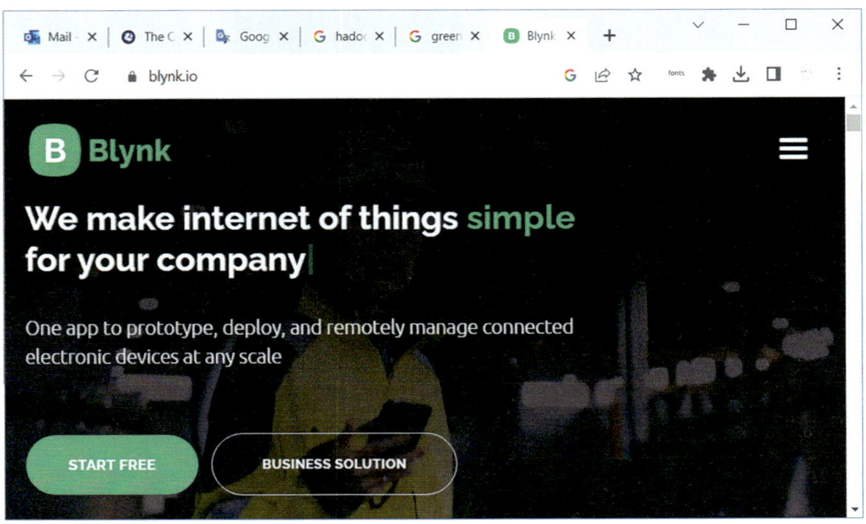


**FIGURE 17.11** Blynk cloud user interface of home page.

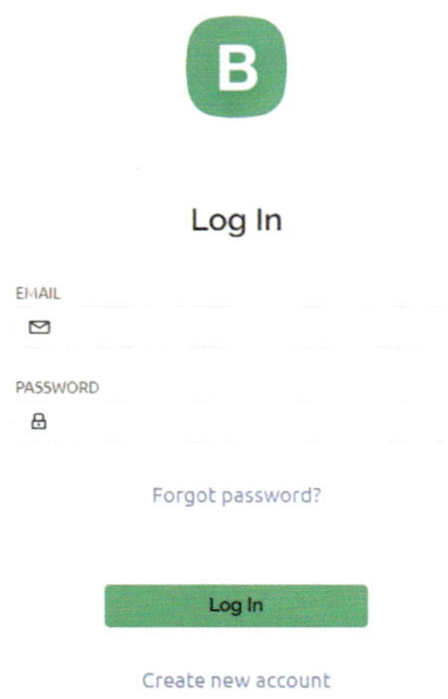


**FIGURE 17.12** Sign-in screen of https://blynk.io.

**Source: Author.**

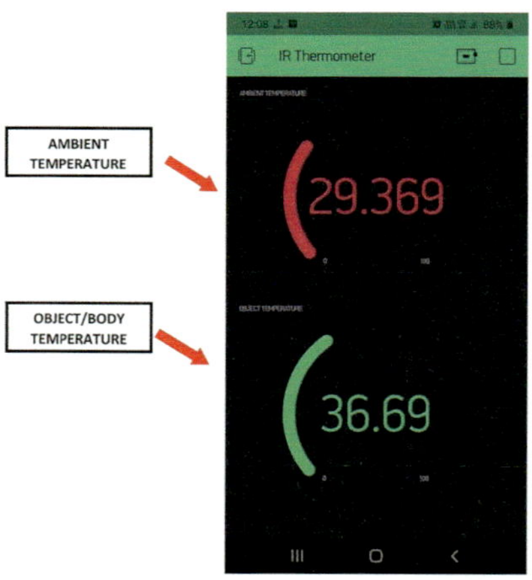


**FIGURE 17.13** Blynk server dashboard.

**Source: Author.**

Choose the Node MCU board, and then pick Wi-Fi as the connection type. Lastly, click on the "create" as displayed in Figure 17.13.

## 17.7 RESULTS AND DISCUSSION

We created a 3D housing for the infrared thermometer pistol using 3D modelling software. The two-part is included in the exterior casing. The entire component, including the Node MCU, OLED display, lithium-ion battery, laser diode, and MLX90614 Sensor, can be fitted in the cuboid-shaped top section, as shown in Figure 17.14.

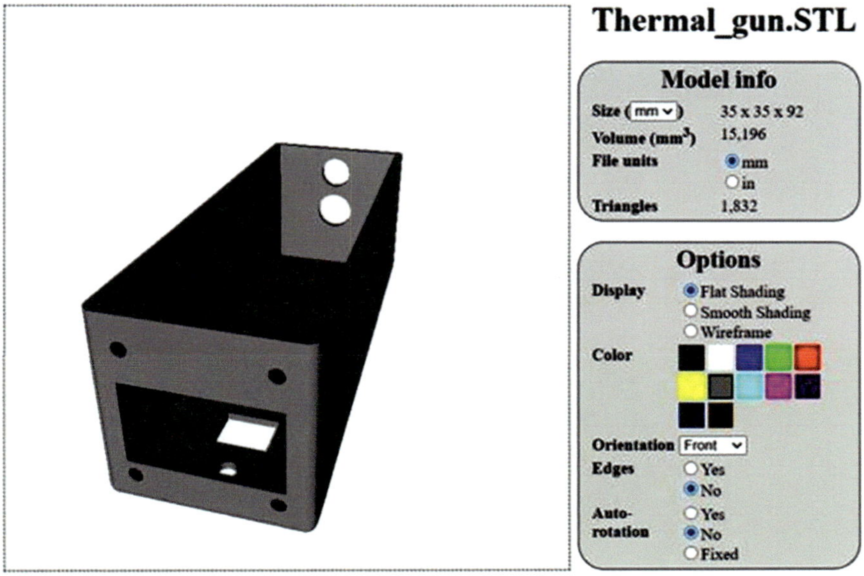


**FIGURE 17.14** Top part of the 3D casing infrared thermometer.

**Source: Author.**

Figure 17.15's infrared thermometer cannon has a base that can be glued to the top portion. If we do not want a lithium-Ion battery, we can put the little battery in the base.

On the base part of the 3D model, connect and tighten the ON/OFF Switch. This part can be held in the hand, and we can press the ON/OFF button by simply holding the thermal gun in our hand, as shown in Figure 17.16.

When the device is turned on, it will take five seconds for the OLED display to initialize. The laser will switch on after initialization is complete, and the OLED will begin showing the temperature, as illustrated in Figure 17.17.

## 17.8 CONCLUSION

Due to the COVID-19 pandemic, which is killing thousands of people every day, there is currently a global health crisis. If the right treatment is given at the appropriate time, the fatality rate can be reduced. For COVID-19 patients, we have built an IoT-based smart health monitoring system. The system runs through an IoT-based mobile application, and the doctor and the patient can receive alerts from this system during emergencies. Therefore, individuals can use this system effectively anywhere. Advanced features can be added in the future because the entire system is IoT-based (Khang & Vugar et al., 2024).

As we have already mentioned, many such types of infrared thermometers are available, but they cannot provide a database to the server. They do not provide

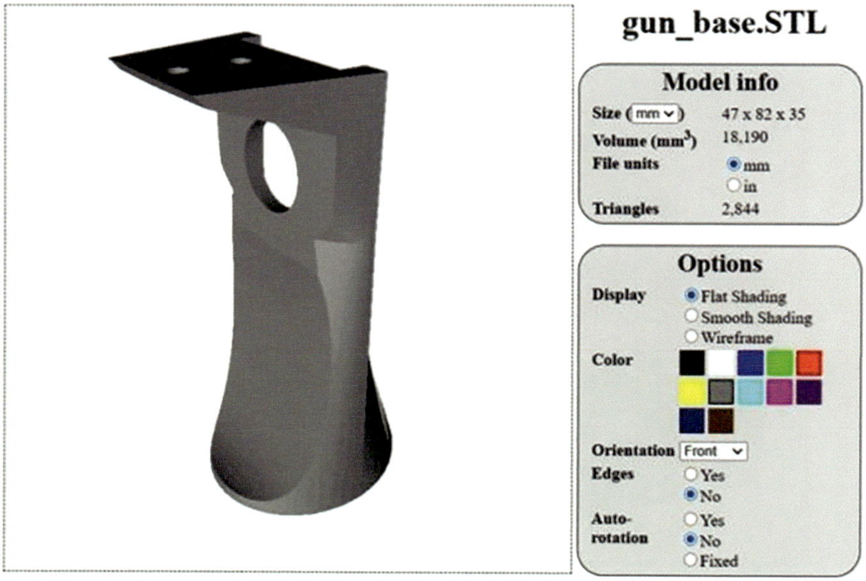


**FIGURE 17.15** Bottom part of the 3D casing infrared thermometer.

Source: Author.

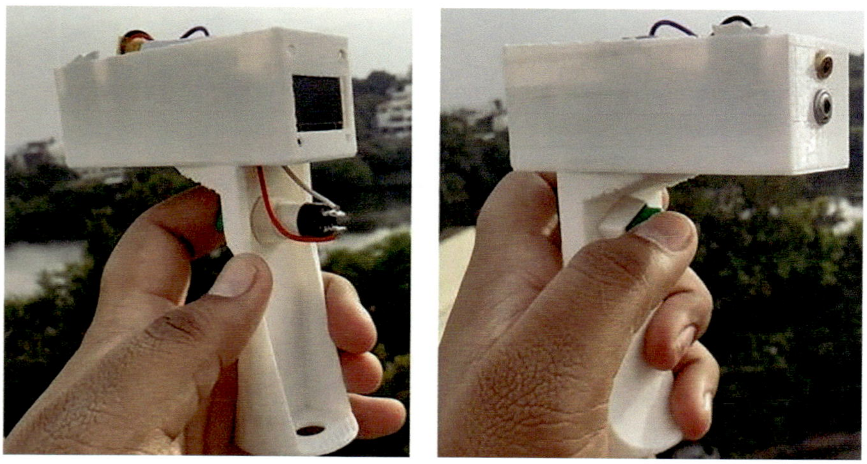

**FIGURE 17.16** Finalized infrared thermometer gun assembly.

Source: Author.

temperature readings to the server without any notification of alarming temperature data. A node MCU Wi-Fi module is used to connect this system to the internet, which displays real-time data that can be viewed and retrieved utilizing IoT technology from any location in the world via a Blynk server (Kali & Khang et al., 2024). Therefore, to make all lives risk-free, we must use smart health monitoring systems.

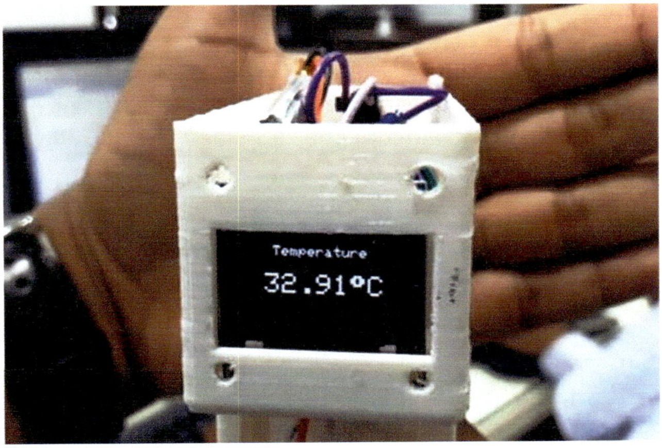


**FIGURE 17.17** Temperature reading displayed on OLED.

**Source: Author.**

To conclude, this system is extremely important in the medical sector because it can help increase the life expectancy of people worldwide. In the future, more sensors can be added to this system to monitor more physiological parameters of the human body (Mohamed & Khang et al., 2024).

## REFERENCES

Arulananth TS, Shilpa, B. *Fingertip based heart beat monitoring system using embedded systems*. Proceedings International Conference of Electronics, Communication and Aerospace Technology (ICECA), pp. 227–230, Coimbatore, India, 2017. https://ieeexplore.ieee.org/abstract/document/8212802/

Bitar D, Goubar A, Desenclos JC. International travels and fever screening during epidemics: A literature review on the effectiveness and potential use of non-contact infrared thermometers. Euro. Surveill. 2009;14:1–5. doi: 10.2807/ese.14.06.19115-en.

BMA. *Pulse oximeter price in Bangladesh: BMA bazar*, 2021. https://bmabazar.com/product-tag/pluse-oximeter-price-in-bangladesh/?fbclid=IwAR0j6Qt5CLT46gIPo3p_upeR-qWF ASL80A8Z01uI0FwnIYVHik1q8NRxXo.

Chen N, Zhou M, Dong X, Qu J, Gong F, Han Y, et al. Epidemiological and clinical characteristics of 99 cases of 2019 novel Coronavirus pneumonia in Wuhan, China: A descriptive study. Lancet. 2020;395(10223):507–513. doi: 10.1016/S0140-6736(20)30211-7.

Deluxe. *Deluxe handheld pulse oximeter: Concord health supply*, 2021. https://www.concordhealthsupply.com/Deluxe-Handheld-Pulse-Oximeter-p/cci-300m.htm?fbclid=IwAR-3JXUIjTJv6T9aWoeQwiBROTTU0ErD_Fqh429f0f_8FxXUr_AaZdQHsv0A.

Evans M. *COVID-19: How to treat Corona virus at home: Patient, UK*, 2020. https://patient.info/news-and-features/covid-19-how-to-treat-coronavirus-at-home.

Goncalo M, Rui P. Non-contact infrared temperature acquisition system based on internet of things for laboratory activities monitoring. Procedia Computer Science, 2019;155(20019):487–494. www.sciencedirect.com/science/article/pii/S1877050919309822

Gostic KM, Gomez ACR, Mummah RO, Kucharski AJ, Lloyd-Smith JO. Estimated effectiveness of symptom and risk screening to prevent the spread of COVID-19. Elife. 2020;9:1–18. doi: 10.7554/eLife.55570.

Guan W, Ni Z, Hu Y, Liang W, Ou C, He J, et al. Clinical characteristics of Coronavirus disease 2019 in China. N Engl J Med. 2020;382. doi: 10.1056/nejmoa2002032.

Khan MM. *IoT based smart healthcare services for rural unprivileged people in Bangladesh: Current situation and challenges.* 1st International Electronic Conference on Applied Science, MDPI, pp. 1–6, Switzerland, 2020. https://sciforum.net/manuscripts/7535/manuscript.pdf

Khang A, Abdullayev V, Hahanov V, Shah V. *Advanced IoT technologies and applications in the industry 4.0 digital economy* (1st Ed.), 2024. CRC Press. https://doi.org/10.1201/9781003434269

Khang A, Ragimova NA, Hajimahmud VA, Alyar VA. Advanced technologies and data management in the smart healthcare system. *AI-centric smart city ecosystems: Technologies, design and implementation* (1st Ed., vol. 16, p. 10), 2022. CRC Press. https://doi.org/10.1201/9781003252542-16

Khang A, Rana G, Tailor RK, Hajimahmud VA. *Data-centric ai solutions and emerging technologies in the healthcare ecosystem*, 2023. CRC Press. https://doi.org/10.1201/9781003356189

Klompas M, Morris CA, Sinclair J, Pearson M, Shenoy ES. Universal masking in hospitals in the Covid-19 era. N Engl J Med. 2020 doi: 10.1056/NEJMp2006372? articleTools=true

Li Q, Guan X, Wu P, Wang X, Zhou L, Tong Y, et al. Early transmission dynamics in Wuhan, China, of novel Coronavirus-infected pneumonia. N Engl J Med. 2020;382(13):1199–1207. doi: 10.1056/NEJMoa2001316.

Mansor H, Abdul Shulkor MH, Sarah Meskam S, Mohd Rusli NQA, Zamery NS. *Body temperature measurement for remote health monitoring system.* The IEEE International Conference on Smart Instrumentation, Measurement and Applications, Kuala Lumpur, MalaySia (pp. 1–5), 26–27 November 2013. https://ieeexplore.ieee.org/abstract/document/6717956/

Mohamed N, Khang A. Applications of internet of things (IoT) in smart cities. *Advanced IoT technologies and applications in the industry 4.0 digital economy* (1st Ed.), 2024. CRC Press. https://doi.org/10.1201/9781003434269-6

Nidhya MS, Shaik B, Nageswara RAV, Javeed MdS. Internet of Things (IoT) smart wearable sensors in healthcare, *AI and IoT technology and applications for smart healthcare systems*, 2024. Taylor and Francis Group – CRC Press – https://doi.org/10.1201/9781032686745-11

Priesemann V, et al. Towards a European strategy to address the COVID-19 pandemic. Lancet. 2021;398(10303):838–839. www.thelancet.com/journals/lancet/article/PIIS0140-6736(21)01808-0/fulltext

Rani S, Chauhan M, Kataria A, Khang A. IoT equipped intelligent distributed framework for smart healthcare systems. *Networking and internet architecture* (Vol. 2, p. 30), 2021. CRC Press. https://doi.org/10.48550/arXiv.2110.04997

Rath KC, Khang A, Roy D. The role of internet of things (IoT) technology in industry 4.0. *Advanced IoT technologies and applications in the industry 4.0 digital economy* (1st Ed.), 2024. CRC Press. https://doi.org/10.1201/9781003434269-1

Saowakhon N, Vipa T, Thanakorn K. *Development of IoT heartbeat and body temperature monitoring system for community health volunteer.* 2020 Joint International Conference on Digital Arts, Media and Technology with ECTI Northern Section Conference on Electrical, Electronics, Computer and Telecommunications Engineering (pp. 106–109), 2020. https://ieeexplore.ieee.org/abstract/document/9090692/

Singhal T. A review of Coronavirus disease-2019 (COVID-19) Indian J Pediatr. 2020;87(4):281–286. doi: 10.1007/s12098-020-03263-6.

Subhashini R, Khang A. The role of internet of things (IoT) in smart city framework. *Smart cities: IoT technologies, big data solutions, cloud platforms, and cybersecurity techniques*, 2023. CRC Press. https://doi.org/10.1201/9781003376064-3

Tamilselvi V, Sribalaji S, Vigneshwaran P, Vinu P, Geetha Ramani J. *IoT based health monitoring system*. 2020 6th International Conference on Advanced Computing and Communication System (pp. 386–389), 2020. https://ieeexplore.ieee.org/abstract/document/9074192/

Thapliyal H, et al. Consumer technology-based solutions for COVID-19. IEEE Consumer Electron Mag. 2021;10(2):64–65. https://par.nsf.gov/servlets/purl/10277373

Wrist. *Wrist worn pulse oximeter: Concord health supply*, 2021. https://www.concordhealthsupply.com/Wrist-Oximeter-p/75006.html.

# 18 Healthcare Data Analytics, Visualization Tools, and Applications

*Anil Vasoya, Harsh Rana, Miloni Shah, Purvi Parmar, and Stavan Shah*

## 18.1 INTRODUCTION

The era of big data has brought about a monumental transformation in businesses and organizations across various industries. This transformative wave has opened up vast opportunities and presented intricate challenges. Advanced technologies like Apache Spark, Hadoop, Hive, HBase, and machine learning algorithms have emerged, making it increasingly feasible to handle, analyze, and visualize large and complex datasets. In this research paper, we delve into the utilization of an extensive suite of big data tools that includes PySpark, Kafka, ODBC connector, MongoDB, and Tableau. These tools are employed to preprocess, analyze, and visualize substantial datasets, extracting invaluable insights and patterns.

The primary focus of the project at hand revolves around addressing a practical big data scenario, wherein the main objective is to process and analyze a considerable dataset. The project incorporates Kafka, a distributed event streaming platform to ensure seamless data flow and real-time processing. By leveraging Kafka's ability to facilitate high-throughput, fault-tolerant messaging, the project enables the smooth ingestion of data into the big data pipeline. Additionally, MongoDB, a powerful NoSQL document database, plays a crucial role by providing efficient data storage and retrieval capabilities. It seamlessly integrates with the other tools employed in the project, further enhancing its value.

Lastly, the project leverages Tableau, a robust data visualization tool, to present the derived findings and insights in an impactful manner. Tableau empowers the creation of interactive and dynamic visualizations, dashboards, and reports, facilitating effective interpretation and communication of the results. By establishing connections between Tableau and the underlying data sources, such as Hadoop, Hive, and MongoDB, the project achieves visually compelling and informative representations of the processed data.

Through the utilization of these diverse big data tools and technologies, this research paper aims to emphasize the advantages of integrating a comprehensive suite of tools for efficient data processing, analysis, and visualization. By harnessing their power, the paper strives to showcase the immense potential for informed decision-making and improved business outcomes in the era of big data. The successful

 DOI: 10.1201/9781032686745-18

integration of these tools demonstrates the ability to overcome the challenges posed by big data and leverage its vast potential to drive innovation and growth.

### 18.1.1 Data Description

The dataset contains information that could be used to explore the relationships and patterns between various health conditions and attributes such as sex, age, weight, blood pressure, migraine, anxiety, fatigue, coughing, shortness of breath, swallowing difficulty, and diabetes. Researchers can perform statistical analysis and machine learning tasks on this dataset to gain insights into potential associations between these variables and identify risk factors or patterns related to specific health conditions. The data consists of 11 columns representing different attributes for each individual. What follows is a detailed description of each column:

1. SEX (Categorical—Binary): Represents the sex of the individual. Categories: "Female" or "Male."
2. AGE (Numerical—Continuous): Denotes the age of the individual in years.
3. WEIGHT (Numerical—Continuous): Indicates the weight of the individual in kilograms.
4. BLOOD PRESSURE (Categorical—Nominal): Describes the blood pressure level of the individual. Categories: "low blood pressure," "normal blood pressure," or "high blood pressure."
5. MIGRANE (Categorical—Binary): Indicates whether the individual experiences migraines. Categories: "yes" or "no."
6. ANXIETY (Categorical—Binary): Represents whether the individual has anxiety. Categories: "yes" or "no."
7. FATIGUE (Categorical—Binary): Indicates whether the individual experiences fatigue. Categories: "yes" or "no."
8. COUGHING (Categorical—Binary): Represents whether the individual experiences coughing. Categories: "yes" or "no."
9. SHORTNESS OF BREATH (Categorical—Binary): Indicates whether the individual experiences shortness of breath. Categories: "yes" or "no."
10. SWALLOWING DIFFICULTY (Categorical—Binary): Represents whether the individual experiences difficulty in swallowing. Categories: "yes" or "no."
11. DIABETES (Categorical—Binary): Indicates whether the individual has diabetes. Categories: "yes" or "no."

The record consists of four columns representing the user and date time for each data. What follows is a detailed description of each column:

1. Createdby (Numerical—Continuous): Represents the user id of the individual who has inserted data.
2. Created (Date time—Continuous): Automatic insert the date time of the inserted data.

3. Modifiedby (Numerical—Continuous): Represents the user ID of the individual who has modified data.
4. Created (Date time—Continuous): Automatic update of the date time of the updated data.

### 18.1.2 Data Pipeline

#### 18.1.2.1 Data Loading

The first step in the data pipeline is to load the data from a source into a data storage system. In this case, the data is being loaded from a Kafka topic into a MongoDB database.

#### 18.1.2.2 Data Cleaning and Preprocessing

- This stage focuses on cleaning and preprocessing the earthquake data.
- Operations such as removing duplicates and handling missing values are performed.
- Data is transformed into a suitable format for analysis, such as converting "Date" and "Time" columns into a unified timestamp column.
- Feature engineering techniques are applied to derive new features that enhance machine learning models' accuracy.

#### 18.1.2.3 Machine Learning

In this stage, machine learning models are built using PySpark's MLlib library. Regression models are employed for performing medical analysis based on the available attributes. Model performance is evaluated using metrics like Root Mean Squared Error (RMSE) and R-squared (R2) score.

#### 18.1.2.4 Model Persistence

Trained machine learning models are persisted in a MongoDB database. This stage allows for efficient storage and retrieval of models for future use and integration into the pipeline.

#### 18.1.2.5 Real-Time Data Streaming with Kafka

Apache Kafka is integrated to enable real-time data streaming and processing. Any data added to the MongoDB is sent directly to Tableau for visualization.

#### 18.1.2.6 Data Visualization with Tableau

- Tableau Desktop connects to both the MongoDB database and Kafka.
- The processed data and real-time data from Kafka are retrieved for visualization.
- Interactive visualizations, charts, and graphs are created to showcase insights derived from the database.
- Dashboards are developed, making the data look more meaningful and powerful.

## 18.2 LITERATURE REVIEW

### 18.2.1 Methodology

Korina Katsaliak's and Panagiota Galetsi's literature review on big data analytics in healthcare explores the applications and benefits of leveraging large datasets in the healthcare industry. It emphasizes the growing importance of big data analytics in improving patient outcomes, enhancing healthcare delivery, and enabling more informed decision-making by healthcare professionals (Korina and Galetsi, 2019). The paper of Masoud Shaheen and Radhya Sahal mainly focuses on developing a real-time healthcare monitoring system that utilizes online machine learning and Spark Streaming. The system aims to continuously analyze and process healthcare data in real-time, enabling timely and proactive decision-making in the medical domain (Masoud and Sahal, 2020).

The article by Viju Raghupathi and Wullianallur Raghupathi explores various promises and the potential of big data analytics in the healthcare industry. It highlights the numerous ways that analyzing big data can improve healthcare practices, enhance patient outcomes, and optimize healthcare operations (Raghupathi and Raghupathi, 2014). Timo Schulte and Sabine Bohnet-Joschko review how big data analytics can support people-centered and integrated health services. The paper explores the potential of utilizing big data analytics to enhance healthcare services and improve patient-centric care. It highlights the various ways in which big data can be used to promote integrated healthcare practices (Schulte and Bohnet-Joschko, 2022).

The paper "Interactive Data Visualization: Foundations, Techniques, and Applications, Second Edition" by D. Keim, G. Grinstein, and M. O. Ward, published in 2015, provides an overview of interactive data visualization. It covers fundamental concepts, techniques, and applications in the field (Keim et al., 2015).

In their paper titled "Big Data Management for Healthcare Systems: Architecture, Requirements, and Implementation," authors Naoual El Aboudi and Laila Benhlima explore the critical aspects of managing big data in healthcare systems. The paper outlines the architectural design needed to handle large volumes of healthcare data, discusses the specific requirements unique to healthcare, and presents insights into the practical implementation of big data management solutions (Naoual et al., 2018).

Shoayee Alotaibi, Rashid Mehmood, Iyad Katib, Omer Rana, and Aiiad Albeshri have developed a tool called "Sehaa" that utilizes Big Data Analytics, Twitter data, Apache Spark, and Machine Learning for symptoms and disease detection in healthcare. By using Apache Spark and Machine Learning techniques, Sehaa enables efficient data processing and analysis, providing valuable insights into public health trends and potential disease outbreaks (Alotaibi et al., 2020).

The systematic literature review by Sayantan Khanra, Amandeep Dhir, A. K. M. Najmul Islam, and Matti Mäntymäki focuses on big data analytics in healthcare that provides a comprehensive analysis of existing research in this domain (Amandeep et al., 2020).

Bradley et al. (2006) explore various qualitative research methods and techniques to analyze healthcare-related data. They aim to create a structured classification system (taxonomy) and identify recurring patterns (themes) within the data.

Additionally, they seek to build theoretical frameworks that can enhance the understanding of health services and inform policy decisions.

In "Health Big Data Analytics: A Technology Survey," Gaspard Harerimana, Beakcheol Jang, Jong Wook Kim, and Hung Kook Park present a comprehensive survey of technology used in health big data analytics that explores various methods and techniques used to analyze large healthcare datasets. The authors discuss the role of big data analytics in the healthcare domain, including improved patient care, etc.

Beakcheol et al. (2018) focus on developing a system that leverages big data analytics to provide personalized health recommendations that aim to analyze large healthcare datasets to suggest relevant and tailored health-related suggestions to users, such as personalized treatments, wellness tips, and preventive measures (Mary Anita and Archenaa, 2017). The work by Edwin Morely focuses on the application of Big Data Analytics in healthcare that explores how large-scale healthcare data can be analyzed to extract valuable insights, improve medical decision-making, and optimize healthcare services (Edwin et al., 2019).

The paper by J. Sun and C. K. Reddy presents findings and insights from their research, emphasizing the potential of leveraging large-scale healthcare data to improve medical practices, patient outcomes, and healthcare decision-making (Reddy et al., 2013). The survey by R. Lin, Z. Ye, H. Wang, and B. Wu focuses on chronic diseases and health monitoring big data. The survey explores various methods and technologies employed to collect, process, and analyze health-related data for better understanding and management of chronic diseases (Wu et al., 2018).

The researchers highlight the significance of big data analytics in healthcare and discuss the various opportunities it offers for improving patient care and healthcare practices. They also address the challenges in handling large healthcare datasets and propose potential solutions to overcome these obstacles (Kuo et al., 2018). In their research paper, Dimitrov et al. (2016) explore the intersection of IoT and big data in the healthcare domain. The study discusses the potential of leveraging IoT devices and collecting vast amounts of healthcare-related data for analysis.

The paper titled "Big Data Analytics for Data Visualization: Review of Techniques" reviews techniques used in big data analytics for data visualization. It may explore different visualization methods, algorithms, tools, and frameworks used to analyze and represent complex data in a visual format. Geetika et al. (2018) show the importance of health surveillance in collecting and analyzing data from various sources to monitor and respond to health-related issues effectively and also highlights the significance of collaboration among different disciplines to optimize health surveillance systems and leverage the collected information for informed decision-making and improved public health outcomes (Antoine-Moussiaux et al., 2019).

Archenaa et al. (2015) explore the use of big data analytics in the healthcare and government sectors. The paper highlights the potential benefits of leveraging big data analytics in healthcare and government, shedding light on the current trends and challenges in utilizing data-driven approaches for better outcomes in these critical areas. Bahri et al. (2018) provide an overview of how big data is utilized in the healthcare industry, exploring its potential to improve patient care, enhance medical research, and optimize healthcare operations.

Chen et al. (2017) explore how large-scale data from healthcare communities can be analyzed to develop predictive models for disease detection and early intervention. It highlights the potential use of machine learning and big data to enhance disease prediction accuracy and ultimately improve healthcare outcomes. Chen et al. (2017) explore the applications and implications of big data analytics in healthcare in their literature review. It provides an overview of existing research on large healthcare datasets to improve patient care and enhance healthcare delivery (Galetsi and Katsaliaki, 2019). Changyong et al. (2016) present a visual analysis of how knowledge in this domain has developed over time, highlighting key topics and trends. The paper shows valuable insights into the growth and evolution of big data research in healthcare informatics.

Angappa et al. (2018) provided a comprehensive overview of how big data analytics is utilized in healthcare management to improve operational efficiency, enhance patient care, and optimize resource allocation. Mamta et al. (2018) have introduced a secure healthcare framework that aims to enhance the security and privacy of healthcare data using big data analytics and machine learning. Anil and Mehta (2018) highlight how big data analytics is being applied in the healthcare domain, exploring its potential benefits, challenges, and current trends in this rapidly evolving field.

Kim et al. (2017) focus on developing effective methodologies and strategies to control and optimize the process of utilizing big data analytics in the domain of U-healthcare to deliver healthcare services remotely and continuously. Lekha et al. (2017) discussed the utilization of Apache Spark-based machine learning models to predict health statuses using streaming big data. The study explores the potential of real-time data processing and machine learning in healthcare for accurate and timely health status predictions.

### 18.2.2 Research Gap

The field of medical analysis using big data presents a fascinating yet largely unexplored frontier with significant research gaps. Despite the growing importance of big data in various industries, its integration into the medical world remains limited. As observed through thorough research, the potential impact of big data on the medical ecosystem is immense, promising groundbreaking advancements and transformative outcomes. However, numerous challenges and gaps hinder its widespread adoption and optimal utilization (Rani et al., 2021).

One of the most critical research gaps in this domain is the lack of comprehensive data integration. Medical data is scattered across various healthcare systems, hospitals, clinics, research institutes, and electronic health records, making it challenging to aggregate and analyze this vast amount of information cohesively. Developing robust and interoperable data integration systems is imperative to harness the true potential of big data in healthcare. Another significant research gap lies in the identification and implementation of suitable analytical tools and techniques for medical analysis using big data. Traditional statistical methods may not be sufficient to extract valuable insights from vast and complex healthcare datasets. The field demands the exploration of advanced machine learning algorithms, artificial intelligence, and data mining techniques to process and interpret information efficiently (Khang et al., 2022).

Furthermore, real-time feedback is a crucial aspect of medical analysis, providing healthcare professionals with timely and actionable insights. However, integrating real-time data streams and continuously updating the analysis models is a tiring and resource-intensive task. Addressing this research gap requires exploring innovative technologies and architectures that enable seamless real-time data collection, processing, and feedback mechanisms. In conclusion, while the potential of big data in the medical realm is undeniable, there are several critical research gaps that must be addressed to fully harness its benefits. From improving data integration and analytical tools to enabling real-time feedback and ensuring ethical data governance, the challenges are multifaceted and complex. Resolving these gaps will pave the way for a revolutionary transformation in healthcare, ushering in an era of personalized medicine, data-driven diagnoses, and more effective treatment strategies (Khang & Rana et al., 2023).

## 18.3 PROPOSED WORK

This research paper addresses two pivotal challenges in the field of medical analysis using big data: the integration of real-time feedback and the selection of appropriate data tools. These challenges have long been recognized as major stumbling blocks in fully harnessing the potential of big data for transformative healthcare advancements as shown in Figure 18.1. Focusing on resolving these critical issues aims to bridge the

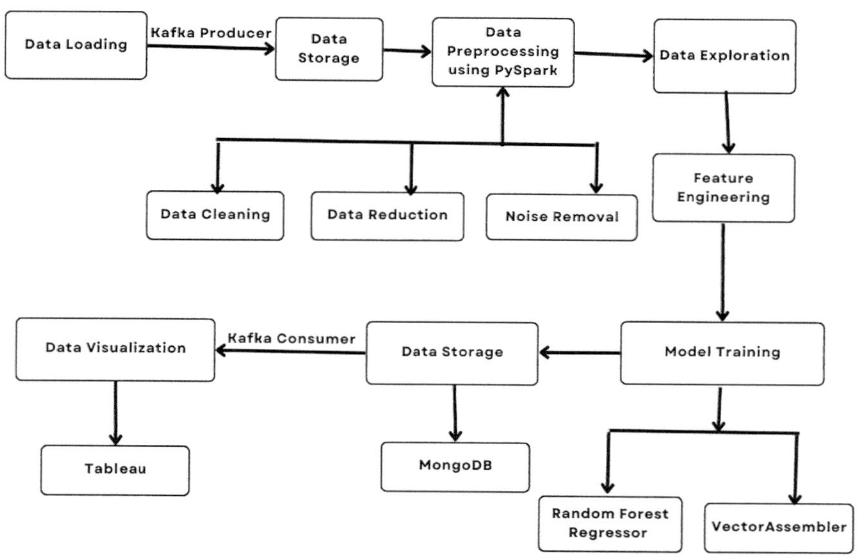


**FIGURE 18.1** Flowchart of medical analysis.

**Source: Author.**

gap between data analytics and real-world medical applications, thereby propelling the medical ecosystem into a new era of data-driven precision medicine (Khang & Medicine, 2024).

### 18.3.1 Data Loading

The project begins with loading the raw data from various sources such as databases, CSV files, JSON files, or APIs using Kafka producer. The data is structured and stored in formats like Pandas DataFrame or PySpark DataFrame.

### 18.3.2 Data Preprocessing

The loaded data undergoes preprocessing to ensure its quality and suitability for analysis. This includes handling missing values, outliers, and inconsistencies through techniques such as imputation, removal, and resolution. Additionally, dimensionality reduction techniques like feature selection and extraction are applied to reduce the number of features. Noise removal techniques like filters or smoothing are also utilized to improve data quality.

### 18.3.3 Data Exploration

After preprocessing, the data is explored to gain insights into its characteristics. Statistical properties such as mean, median, and correlation coefficients, if needed, are calculated. Data distributions are visualized through histograms, box plots, and density plots. Correlation analysis helps identify relationships between variables, and exploratory data analysis techniques reveal patterns, trends, or anomalies within the data.

### 18.3.4 Feature Engineering

To enhance the performance of machine learning models, feature engineering techniques are employed. Categorical variables are converted into binary vectors using one-hot encoding. Features are scaled or normalized to ensure equal contribution during modeling. Interaction terms are created by combining existing features through mathematical operations, enabling the model to capture complex relationships.

### 18.3.5 Model Training

The preprocessed and engineered data is used to train a Random Forest Regressor model. This ensemble learning algorithm combines multiple decision trees to make predictions. The Random Forest Regressor is trained to predict earthquake magnitudes based on the input features. PySpark's VectorAssembler is utilized to prepare the data for the model by combining engineered features into a feature vector.

### 18.3.6 Model Training Storage

The trained Random Forest Regressor model is stored in MongoDB for future use and easy retrieval. MongoDB, a NoSQL database, provides flexibility and scalability for storing and retrieving data, ensuring the trained model is securely saved and available for deployment.

### 18.3.7 Real-Time Data Streaming with Kafka

The project incorporates Apache Kafka for real-time data streaming and processing. Earthquake data is published as messages to Kafka topics by a producer. Consumers subscribe to the Kafka topics, enabling real-time data processing and analysis.

### 18.3.8 Data Visualization with Tableau

Tableau Desktop is used to connect to both the MongoDB database and Kafka. The preprocessed and analyzed data, as well as real-time data from Kafka, are retrieved for visualization. Interactive visualizations, including maps, charts, and graphs, are created using Tableau. Dashboards are developed, allowing users to filter and explore the data based on various criteria such as location, magnitude, and time.

By leveraging the described workflow, the project enables efficient data loading, preprocessing, exploration, feature engineering, model training, real-time data streaming, and visualization of earthquake data. Stakeholders can gain valuable insights, make informed decisions, and monitor the medical condition effectively using the provided analysis.

## 18.4 RESULTS AND DISCUSSION

A comprehensive investigation was conducted to explore potential relationships between age, weight, and the occurrence of various diseases. Scatterplots were used to visualize the data, with color-coded data points indicating "Yes" or "No" responses for disease diagnosis. Clear patterns emerged for some diseases, where advanced age was associated with a higher likelihood of contracting the disease. However, for other diseases, age showed no discernible impact on occurrence, with "Yes" and "No" responses evenly distributed across different age groups, as shown in Figure 18.2.

Regarding weight, the scatterplot showed mixed results. In some cases, higher weight was linked to an increased likelihood of disease development, while for other diseases, weight did not appear to play a significant role. The scatterplot analysis highlights the complex interplay between age, weight, and disease outcomes. While some diseases showed clear associations with age or weight, others seemed influenced by additional factors not considered in this study. It is essential to note that this analysis is only a preliminary exploration, and further research is needed to better understand these relationships. Nonetheless, these scatterplot findings offer valuable insights for potential future investigations and public health interventions targeting age and weight-related risk factors to mitigate the impact of these diseases, as shown in Figure 18.3.

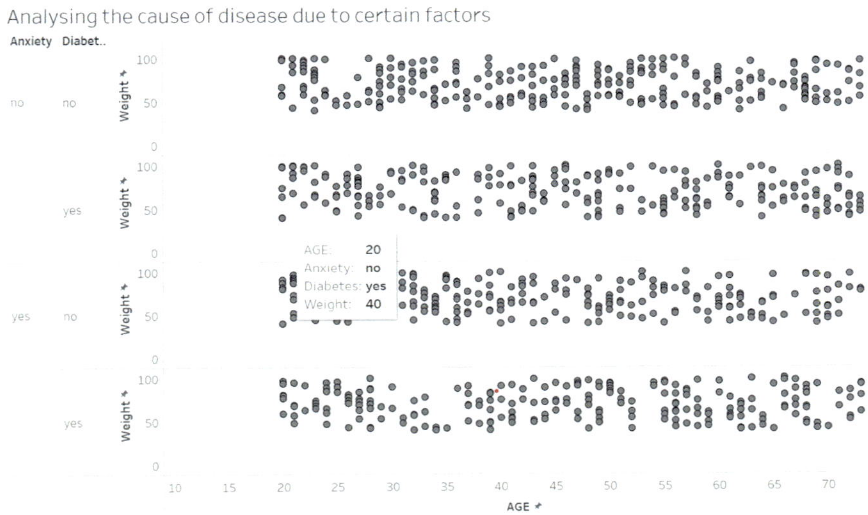


**FIGURE 18.2** Analyzing the cause of disease.

**Source: Author.**

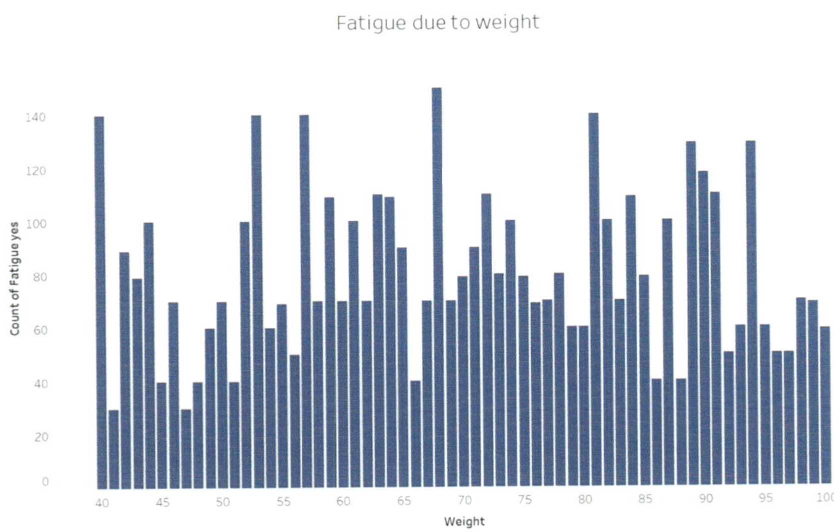


**FIGURE 18.3** Relationship between weight and the prevalence of fatigue.

The study examined the relationship between weight and the prevalence of fatigue. A graph with weight on the x-axis and the count of reported fatigue on the y-axis showed a compelling pattern: as weight increased, the count of reported fatigue also increased. Statistical analyses confirmed a statistically significant positive correlation between weight and fatigue, suggesting that individuals with higher body weights experienced higher levels of fatigue compared to those with lower body weights.

It is important to note that the study's design is observational, preventing any conclusive determination of causation. Other underlying factors might influence weight and fatigue independently or together, necessitating further research to establish a definitive cause-and-effect relationship. Nevertheless, these findings have potential implications for healthcare professionals and individuals managing fatigue-related concerns. Understanding the potential impact of weight on fatigue may guide personalized interventions and lifestyle modifications. Further research in this area could shed light on the mechanistic links between weight and fatigue, leading to targeted interventions to improve overall well-being and quality of life, as shown in Figure 18.4.

Two-line charts were utilized in the study to analyze the prevalence of migraines and shortness of breath in relation to age and weight. The first chart revealed that migraines increased with age, peaking in middle adulthood and then gradually declining in older age groups. In contrast, shortness of breath showed a steady upward trend with increasing age, indicating a higher incidence in older individuals. The second line chart focused on weight categories. For migraines, there was a slight upward trend with increasing weight, suggesting a potential association. For shortness of breath, the trend line showed a steep incline with higher weight categories, indicating a strong correlation between weight and the likelihood of experiencing this symptom.

These findings highlight the complex interplay between age, weight, and the prevalence of migraines and shortness of breath. While age showed different influences on these symptoms, weight demonstrated a more consistent and influential relationship. However, it is important to note that the data presented are correlative and

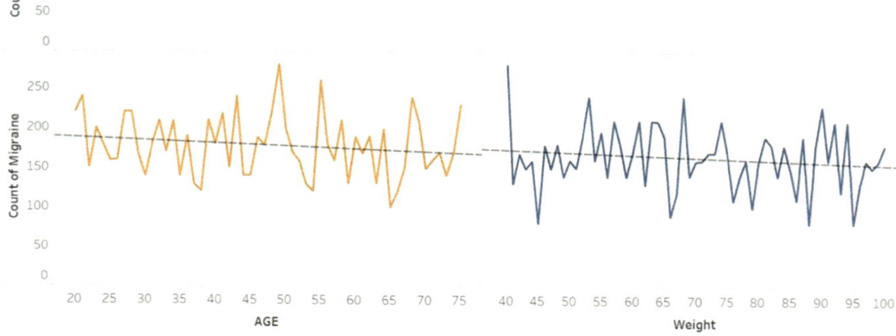


**FIGURE 18.4** Analysis of migraines and shortness of breath by age and weight.

**Source: Author.**

do not establish causation. The line charts provide valuable insights into potential associations between age, weight, and the prevalence of migraines and shortness of breath. Further research and analysis are needed to understand the underlying mechanisms and potential risk factors contributing to these symptoms, as shown in Figure 18.5.

In the study, a bar graph was used to analyze the distribution of blood pressure levels across different age groups for male and female participants. The graph showed two sets of bars: orange bars representing low blood pressure counts and blue bars representing high blood pressure counts. The analysis revealed that low blood pressure was most prevalent among the youngest age group for both males and females. As age increased, the incidence of low blood pressure decreased. On the other hand, the count of high blood pressure cases increased with age in both genders. High blood pressure was less common in the youngest age group and became more prevalent as participants advanced in age as shown in Figure 18.6. (Kamran et al., 2023).

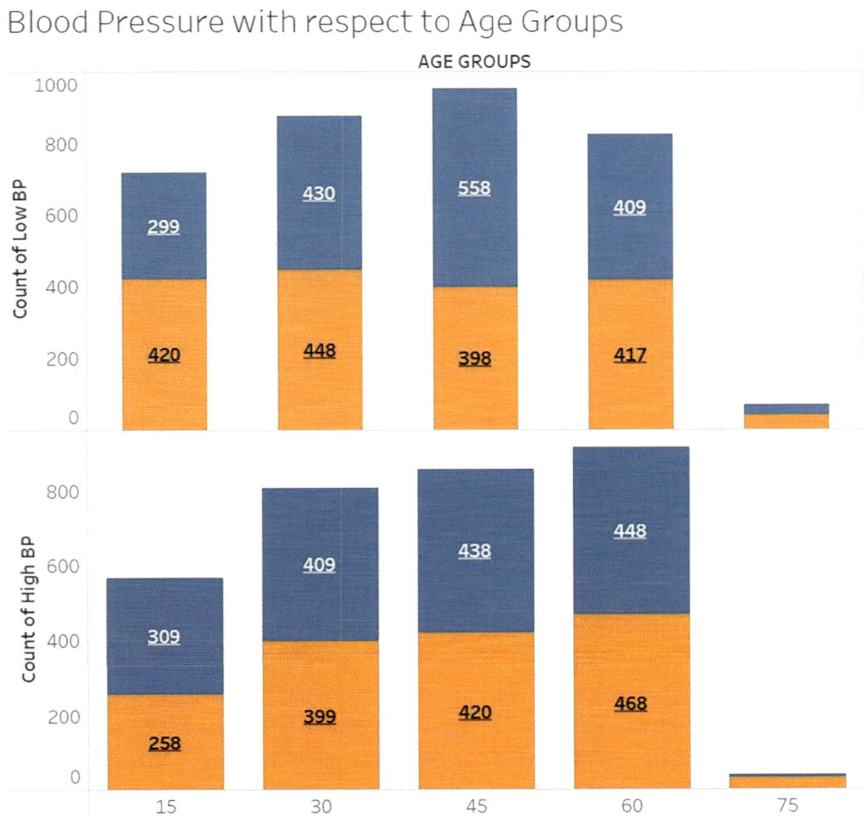


**FIGURE 18.5** Blood pressure with respect to age groups.

**Source: Author.**

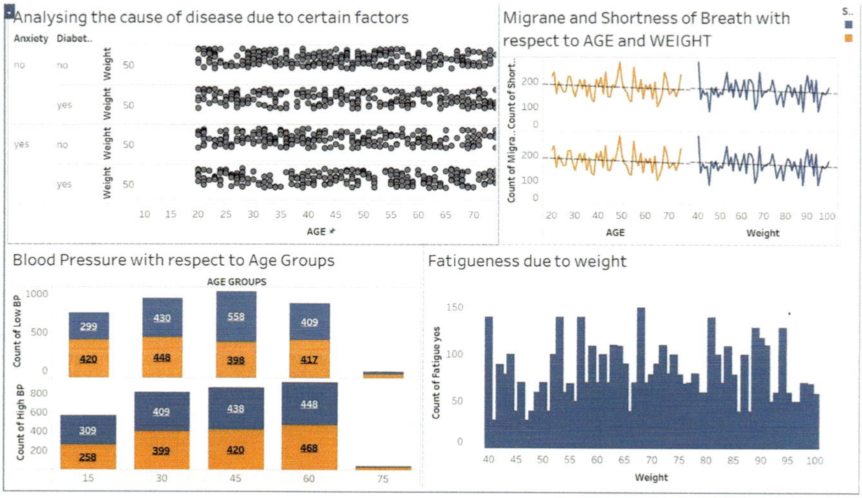


**FIGURE 18.6** Comprehensive health analysis dashboard.

**Source: Author.**

Comparing the orange and blue bars suggested potential gender differences in blood pressure distribution, with similar trends in both males and females. However, there might have been variations in the absolute counts between genders, warranting further statistical analysis to explore these gender-specific differences. These insights provide valuable information for healthcare professionals and researchers, guiding targeted cardiovascular health interventions based on age-related patterns of low and high blood pressure. Additionally, recognizing potential gender disparities in blood pressure levels can inform tailored strategies for blood pressure management.

In the final phase of the study, we developed a comprehensive dashboard that visually represents the relationships between age, weight, disease occurrence, migraines, shortness of breath, and blood pressure levels. The dashboard includes a scatterplot to explore correlations between age, weight, and diseases, two line charts to observe trends in migraines and shortness of breath with age and weight, and a bar graph to understand blood pressure distribution across different age groups. This integrated dashboard provides valuable insights for healthcare professionals and researchers, facilitating data-driven decision-making and the development of targeted interventions to improve public health outcomes. However, further analyses and considerations may be required to establish more definitive conclusions from the dashboard's findings. The dashboard provides a comprehensive overview of the analysis and allows users to interact with the data to explore different aspects of the health domain (Vrushank & Khang, 2023).

## 18.5 CONCLUSION

In conclusion, the health data analysis project represented a groundbreaking and highly impactful endeavor that revolutionized how we approach health-related data.

By seamlessly integrating cutting-edge technologies such as PySpark, MongoDB, Tableau Desktop, and Apache Kafka, we constructed an intricate and sophisticated data pipeline encompassing various stages of data processing, feature engineering, machine learning, and real-time data streaming. One of the key highlights of this project was the seamless integration of Apache Kafka, which played a crucial role in enabling real-time data streaming capabilities. This dynamic and fault-tolerant messaging system allowed for the continuous and timely processing of health data as it was generated, opening up new horizons for the acquisition of instantaneous insights and informed decision-making in the realm of healthcare (Khang & Smart Healthcare, 2023).

The scalability and adaptability offered by this data pipeline empowered us to analyze vast volumes of health data efficiently, unveiling critical health trends, disease patterns, and risk factors. By harnessing the potential of big data analytics and machine learning, we were able to extract hidden patterns and correlations within the data, enriching our understanding of complex health phenomena and unlocking opportunities for preventive measures and optimized healthcare resource allocation. Furthermore, the data visualization capabilities provided by Tableau Desktop allowed us to transform raw data into insightful and visually appealing representations. This facilitated effective communication of our findings to stakeholders, healthcare professionals, and policymakers, making the project's impact more far-reaching and actionable (Anh et al., 2024).

Overall, the successful implementation of this health data analysis project showcases the tremendous potential of data-driven solutions in revolutionizing the healthcare landscape. The project's outcomes underscore the importance of leveraging advanced technologies to drive evidence-based decision-making, improve patient care, and enhance public health initiatives. As we continue to explore the boundless possibilities of big data analytics, real-time data streaming, and interactive data visualization, the future of healthcare appears brighter than ever, with data leading the way toward healthier communities and improved well-being (Khang & Muthmainnah et al., 2023).

## 18.6 FUTURE SCOPE OF WORK

In the medical domain, in addition to the existing methodology, further advancements can be made to incorporate multimodal data analysis, where different types of medical data, such as images, text, and time series, are combined for more comprehensive insights. Integration of advanced deep learning techniques, like CNNs and RNNs, can enable accurate medical image analysis, disease progression prediction, and natural language processing for clinical notes and reports (Khang et al., 2024). Additionally, the methodology can be extended to support real-time patient monitoring, enabling early detection of anomalies and timely interventions. To enhance model interpretability, attention mechanisms, and explainable AI techniques can be explored, aiding medical professionals in understanding the rationale behind the model's predictions. By collaborating with domain experts and conducting thorough clinical validation, the methodology's applications can be adapted to support evidence-based decision-making and personalized patient care (Khang & Rana et al., 2023).

## REFERENCES

Alotaibi Shoayee, Rashid Mehmood, Iyad Katib, Omer Rana and Aiiad Albeshri, "Sehaa: A Big Data Analytics Tool for Healthcare Symptoms and Diseases Detection Using Twitter, Apache Spark, and Machine Learning," Appl. Sci., vol. 10, p. 1398, 2020, DOI:10.3390/app10041398

Amandeep Dhir, A. K. M. Najmul Islam, Matti Mäntymäki and Sayantan Khanra, "Big data analytics in healthcare: A systematic literature review," Enterprise Information Systems, vol. 14 (7), 2020, DOI:https://doi.org/10.1080/17517575.2020.1812005

Angappa Gunasekaran, Jaswant Manda, Milind Goswami and Sachin S. Kamble, "A systematic perspective on the applications of big data analytics in healthcare management," Int. J. Health. Manage., vol. 12 (3), pp. 226–240, 2018, DOI:10.1080/20479700.2018.1531606

Anh P. T. N., Vladimir Hahanov, Triwiyanto, Ragimova Nazila Ali, Rashad İsmibeyli, Vugar Abdullayev and Abuzarova Vusala Alyar. "AI models for disease diagnosis and prediction of heart disease with artificial neural networks," *Computer vision and AI-integrated IoT technologies in medical ecosystem* (1 Ed.), 2024. CRC Press. https://doi.org/10.1201/9781003429609-9

Anil Pandit and Nishita Mehta, "Concurrence of Big data analytics and healthcare: A systematic review." Int. J. Med. Inform., vol. 114, pp. 57–65, 2018, DOI:10.1016/j.ijmedinf.2018.03.013

Antoine-Moussiaux N., A. Ravel, C. Aenishaenslin, M. Peyre, M. Roche, O. Vandenberg and Z. Kozlakidis, "Valuing health surveillance as an information system: Interdisciplinary insights," Front. Public Health, vol. 7, p. 138, 2019, DOI:10.3389/fpubh.2019.00138

Archenaa J. and E. M. Anita, "A survey of big data analytics in healthcare and government," Proc. Computer Sci., vol. 50, pp. 408–413, 2015, DOI:10.1016/j.procs.2015.04.021

Bahri S., N. Zoghlami, M. Abed and J. M. R. Tavares, "Big data for healthcare: A survey." IEEE Access, vol. 7, pp. 7397–7408, 2018, DOI:10.1109/ACCESS.2018.2889180

Beakcheol Jang, Gaspard Harerimana, Hung Kook Park and Jong Wook Kim, "Health big data analytics: A technology survey", date of current version November 30, 2018, Health Services Research, vol. 42 (4), DOI:10.1109/ACCESS.2018.2878254

Bradley Elizabeth H, Kelly J. Devers and Leslie A. Curry. 2006, "Qualitative data analysis for health services research: Developing taxonomy, themes, and theory", Health Services Research, vol. 42 (4). DOI:10.1111/j.1475–6773.2006.00684.x

Changyong Liang, Dongxiao Gu, Jingjing Li, Xingguo Li, "Visualizing the knowledge structure and evolution of big data research in healthcare informatics," Int. J. Med. Inform., 98, pp. 22–32, DOI:10.1016/j.ijmedinf.2016.11.006

Chen K. L. Hwang, M. Wang and Y. Hao, "Disease prediction by machine learning over big data from healthcare communities." IEEE Access, vol. 5, pp. 8869–8879, 2017, DOI:10.1109/ACCESS.2017.2694446

Dimitrov D. V., "Medical Internet of Things and big data in healthcare," Healthcare Inform. Res, DOI:10.4258/hir.2016.22.3.156

Edwin Morely, "Big Data Analytics in healthcare", Date Added to IEEE Xplore: 23 December 2019, ISBN:978-1-7281-0353-2, DOI:10.1109/ICoAC44903.2018.8939061

Galetsi P. and K. Katsaliaki, "A review of the literature on big data analytics in healthcare," J Oper. Res. Soc., pp. 1–19, 2019, DOI:10.1080/01605682.2019.1630328

Geetika Chawla, Rekha Khatana and Savita Bamal, "Big Data Analytics for Data Visualization: Review of Techniques", Int. J. Comput. Appl. (0975–8887), vol. 182 (21), October 2018, DOI:10.5120/ijca2018917977

Kim Haeng-Kon, M. G. Zaragoza and Youn-ky Chung, "U-healthcare big data analytics process control," Int. J. Control Automat., vol. 10 (11), pp. 165–174, DOI:10.14257/ijca.2017.10.11.15

Kamran Ikram, Noman Ali Buttar, Muhammad Mohsin Waqas, Muthmainnah, Muhammad Mubashar Omer, Yasir Niaz, Khang A., "Robotic innovations in agriculture: Maximizing Production and sustainability." *Advanced technologies and AI-equipped IoT applications in high-tech agriculture* (1st Ed.), pp. 131–154, 2023. IGI Global Press. https://doi.org/10.4018/978-1-6684-9231-4.ch007

Keim D., G. Grinstein and M. O. Ward, *Interactive data visualization: Foundations, techniques and applications* (2nd Ed.), 2015. A. K. Peters, Ltd. ISBN 9781032530727, https://doi.org/10.1201/b18379

Khang A. (Ed.), *AI and IoT-based technologies for precision medicine*, 2024. ISBN: 9798369308769. IGI Global Press. https://doi.org/10.4018/979-8-3693-0876-9

Khang A., V. A. Abdullayev, Olena Hrybiuk and Arvind Kumar Shukla. *Computer vision and AI-integrated iot technologies in medical ecosystem* (1 Ed.), 2024. CRC Press. https://doi.org/10.1201/9781003429609

Khang A., V. Hahanov, G. L. Abbas and V. A. Hajimahmud, "Cyber-physical-social system and incident management," *AI-centric smart city ecosystems: technologies, design and implementation* (1st Ed., vol. 2 (15)), 2022. CRC Press. https://doi.org/10.1201/9781003252542-2

Khang A., Muthmainnah, Prodhan Mahbub Ibna Seraj, Ahmad Al Yakin, Ahmad J. Obaid and Manas Ranjan Panda. "AI-aided teaching model for the education 5.0 ecosystem" *AI-based technologies and applications in the era of the metaverse* (1 Ed.), pp. 83–104, 2023. IGI Global Press. DOI:https://doi.org/10.4018/978-1-6684-8851-5.ch004

Khang A., G. Rana, Tailor, R. K. and V. A. Hajimahmud (Eds.), *Data-centric AI solutions and emerging technologies in the healthcare ecosystem*, 2023. CRC Press. https://doi.org/10.1201/9781003356189

Korina Katsaliak's and Panagiota Galetsi, "A review of the literature on big data analytics in healthcare", 2019, ISSN: 0160–5682 1476–9360, https://doi.org/10.1080/01605682.2019.1630328

Kuo M.H., T. Sahama, A. W. Kushniruk, E. M. Borycki and D. K. Grunwell, "Health big data analytics: Current perspectives, challenges and potential solutions," Int. J. Big Data Intell., 2018, DOI:10.1109/RBME.2018.2829704

Lekha R. Nair, S. Shetty and Siddhanth D. Shetty, "Applying spark based machine learning model on streaming big data for health status prediction," Comput. Electr. Eng, 2017, DOI:10.1016/j.compeleceng.2017.03.009

Mamta M., M. Sharma and P. Kaur, "Big data and machine learning based secure healthcare framework," Proc. Comput. Sci., vol. 132, pp. 1049–1059, 2018, DOI:10.1016/j.procs.2018.05.020.

Mary Anita E.A. and J. Archenaa, "Health recommender system using big data analytics," J. Manage. Sci. Bus. Intell., vol. 2 (2), 2017, ISBN 2472–9264 (Online), 2472–9256 (Print), DOI:10.5281/zenodo.835606

Masoud S. and R. Sahal, "Real-time healthcare monitoring system using online machine learning and spark streaming," Int. J. Adv. Comput. Sci. Appl., vol. 11 (9), September 2020, DOI:10.14569/IJACSA.2020.0110977

Naoual E.A. and L. Benhlima, "Big data management for healthcare systems: Architecture, requirements, and implementation", Adv. Bioinfor., vol. 2018, 2018, Article ID 4059018, 10 pages, DOI: https://doi.org/10.1155/2018/4059018

Rani S., M. Chauhan, A. Kataria and A. Khang, "IoT equipped intelligent distributed framework for smart healthcare systems," *Networking and internet architecture* (vol. 2), p. 30, 2021. CRC Press. https://doi.org/10.48550/arXiv.2110.04997

Reddy C. K. and J. Sun, "Big data analytics for healthcare," in *Proc. 19th ACM SIGKDD Int. Conf. Knowl. Discovery Data Mining*, 2013, p. 1525, https://doi.org/10.1145/2487575.2506178

Raghupathi V. and W. Raghupathi, "Big data analytics in healthcare: Promise and potential," Health Inf. Sci. Syst., vol. 2, 2014, Article Number 3, DOI:10.1186/2047-2501-2-3

Schulte T. and S. Bohnet-Joschko. "How can big data analytics support people-centred and integrated health services: A scoping review," Int. J. Integr. Care, vol. 22, 2022, DOI:10.5334/ijic.5543

Vrushank S. and A. Khang, "Metaverse-enabling IoT technology for a futuristic healthcare system," *AI-based technologies and applications in the era of the metaverse* (1st Ed.), 2023. IGI Global Press. https://doi.org/10.4018/978-1-6684-8851-5.ch008

Wu B., H. Wang, R. Lin and Z. Ye, "Chronic diseases and health monitoring big data: A survey," IEEE Rev. Biomed. Eng., vol. 11, pp. 275–288, 2018, DOI:10.1109/RBME.2018.2829704

# 19 Applications of Internet of Things (IoT) Technologies in the Fields of Business and Healthcare

*Tanmay Gupta, Rajat Verma, and Namrata Dhanda*

## 19.1 INTRODUCTION

The Internet of Things (IoT) (Li et al., 2014; Verdouw et al., 2013) has emerged as a game-changing technology that has completely changed how companies conduct business and manufacture things. The ability of IoT devices to gather and analyze data in real-time allows companies to streamline operations, automate procedures, and develop new business models. Businesses across industries are spending extensively on IoT as a result of the broad use of IoT technology to stay ahead of the curve. In this chapter, the authors will examine how the Internet of Things (IoT) affects business and manufacturing, with a particular emphasis on supply chain management, predictive maintenance, and product innovation.

The authors will also cover the difficulties firms encounter while deploying IoT technologies and offer suggestions for overcoming these difficulties. Businesses may increase productivity, cut expenses, and generate new revenue streams by using the power of IoT, which will eventually spur growth and success in today's competitive business environment. The chapter discusses IoT, IIoT, IoT and Cloud, IoT, AI, and diverse use cases of integrating IoT with business and production, which is highlighted in the next sub-sections of the chapter (Khang & Vugar et al., 2024).

## 19.2 INTERNET OF THINGS

IoT stands for "Internet of Things". It is the network of interconnected physical objects, devices, and machines that are embedded with sensors, software, and connectivity capabilities, which allows them to communicate and exchange information with each other and humans over the internet (Perwej et al., 2019; Shackelford et al., 2020). The idea of IoT has been around for decades, but the term IoT only came up in 1999 when it was coined by Kevin Ashton, a British technology pioneer and

DOI: 10.1201/9781032686745-19

entrepreneur. He used the term to describe the interconnection of various physical objects using the internet.

The first internet-connected device was a toaster, which was connected to the internet in 1989 by a group of researchers at Cambridge University (Maple et al., 2017).

In the early 2000s, various advancements were made in wireless communication, sensor technology, and cloud computing, which made it possible to connect a wider range of devices and objects to the internet. This led to the development of the first IoT applications, such as smart home systems, industrial automation, and healthcare monitoring. When there were more internet-connected devices than people on the planet in the 2010s, the idea of IoT began to take off. IoT has since developed and expanded, with new use cases and applications appearing across numerous industries.

IoT is currently seen as a crucial enabler of digital transformation and is anticipated to have a significant impact on society and the economy in the years to come. IoT's major goal is to give everyday objects greater intelligence and responsiveness to carry out automatic operations and give users insightful data.

Numerous industries, including healthcare, industry, transportation, agriculture, and more, can use this technology in a wide range of ways. Smart thermostats, wearable fitness trackers, home security systems, self-driving cars, and industrial robots are a few instances of IoT. These gadgets generate a lot of data that may be analyzed to increase productivity, improve user experiences, and cut expenses.

To ensure the safe and responsible development and deployment of this technology, questions about data privacy, security, and other ethical implications are raised by IoT. IoT has huge potential; it can be used to revolutionize the way people live and work. The connection of devices and objects to the internet will enable the collection and analysis of data in real-time, which will help us make more informed decisions and improve efficiency.

The widespread adoption of IoT will also enable automation, remote control, and access to various everyday objects. For example, in the healthcare industry, IoT technologies, such as wearable fitness trackers and medical sensors, can monitor patients' vital signs and health indicators, enabling doctors and other healthcare professionals to spot potential health issues before they worsen. This can assist in avoiding hospitalization and lowering medical expenses.

IoT devices can be used to monitor and improve production processes in the industrial sector. For example, sensors can be added to machines to monitor performance and forecast maintenance requirements. Increasing productivity and reducing downtime can help the company save money. IoT also has implications for agriculture, smart cities, and transportation. Self-driving automobiles and intelligent traffic systems can potentially increase safety and lessen traffic congestion in the transportation sector. IoT sensors can be used in agriculture to monitor soil conditions and optimize irrigation, resulting in more productive and environmentally friendly farming methods. IoT devices can be used in smart cities to monitor and manage street lighting, public transportation, and traffic flow, creating a more livable and sustainable urban environment. As with any new technology, there are various concerns about data privacy, security, and ethical implications.

IoT devices collect huge amounts of data, which can be sensitive and personal, raising questions about who has access to this data and how it is used. Additionally, the interconnected nature of IoT devices can make them vulnerable to hacking and cyber-attacks, which can have serious consequences for individuals and businesses.

### 19.2.1 IoT Concerns

The absence of security features on IoT devices is one of the main security issues. With default usernames and passwords that are simple to guess, many IoT devices are open to hacking and unauthorized access. Once an attacker has access to a device, they can use it to conduct attacks against other network nodes, steal confidential information, or engage in other harmful activities (Elaine et al., 2004).

IoT developers and vendors must put robust authentication and access control measures in place to solve this, including two-factor authentication, biometric authentication, and encryption of critical data (Mahmoud et al., 2015). IoT devices gather a ton of data, including sensitive and personal data accessible to and usable by unauthorized parties. This presents issues with data privacy and the requirement to put safeguards in place to safeguard personal data and prevent unauthorized access.

IoT developers and providers must use robust encryption technologies, data access controls, and data anonymization techniques to preserve user data privacy. Additionally, users should also receive training on how to safeguard their personal information and prevent sharing it with unauthorized persons. Because IoT devices are frequently connected to bigger networks, such as the internet, they are susceptible to assaults that might bring down the entire network. This covers man-in-the-middle (MITM) (Hwang et al., 2008) attacks that intercept and alter network communication, as well as distributed denial of service (DDoS) (Mirkovic et al., 2004) assaults that can flood the network with traffic.

To address this, IoT developers and producers must use robust network security measures, such as firewalls, intrusion detection and prevention systems, and virtual private networks (VPNs) (Hooper et al., 2007). To separate their IoT devices from other devices on their network, consumers must also segment their networks. Many IoT devices employ proprietary firmware, which could have security flaws that attackers could exploit. Many IoT devices cannot regularly receive updates, putting them at risk of attack. Firmware updates can solve these vulnerabilities.

Firmware updates and security patches must be regularly implemented by IoT suppliers and developers. Users also need to be taught how to upgrade their IoT devices and make sure they have the most recent firmware.

In conclusion, tackling the security concerns posed by IoT calls for a comprehensive strategy incorporating robust security safeguards at every stage of the device lifecycle, from design to deployment. Users also need to be taught how to secure their IoT devices and safeguard their data. Users can ensure that IoT devices are implemented safely and responsibly and that the benefits of IoT may be reaped without jeopardizing security and privacy by putting these measures into place.

### 19.2.2 IoT Future

IoT has a bright future ahead of it, with many industries predicted to be transformed by the technology as it continues to advance. The following are some of the major trends and advancements that are anticipated to influence the IoT in the future (Madhav et al., 2021):

- **5G Networks**: The introduction of 5G networks is anticipated to hasten the adoption of the Internet of Things by enabling faster and more dependable connectivity for IoT devices. This will make it possible to roll out more complex and data-intensive applications, like autonomous vehicles, remote medical care, and smart cities.
- **Artificial Intelligence and Machine Learning**: By making it possible to analyze IoT data in real-time and create predictive models, the combination of IoT, AI, and machine learning (Chamola et al., 2020) is expected to lead to new insights and efficiencies. Businesses will be able to make better decisions as a result, and their operations will be optimized.
- **Edge Computing**: As edge computing enables the processing of IoT data at the network's edge, closer to where the data is created, adoption is anticipated to rise. As a result, the amount of data that needs to be transmitted over the network is decreased, dependability is increased, and latency is decreased (Ma et al., 2019).
- **Interoperability**: As organizations and consumers look to integrate various IoT solutions and provide a smooth user experience, the necessity for interoperability between various IoT devices and platforms is anticipated to increase. To allow various IoT devices to connect, interoperability standards are being developed by standards organizations like the Open Connectivity Foundation (OCF).

Security will continue to be a major concern as IoT use increases. IoT suppliers and developers will need to keep up with the most recent security threats and vulnerabilities while implementing robust security solutions. In conclusion, the IoT has a bright future as several industries are predicted to be transformed by technology as it continues to advance. Businesses and consumers may fully use the potential of IoT and reap its benefits by implementing new technologies such as 5G, AI, and edge computing, as well as addressing security and interoperability problems.

### 19.2.3 Architecture of IoT

The Internet of Things (IoT) architecture typically consists of four basic layers, which are as follows:

- **Perception Layer**: Data from various physical sensors, equipment, and devices must be gathered by this layer. The information could be presented as temperature, humidity, pressure, motion, or any other observable quantity.

Smart sensors, RFID tags, GPS units, and other smart gadgets that can perceive the environment could be among the gadgets in this layer.

- **Network Layer**: It is the job of this layer to send the information gathered from the perception layer to the cloud or the main server. The network layer may transfer data using wired or wireless communication protocols, including cellular networks, Wi-Fi, Bluetooth, ZigBee, or Bluetooth Low Energy.
- **Data Processing Layer**: The data gathered from the perception layer must be processed and analyzed by this layer. Depending on the application, the data may be processed locally on the device or in the cloud. To get actionable insights from the data, the data processing layer may employ a variety of methods, including machine learning, deep learning, and statistical analysis.
- **Application Layer**: This layer is in charge of providing the end-user with the IoT system's ultimate output. The output may take the form of notifications, alerts, reports, or system actions. A dashboard, a web or mobile application, or an API that connects with other systems could all be considered the application layer.

Overall, the IoT architecture is built to facilitate seamless communication and collaboration between various systems and devices, enhancing productivity, automation, and efficiency.

## 19.3 INTERNET OF THINGS AND CLOUD COMPUTING

IoT (Internet of Things) and cloud computing (Dang et al., 2019) are two linked technologies that are frequently used in unison. The Internet of Things (IoT) is a system of physical objects, such as furniture, vehicles, appliances, and other items, which are connected to the internet and have sensors, software, and network connectivity (Munirathinam et al., 2020; Giri et al., 2017).

Data from these sensors can be used for many purposes, such as automation, analysis, and monitoring. On the other side, cloud computing describes the internet-based provision of computing services such as servers, storage, databases, networking, software, and analytics (Armbrust et al., 2010). Users who use cloud computing can access these services from any location with an internet connection and only pay for the services they use.

IoT devices may use the computing power, storage, and scalability of cloud computing to execute complex analytics, machine learning, and AI algorithms when they are linked to the cloud. This makes it possible for businesses to handle and examine the massive amounts of data produced by IoT devices and gain insights that can be applied to operational optimization, product and service improvement, and customer experience improvement (Rana et al., 2021).

Additionally, cloud computing offers a centralized platform for managing and controlling IoT devices, making remote monitoring, configuration, and upkeep of IoT systems possible. This aids in lowering the difficulty and expense of administering extensive IoT deployments (Yarali et al., 2021). IoT and cloud computing are complementary technologies that let businesses use the data produced by IoT devices and gain insightful knowledge from them.

Massive volumes of data are produced by IoT devices frequently in real-time. This information can be utilized to streamline processes, boost effectiveness, and offer insightful information. However, it takes a lot of computational power and storage to analyze this data. Cloud computing can help with this. Organizations may store and analyze enormous amounts of data produced by IoT devices by utilizing cloud services, allowing for real-time data analysis and decision-making. Depending on the amount of data being generated, cloud computing also enables organizations to scale their resources up or down as necessary effortlessly.

Additionally, cloud computing gives IoT devices a centralized platform for management and control. This may involve doing IoT system configuration, monitoring, and maintenance remotely.

For instance, updating the firmware on an IoT device can be done remotely over the cloud without requiring physical access to the device. Enhanced security is a benefit of combining IoT and cloud computing. The majority of cloud service providers have strong security mechanisms in place to safeguard data and thwart unauthorized access (Armbrust et al., 2010).

Organizations may lower their risk of data breaches and guarantee the security of their IoT systems by storing data in the cloud.

Some key pointers about the correlation between IoT and the cloud include:

- **Scalability**: Scalability is one of the key advantages of combining cloud computing with IoT. Cloud computing enables businesses to rapidly scale up their resources as needed to handle and store the enormous volumes of data that IoT devices create (Hashem et al., 2015).
- **Real-Time Data Analysis**: Using cloud computing with IoT has the added advantage of enabling real-time data analysis. Organizations may collect and analyze IoT device data in real-time using cloud computing, which offers insightful information and facilitates prompt decision-making.
- **Centralized Management**: Cloud computing offers a centralized platform for managing and controlling IoT devices. This comprises operations like the remote configuration, monitoring, and upkeep of IoT systems.
- **Cost-Effectiveness**: Organizations can lower the cost of managing extensive IoT deployments by combining cloud computing with IoT. Because they only pay for what they use, businesses no longer need to invest in costly gear and infrastructure thanks to cloud computing.
- **Security**: To safeguard data and stop unauthorized access, cloud service providers often have strong security measures in place (Sabahi, 2011). Organizations may lower their risk of data breaches and guarantee the security of their IoT systems by storing data in the cloud.
- **AI and Machine Learning**: Cloud computing provides the computational capacity required to run sophisticated AI and machine learning algorithms on the data produced by IoT devices. This makes it possible for businesses to get the most out of their IoT data and optimize their operations (Rana et al., 2021).

IoT and cloud computing go hand in hand, with the latter offering the scalability, real-time data analysis, centralized management, cost-effectiveness, security, and computing capacity required for organizations to properly utilize IoT (Botta et al., 2016).

## 19.4 INTERNET OF THINGS AND ARTIFICIAL INTELLIGENCE

Artificial intelligence (AI) and the Internet of Things (IoT) (Gupta and Khattar, 2020) are two rapidly developing technologies that are altering how people connect with the outside world. The phrase "Internet of Things" (IoT) refers to how everyday objects are connected to the internet so they may communicate with one another and with humans.

The creation of intelligent computers that can carry out tasks that frequently need human intelligence, such as learning, thinking, and problem-solving, is known as artificial intelligence (AI). The Internet of Things (IoT) is a system of physical objects, such as furniture, vehicles, appliances, and other goods, which are connected to the internet and have sensors, software, and network connectivity (Merenda et al., 2020).

AI and IoT are complementary technologies that can be used to develop potent and innovative solutions. Large volumes of data are produced by IoT devices, which may be analyzed and processed by AI algorithms to help in decision-making. For instance, temperature, light, and humidity data can be collected by smart home sensors and used by an AI system to modify the environment to suit the tastes of the residents. Similarly, AI can be applied to improve IoT device functionality. An AI-powered camera, for instance, can identify and distinguish faces, enabling it to offer more specialized security features. Additionally, AI can assist IoT devices in learning from user preferences and behavior, enabling them to adjust and advance over time (Khang & Misra et al., 2023).

In general, the fusion of IoT and AI has the potential to revolutionize several industries, including manufacturing, healthcare, transportation, and more. These technologies enable us to build more effective systems that enhance our quality of life and assist us in achieving our objectives. Various businesses can be transformed by IoT and AI together:

- **Healthcare**: IoT and AI are revolutionizing the healthcare sector by enhancing operating efficiency, lowering costs, and improving patient care. IoT gadgets like wearables, remote monitoring tools, and sensors may gather patient data and send it instantly to medical professionals. These data can be analyzed by AI systems to offer individualized treatment strategies, early illness diagnosis, and improved disease management.
- **Manufacturing**: The manufacturing sector is changing thanks to IoT and AI, which enable predictive maintenance, enhance quality assurance, and boost output efficiency. IoT sensors can gather information on machine performance, enabling manufacturers to identify and fix problems before they become life-threatening. Production schedules, waste reduction, and supply chain management can all be improved by AI algorithms.
- **Transportation**: The Internet of Things and artificial intelligence (Gupta and Khattar, 2020) are revolutionizing the transportation sector by enabling

intelligent and autonomous cars, enhancing safety, and enhancing traffic management. Real-time data on weather, road conditions, and traffic flow can be gathered by IoT sensors, which can be utilized to improve routing and ease congestion. To help autonomous vehicles make wise decisions, AI algorithms can also analyze data from cameras and sensors.

- **Agriculture**: By increasing agricultural yields, decreasing waste, and boosting sustainability, IoT and AI are revolutionizing the agriculture sector. To improve irrigation and fertilization, IoT devices like sensors, drones, and robots may gather information on the soil's moisture, temperature, and nutrient content. These data can also be analyzed by AI systems to provide immediate suggestions for planting, harvesting, and pest control.

The combination of IoT and AI is changing how people live and work. It is creating new opportunities for innovation and growth, and it has the potential to improve our lives in countless ways.

### 19.4.1 Benefits of Integrating IoT and AI

People can get the following advantages with the amalgamation of IoT and AI, which are highlighted in what follows:

- **Greater Efficiency**: The combination of IoT and AI can assist businesses in automating procedures, cutting waste, and raising production. IoT device data can be analyzed by AI to find trends that can be used to improve workflows, decrease downtime, and increase quality (Khang & Hajimahmud et al., 2023).
- **Personalized Services**: IoT devices have the potential to provide a sizable amount of data, which AI can then examine to comprehend client behavior and preferences. This study can assist businesses in providing more individualized services, customizing marketing initiatives, and improving consumer satisfaction.
- **Predictive Maintenance**: IoT sensors can find equipment problems before they get serious. To decrease downtime and lengthen the lifespan of equipment, AI systems can analyze this data and find patterns that indicate when maintenance is necessary.

### 19.4.2 Challenges toward Integration of IoT and AI

With the amalgamation of IoT and AI, the following challenges may lead to diverse consequences. They are highlighted in what follows:

- **Security and Privacy**: The system is increasingly susceptible to cyberattacks as more devices are connected to the internet. Making sure AI algorithms and IoT devices are secure and shielded from unauthorized access is a challenge.

- **Complexity**: The fusion of IoT and AI technologies results in a complicated system that calls for a wide variety of design, development, and management abilities. To successfully implement IoT and AI solutions, organizations must invest in the proper skills and technologies.
- **Interoperability**: For the greatest benefit, IoT devices and AI algorithms must operate in unison. Ensuring that gadgets from many manufacturers can connect and cooperate without problems is the difficult part.

In summary, the advantages of merging IoT and AI greatly outweigh the disadvantages. Businesses must, however, be aware of the issues and take action to resolve them. By doing this, they can fully utilize IoT and AI to develop innovative solutions that alter their companies.

## 19.5 INDUSTRIAL INTERNET OF THINGS (IIoT)

The Industrial Internet of Things (IIoT) (Boyes et al., 2018) is the integration of the Internet of Things in the industrial and manufacturing sectors. It utilizes a wide range of interconnected devices, sensors, and systems that collect, analyze, and communicate data in real-time to optimize various operations, increase efficiency, optimize cost, and reduce safety hazards. It is a vital and most important part of the Fourth Industrial Revolution or Industry 4.0 (Lasi et al., 2014).

Industry 1.0 was the first Industrial Revolution in the 1700s, Industry 2.0 was the introduction of assembly lines and electricity, and Industry 3.0 began with the utilization of computers in the manufacturing process (Vinitha et al., 2020). Industry 4.0 utilizes the features of smart devices and real-time data analytics to use the data generated by industrial machines efficiently.

The Industrial Internet of Things premise is that intelligent devices are better at gathering data, analyzing it in real-time, and communicating critical details that may be utilized to make business decisions more successfully (Shrouf et al., 2014). IIoT is expected to revolutionize the industrial landscape, enabling businesses to achieve new levels of operational efficiency and productivity. The components of IIoT vary depending on the specific implementation and application, but some common components include:

- **Sensors and Devices**: These are the physical components or hardware units used to collect data from the environment. These include temperature sensors, pressure sensors, and motion sensors. This layer may also consist of robots, drones, and other machines which may be used to interact with the user and/or perform various tasks.
- **Connectivity**: The sensors and device need to be connected with other components of the IIoT system to carry out further operations. This is done by the connectivity layer, which may include Wi-Fi, Bluetooth, Ethernet, or any other communication protocol through which the devices and sensors are connected to the internet or a private network.
- **Cloud Computing**: The sensors and devices produce massive amounts of data, and to counter this problem, cloud computing is often used to store and

process the data generated. Cloud platforms, such as Amazon Web Services (AWS), Microsoft Azure, and Google Cloud Platform (GCP), offer scalable and flexible computing resources to support IIoT applications.

- **Analytics and Machine Learning**: The data generated by the IIoT system is processed using various analytics and/or machine learning. This may include real-time analysis to detect anomalies or predict equipment failures, as well as advanced analytics to identify patterns and trends over time.
- **Applications and Dashboards**: The insights generated by IIoT analytics must be presented to users in a useful and actionable way. This may involve dashboards, reports, or applications that provide real-time visibility into industrial processes and operations.
- **Security**: Security is a critical component of IIoT systems, as the data collected by sensors and devices can be sensitive and valuable. IIoT security measures may include access controls, encryption, and data protection techniques to ensure data is not compromised.

Overall, the components of IIoT work together to enable real-time monitoring, analysis, and control of industrial processes and operations, ultimately driving greater efficiency, productivity, and profitability.

### 19.5.1 Benefits of IIoT

There are numerous benefits of IIoT. Some of them are:

- **Improved Efficiency**: By delivering real-time data on equipment operation and production output, the IIoT helps optimize industrial processes. It uses this information to locate bottlenecks, lessen downtime, and boost production.
- **Cost Reduction**: As IIoT improves efficiency and reduces maintenance and repair expenses, it helps reduce costs. For example, predictive maintenance based on IIoT data can prevent equipment failures and reduce the need for costly repairs.
- **Enhanced Safety**: Real-time equipment and process monitoring provided by IIoT can increase safety. This can assist in avoiding mishaps and spotting potential dangers.
- **Better Decision-Making**: IIoT offers real-time data and analytics that can assist businesses in making decisions based on data. This may result in more effective resource management, increased operational effectiveness, and more informed strategic planning.
- **New Business Models**: Pay-per-use or subscription-based services are two examples of new business models that IIoT might make possible. These models can boost income and offer customers additional sources of value.
- **Supply Chain Optimization**: The IIoT can also improve the supply chain by giving real-time information on inventory levels, production output, and shipping and delivery schedules. Through the optimized supply chain, businesses can become more efficient and spend less money.

- **Predictive Maintenance**: Predictive maintenance is one of the fundamental advantages of IIoT (Mobley et al., 2002). IIoT can identify equipment problems before they happen by analyzing data from sensors and devices, allowing businesses to undertake maintenance and repairs before expensive downtime occurs.
- **Remote Monitoring and Control**: IIoT enables remote monitoring and control of industrial processes and equipment, allowing businesses to keep an eye on activities from any location in the world. As a result, there may be less need for on-site workers and more flexibility.
- **Environmental Sustainability**: Through maximizing energy use, lowering waste, and boosting efficiency, IIoT can also help environmental sustainability. By doing this, businesses can lessen their impact on the environment and achieve sustainability objectives.
- **Customization and Personalization**: Industrial items can be modified and personalized thanks to IIoT, enabling businesses to offer clients unique solutions. IIoT, for instance, can make it possible to produce personalized goods in small batches, cutting waste and raising consumer satisfaction.
- **Integration with Existing Systems**: Enterprise resource planning (ERP) and manufacturing execution systems (MES) are two examples of existing systems that can be connected with IIoT to provide a more complete picture of industrial operations. Businesses can find areas for improvement and optimize procedures thanks to this.
- **Industry 4.0**: Industry 4.0, a manufacturing trend that stresses using digital technology to optimize industrial operations, includes IIoT as a significant element. IIoT, artificial intelligence, robotics, and augmented reality are examples of industry 4.0 technologies.

IIoT is a fast-developing industry with a wide range of uses and advantages. With the use of data analytics, cloud computing, and connectivity, IIoT may help businesses streamline industrial operations, cut costs, and boost efficiency, which will ultimately lead to higher production and profitability.

### 19.5.2 Challenges to IIoT

While IIoT has many advantages, there are also several difficulties that businesses must overcome to install and operate these systems successfully. Here are a few such problems (Jaidka et al., 2020):

- **Interoperability**: IIoT systems frequently consist of a variety of hardware and software from several suppliers, each of which may adhere to a separate set of communication standards and protocols. A seamless integration of all the components may be challenging as a result.
- **Security**: Because IIoT systems receive and send sensitive data, it is essential to make sure they are secure. The network and cloud infrastructure that are used to store and process data, as well as the devices and sensors themselves, must all be secured.

- **Data Quality**: IIoT systems may collect noisy or incomplete data, which can make it challenging to evaluate and draw conclusions. It makes it necessary to do data normalization and cleansing to guarantee the data's superior quality.
- **Data Governance**: Businesses must create rules and regulations for controlling this data as IIoT systems produce enormous amounts of data. Determining who gets access to the data, how it may be used, and how it is safeguarded is part of this process (Carter et al., 1994).
- **Scalability**: Organizations must make sure they can scale IIoT systems to manage growing amounts of data and devices as these systems grow in size and complexity. More edge computing or cloud computing assets might be required to achieve this.
- **Talent and Skills**: Data analytics, machine learning, and software development are just a few of the technical skills needed to implement and maintain IIoT systems. For some businesses, it might be difficult to find and keep personnel with these skills.
- **Return on Investment (ROI)**: Organizations must ensure they can create a significant return on investment to cover the costs associated with implementing IIoT technologies because doing so can be expensive. It could be necessary to create fresh business plans or revenue sources.

It takes technical knowledge, business sense, and organizational agility to meet these problems. Businesses that can effectively navigate these difficulties will reap the many advantages of IIoT, including improved production, profitability, and efficiency.

### 19.5.3 Future of IIoT

Given how quickly this technology is developing and expanding into new sectors of business, IIoT has a promising future (Rani & Chauhan et al., 2021). Here are some probable changes that could affect IIoT's future:

- **Increased Integration**: IIoT systems are projected to become more connected with other business systems over time, including customer relationship management (CRM) and enterprise resource planning (ERP) systems. Organizations will be able to see their operations more thoroughly and make better decisions as a result.
- **Edge Intelligence**: When real-time analysis and decision-making are closer to the data's source, edge computing is projected to become more significant in IIoT systems. Organizations may benefit from quicker event responses and real-time operational optimization as a result.
- **Artificial Intelligence and Machine Learning**: As IIoT devices generate more data, it is anticipated that the use of artificial intelligence and machine learning algorithms will rise. These technologies can assist companies in locating anomalies, anticipating equipment issues, and continuously enhancing their operations (Das et al., 2015).

- **5G Connectivity**: Once 5G networks are introduced, they are likely to have a considerable influence on IIoT systems since they will allow for quicker, more dependable communication and higher data transmission rates. Businesses may upgrade their operations and adopt more advanced IIoT systems by using 5G.
- **Autonomous Operations**: As IIoT systems improve, it is anticipated that more autonomous operations will be possible. This could involve the deployment of robots and autonomous vehicles, which can function more safely and effectively than human operators.
- **Continued Innovation**: The IIoT market is expected to keep innovating and developing, with modern technologies and applications appearing often. This will give businesses fresh chances to enhance their processes and achieve a competitive edge.

Overall, greater integration, edge intelligence, artificial intelligence, machine learning, 5G connection, autonomous operations, and ongoing innovation are likely to characterize the future of IIoT. These technologies will allow businesses to streamline processes, cut costs, and boost their competitiveness as they continue to develop and mature.

## 19.6 USE-CASES OF IOT IN BUSINESS AND PRODUCTION

IoT is set to play an essential role in the evolution and modernization of businesses. Let us look at some examples where IoT can play a significant role in business and production.

### 19.6.1 IoT in Manufacturing

The manufacturing sector could transform thanks to the Internet of Things (IoT), which will boost operational effectiveness, cut costs, and boost overall production. (Shrouf et al., 2014).

Through connected devices, sensors, and software applications, the Internet of Things (IoT) is used in manufacturing to collect and analyze data from various machines, equipment, and processes. There are numerous ways IoT may be used in manufacturing to boost output, cut costs, and improve efficiency.

- **Predictive Maintenance**: Using IoT in manufacturing to execute predictive maintenance is one of the most important advantages. Manufacturers can track the condition of their equipment and forecast when maintenance will be necessary before a problem occurs by employing sensors and real-time data analytics. This strategy can save maintenance expenses and help prevent unplanned downtime by scheduling maintenance only when necessary.
- **Quality Control**: By giving real-time information on the manufacturing process, IoT can enhance quality control. For instance, sensors can be used to keep an eye on the temperature and humidity levels during production to make sure that the necessary conditions are met for product production. IoT

can also aid in the detection of product flaws throughout the manufacturing process, preventing them from reaching the market.

- **Supply Chain Management**: The Internet of Things (IoT) can assist firms in tracking the transfer of products and raw materials across the supply chain, lowering the risk of loss or theft. Products or containers can be equipped with sensors, enabling producers to track their position and state in real-time. Utilizing this information can streamline the supply chain, lower inventory levels, and increase shipment effectiveness.
- **Energy Efficiency**: By locating energy-wasting locations, IoT can assist manufacturers in maximizing energy utilization. For instance, sensors can be used to track how machinery and equipment are used, allowing producers to spot wasteful procedures and reduce energy use. The use of this strategy can lower energy expenditures and increase sustainability.
- **Increased Productivity**: By automating procedures and lowering manual labor, IoT can increase productivity. Robotics and automation, for instance, can be used by factories to carry out monotonous activities, freeing up staff members to work on more difficult jobs. Production schedules and workflows can also be optimized using IoT to cut downtime and boost efficiency.

IoT system implementation in manufacturing, however, can be difficult and expensive. To install and manage IoT systems, manufacturers must carefully weigh the advantages and disadvantages of IoT. To guard against data breaches and other security concerns, it is also necessary to carefully manage cybersecurity risks.

### 19.6.2 IoT in Supply Chain Management

The Internet of Things (IoT) has become increasingly important in supply chain management as it allows for real-time tracking of goods, equipment, and vehicles. Companies can optimize their supply chain operations, cut costs, and boost efficiency thanks to this technology. The use of sensors and RFID tags to track the movement and location of commodities in real-time is one example of IoT in supply chain management. The time and expense involved in supply chain activities can be decreased by using this information to optimize delivery and transportation schedules.

IoT can be used to keep an eye on the state of cargo as it is being transported. For instance, sensors can assess vibration, humidity, and temperature to make sure that fragile items are handled carefully and perishable commodities are maintained at the optimum temperature. IoT can also be used to monitor the efficiency of the machinery and vehicles employed in the supply chain. Sensor data can be utilized to anticipate issues, allowing businesses to do preventative maintenance and minimize downtime. Overall, IoT has many advantages for supply chain management, including boosted productivity, enhanced visibility, and cost savings. It is possible that as this technology develops, the supply chain sector will see even more innovative IoT applications.

- **Predictive Maintenance**: IoT devices can assist businesses in determining when equipment and vehicle maintenance or repairs are required, lowering the risk of breakdowns and raising overall productivity.

- **Inventory Management**: With the help of IoT devices, businesses can monitor inventory levels in real-time to make sure they always have the proper amount of product on hand. This can aid in lowering waste, raising accuracy, and maximizing available storage.
- **Supply Chain Visibility**: From manufacturing to distribution, IoT devices may offer real-time visibility into every step of the supply chain. This can assist businesses in identifying potential problems, such as bottlenecks or delays, and taking steps to alleviate them.
- **Better Customer Service**: Businesses can offer consumers real-time updates on the status of their orders, including when they will be delivered and whether there are any delays, by utilizing IoT data. This may enhance client loyalty and satisfaction.
- **Sustainability**: Businesses may monitor their environmental impact and take action to lessen their carbon footprint by using IoT devices to track environmental variables like air quality and carbon emissions.

Overall, IoT is revolutionizing supply chain management by enabling businesses to streamline processes, cut costs, and enhance customer satisfaction. Users may anticipate seeing even more innovative IoT applications in the supply chain sector as this technology develops.

### 19.6.3 IoT in Agriculture

IoT integrates robots, drones, sensors, and computer imaging with agriculture. These, along with analytical tools, provide insights and help monitor the farms. IoT in agriculture works by integrating physical hardware and analytical software. The analytical dashboard mostly consists of software that is used to process information gathered by the various smart devices. However, the efficient integration of IoT in agriculture requires pre-requisite knowledge of robotics and computer-based intelligence.

Agricultural productivity has increased at a lesser cost thanks to the Industrial IoT (Hassoun et al., 2022). IoT-powered smart solutions will become more prevalent in agriculture operations during the coming years. In fact, according to a few recent reports, the agriculture sector would have an IoT device installation growth rate of 20% CAGR. And by 2024, there will be 225 million connected agricultural devices, up from 13 million in 2014.

According to recent statistics, the global population is expected to reach 9.6 billion by 2050. This will result in more demand for food. The agriculture industry needs to increase production to meet this huge demand. The challenges to this increased production are extreme weather conditions, climatic changes, environmental impact, and inefficient farming. The eradication of these problems can be easily achieved by using IoT. The following are the use cases of IoT in agriculture.

#### 19.6.3.1 Climate Conditions

Climatic conditions play a vital role in farming. Knowing about these climatic changes can reduce losses due to a lack of awareness of climatic changes, such as sudden changes in humidity, rainfall, and temperature. IoT enables real-time monitoring of weather conditions with the help of sensors placed in and around the agricultural field. It can also incorporate weather forecast data and alert the farmers about any disturbing condition if and when such is encountered. This can eliminate the need for a human to monitor the weather conditions, provide better analysis of climatic conditions to suggest crops that give better yields, and also reduce losses due to climatic changes.

#### 19.6.3.2 Smart Greenhouse

With the help of various IoT-based sensors, greenhouses can be made smart by enabling autonomous weather tracking. Adopting IoT in greenhouses eliminates the need for human intervention, thus reducing the cost of running greenhouses at the same time increasing accuracy. These sensors can adjust the conditions to maintain the weather conditions as per the set of instructions. The sensors collect real-time data, analyze it, and perform the necessary actions. It can also help monitor water levels and enable better automatic irrigation.

#### 19.6.3.3 Data Analytics

IoT-based agriculture uses a large number of sensors. These sensors create vast amounts of data that can be analyzed to achieve better results. However, the conventional storage of such large data is impractical, so cloud-based storage can be incorporated with IoT to enable better data analytics. The collected data can be used for leveraging technological advancements. Predictive analysis can be done to make better decisions about harvesting. Analyzing the weather trends can help farmers make more productive decisions about their crops, thus ensuring high efficiency and increasing the yields of the crop.

#### 19.6.3.4 Agricultural Drones

Drones can be used on the ground or in the air to inspect crops, monitor crops, plant seeds, apply fertilizer, and analyze fields (Ahirwar et al., 2019). Drone technology has transformed the agriculture industry by giving it a high-rise makeover with proper strategy and planning based on real-time data. Drones with thermal or multispectral sensors can quickly determine which regions need watering. Additionally, they analyze fertilizer needs, allowing for optimal use and minimizing waste, which not only lowers costs but also stops chemical seepage into groundwater.

#### 19.6.3.5 Crop Monitoring and Precision Farming

IoT sensors may also be used to keep an eye on the development and health of crops, spotting pests and diseases before they cause damage and allowing farmers to take precise preventative action. Real-time data on soil moisture, temperature, humidity, and other elements that impact crop growth can be gathered via IoT sensors and devices. This knowledge can be applied to improve irrigation, fertilization, and other farming methods, increasing yields and lowering expenses.

#### 19.6.3.6 Supply Chain Management

IoT sensors can be used to follow products from the farm to the market, giving current details on the whereabouts and state of the goods. Guaranteeing that goods are delivered to clients in the best condition possible can assist in optimizing logistics and reducing waste.

IoT, with the help of its various use cases, has enabled higher production while maintaining the quality of the yield. The data collected from various sensors ensure swift action and lesser damage to crops. IoT technology may support agriculture in a variety of ways, including supply chain management, precision farming, and animal and crop monitoring. Farmers may improve their procedures and cut expenses by deploying IoT sensors and devices to gather real-time data on soil moisture, temperature, humidity, animal movement, feeding patterns, and other things. IoT can also aid early pest and disease detection, better logistics, waste reduction, and higher productivity.

### 19.6.4 IoT in Poultry Farming

IoT, or the Internet of Things, like many other businesses, can be used in poultry farming as well. Integration of IoT in poultry farming can improve efficiency and productivity. It can also automate various processes like feeding. It can also alert farmers about the temperature, humidity, and air quality of the chicken coops if the conditions become unfavorable. Additionally, IoT can be used to keep an eye on the health and location of individual chickens, which enables quick and easy isolation and selection of infected birds (Khang et al., 2023).

#### 19.6.4.1 Environmental Monitoring

IoT sensors can be placed in chicken coops to monitor temperature, humidity, and air quality. This helps maintain optimal conditions for the well-being and health of chickens. It can alert the farmers to unfavorable conditions and can even take action to correct the problems.

#### 19.6.4.2 Automatic Feeding and Watering Systems

IoT can automate the process of feeding and watering livestock. IoT also helps analyze the eating and drinking habits of the chickens and can help easily find any irregularities. This way, farmers can schedule feedings and watering. Also, it can be done with the help of sensors that can detect the water and food levels to refill them whenever required automatically.

#### 19.6.4.3 Livestock Tracking

IoT-based trackers such as RFID tags can be attached to individual chickens to track their location and monitor their health. This can help farmers identify and isolate sick birds quickly, reducing the risk of disease spreading throughout the flock.

#### 19.6.4.4 Predictive Maintenance

IoT's biggest usage today is predictive maintenance, and it can be implemented in Poultry farming as well. Predictive maintenance can be used to predict when servicing of equipment will be required and will prevent the sudden failure of machinery.

#### 19.6.4.5 Automated Decision Making

The data collected from these sensors can be analyzed by AI algorithms, which can help farmers make more informed decisions about their flocks, such as optimal feeding schedules, ideal temperature and humidity levels, and other factors that impact the health and productivity of chickens.

#### 19.6.4.6 Automated Egg Collection

IoT sensors and cameras can detect if a chicken has laid an egg, which can then trigger the action for the collection of eggs. It can reduce the risk of broken eggs and reduce human involvement in the process.

#### 19.6.4.7 Lighting Control

IoT sensors can sense the light levels inside the chicken coops and adjust the artificial light accordingly. This can avoid any problems occurring due to lack of natural light, which is then compensated by artificial light (Khang & Rani et al., 2022).

#### 19.6.4.8 Remote Monitoring

IoT can enable remote monitoring of the poultry farm from anywhere by using mobile devices or computers. This can also enable automated feeding and watering, livestock tracking, and even automated egg collection.

#### 19.6.4.9 Biosecurity

Sensors and cameras can detect the movement of people and vehicles in and out of farms. This can help maintain biosecurity protocols and prevent the spread of diseases by tracking and controlling the movements of people and vehicles. All of these usage cases can help farmers improve the efficiency, productivity, and overall management of their poultry farm operations and help ensure the well-being of their chickens.

### 19.6.5 IoT in the Automotive Industry

IoT has helped evolve several sectors, including the automotive. Connectivity, smart sensors and gadgets, edge computing, and mobile apps have revolutionized the way people interact with and use our automobiles (Vrushank & Khang et al., 2023). With the help of IoT, the automotive industry has created innovations such as Advanced Driver-Assistance Systems (ADAS), advanced navigation and telematics solutions, and predictive maintenance solutions, among various others. With the help of IoT-based sensors, better traffic management can be achieved. Using sensors and the data they generate, services such as Google Maps can tell about the traffic density of any location, and this data can also be used by various administrative authorities, such as the traffic police, to manage traffic effectively. These sensors can also detect if the driver is driving rashly and alert the police to act against the traffic rule violator and the nearby drivers to be cautious of the vehicle (Shukla et al., 2023) (Verma et al., 2023).

IoT can also help reduce vehicle accidents by implementing various sensor-based applications such as pedestrian detection, automatic lane assist, traffic sign recognition, and automatic emergency braking. Features of modern-day vehicles such as Adaptive Cruise Control not only make driving convenient but also make it safer by adjusting the vehicle's speed depending on the actions of other objects in the immediate area. Adaptive Light control is another feature that changes the vehicle's light depending on the external lighting conditions and prevents other road users from being temporarily blinded by the high-intensity light beams. Features such as parking assist make the life of drivers easier as the sensors and cameras placed all around the car make it easy to park. Some manufacturers even have introduced autonomous parking through which the vehicle can park itself autonomously park itself with little or no human intervention (Sakthivel & Shashi et al., 2022).

Improved navigation systems have voice-activated prompts and instructions that make it easier for drivers to follow a route and keep their eyes on the road. Even heads-up displays are available in advanced systems to lessen driver attention. Vehicles nowadays also come with advanced sensors that enable night vision, which enables the drivers to have a better view of the otherwise difficult-to-see environment at night. They use infrared imaging and rely on thermal energy emitted by cars, animals, and other objects. Automatic emergency braking senses if the vehicle is going to collide with another object. This can alert the driver, reduce speed, tighten seat belts, and, in some cases, even apply brakes to help avoid collisions. IoT can also assist with the identification of driver tiredness. Sensors can detect this by examining the driver's head movement and pulse rate to see whether they indicate drowsiness (Verma et al., 2022; Junaid et al., 2023).

Smart apps and mobile networks have now enabled users to unlock and lock their vehicles using their smartphones. IoT also enables predictive maintenance. Various sensors installed in the vehicle can tell when a part needs to be serviced and when a part needs to be replaced. This not only reduces maintenance costs but also prevents major mishaps. These sensors also measure performance variables such as temperature, speed, and electrical systems. The data generated can also be used by the servicing agency to allow better diagnosis and faster repairs (Suresh & Bala et al., 2023).

### 19.6.6 IoT in Healthcare

IoT has numerous applications, including healthcare. IoT enables remote monitoring and allows faster and more accurate diagnosis than ever before. Before the introduction of IoT in healthcare, doctors were limited to visits and telecommunications to interact with patients. Moreover, to accurately diagnose, patients had to stay in hospitals for multiple days, which not only increased medical expenses but also strained the already underdeveloped healthcare sector (Khang, 2023).

The Internet of Things has introduced various revolutionary features, such as remote monitoring, which gives doctors better insight into various medical parameters such as heart rate, blood pressure, blood glucose, and spO2. Not only are these results more accurate, but they are so easy to conduct that they can be performed at home without the help of specially trained medical staff. Not only this, but the availability of smart devices such as fitness bands has made people conscious of their lifestyle and forced them to improve their lifestyle and lead healthier lives (Khang & Abdullayev et al., 2024).

IoT also enables remote medical assistance, which is not only revolutionary for the rural population that does not have access to good healthcare but also for the urban population, which at times may find it difficult to pay a visit to a doctor or, in case of an emergency where a doctor's advice is required urgently but the doctor is kilometers away. By altering how equipment and people interact while delivering healthcare solutions, IoT is, without a doubt, revolutionizing the healthcare sector. IoT healthcare applications benefit patients, families, physicians, hospitals, and insurance providers (Kumar et al., 2022).

IoT devices such as wirelessly connected heart rate monitoring cuffs, glucometers, and wearables like fitness bands can be tuned to alert patients, concerned health providers, and their relatives of any disturbance in their health conditions so that quick action can be taken. The application of IoT in healthcare comes with many benefits, such as reducing medical expenses, enabling real-time patient monitoring, and minimizing the need to visit doctors and hospital stays (Vrushank & Vidhi et al., 2023).

IoT also allows better treatment as intricate surgeries can be aided by smart devices, also, the data collected from various health sensors can be used to make evidence-based diagnoses. It also makes diagnosis easier and faster, which can save people from fatal medical conditions by detecting them in an early stage or even before they develop based on the symptoms. IoT can also be utilized to improve equipment and drug management by implementing better inventory and supply change management, maintaining the essential conditions for the storage of various drugs that have to be stored under specific environmental conditions (Verma et al., 2021; Verma al., 2022).

However, healthcare IoT has its challenges, the major being data security, as these sensors produce substantial amounts of data, which include sensitive information and give rise to concerns about data security. Better device integration is also required because there is no agreement among device manufacturers on communication protocols. Having various protocols complicates the communication process and even creates compatibility issues among the various devices. It is important to take the proper security precautions (Khang & Ragimova et al., 2022).

Through real-time health monitoring and access to patient health data, IoT explores new patient care facets. (Benharref and Serhani, 2014). This information can be used by those involved in the healthcare industry to improve patient satisfaction and health, open up new commercial prospects, and raise operational effectiveness. Knowing how to employ this digital power successfully would set you apart in a world that is becoming more connected.

## 19.7 CONCLUSION

In conclusion, the Internet of Things (IoT) is a game-changing technology altering how organizations conduct business and manufacture things. IoT devices can gather and analyze data in real-time, allowing organizations to streamline operations, automate procedures, and develop new business models. IoT can further improve corporate outcomes by enabling more complex data analysis and decision-making when paired with AI and cloud computing (Muthmainnah et al., 2023).

IoT has several applications in many different industries and is not just used by corporations. Precision farming may increase productivity and decrease waste in agriculture with the help of IoT. By providing remote monitoring and in-the-moment data analysis in healthcare, IoT can enhance the treatment of patients. IoT can enhance quality control and enable predictive maintenance in the manufacturing industry. IoT can provide real-time tracking of commodities in supply chain management, increasing productivity and lowering costs. IoT can monitor environmental factors and bird health in poultry production, allowing farmers to optimize feed and water use and cut waste. However, businesses must overcome several challenges when implementing IoT technologies, including security risks, data privacy concerns, and the need for new skills and expertise. Nevertheless, IoT has the potential to enable businesses to enhance efficiency, reduce costs, and create new revenue streams, driving growth and success in today's dynamic business environment (Anh & Vladimir et al., 2024).

## REFERENCES


Ahirwar S., R. Swarnkar, S. Bhukya, and G. Namwade, "Application of Drone in Agriculture." Int. J. Curr. Microbiol. Appl. Sci., vol. 8, no. 1, pp. 2500–2505, 2019, doi: 10.20546/ijcmas.2019.801.264.

Anh P. T. N., Vladimir Hahanov, Triwiyanto, Ragimova Nazila Ali, Rashad İsmibeyli, Vugar Abdullayev, Abuzarova Vusala Alyar. "AI Models for Disease Diagnosis and Prediction of Heart Disease with Artificial Neural Networks," *Computer Vision and AI-integrated IoT Technologies in Medical Ecosystem*. (1 Ed.) (2024). CRC Press. https://doi.org/10.1201/9781003429609-9

Armbrust M., "A View of Cloud Computing." Communications of the ACM, vol. 53, no. 4, pp. 50–58, 2010, doi: 10.1145/1721654.1721672.

Benharref A. and M. A. Serhani, "Novel Cloud and SOA-Based Framework for E-Health Monitoring Using Wireless Biosensors." IEEE Journal of Biomedical and Health Informatics, vol. 18, no. 1, pp. 46–55, 2014, doi: 10.1109/jbhi.2013.2262659.

Botta A., W. De Donato, V. Persico, and A. Pescapé, "Integration of Cloud Computing and Internet of Things: A Survey." Future Generation Computer Systems, vol. 56, pp. 684–700, 2016, doi: 10.1016/j.future.2015.09.021.

Boyes H., B. Hallaq, J. Cunningham, and T. Watson, "The Industrial Internet of Things (IIoT): An Analysis Framework." Computers in Industry, vol. 101, pp. 1–12, 2018, doi: 10.1016/j.compind.2018.04.015.

Carter N. P., S. W. Keckler, and W. J. Dally, "Hardware Support for Fast Capability-Based Addressing." ACM SIGOPS Operating Systems Review, vol. 28, no. 5, pp. 319–327, 1994, doi: 10.1145/381792.195579.

Chamola V., V. Hassija, V. Gupta, and M. Guizani, "A Comprehensive Review of the COVID-19 Pandemic and the Role of IoT, Drones, AI, Blockchain, and 5G in Managing Its Impact." IEEE Access, vol. 8, pp. 90225–90265, 2020, doi: 10.1109/access.2020.2992341.

Dang L. M., M. J. Piran, D. Han, K. Min, and H. Moon, "A Survey on Internet of Things and Cloud Computing for Healthcare." Electronics, vol. 8, no. 7, p. 768, 2019, doi: 10.3390/electronics8070768.

Das S., A. Dey, A. Pal, and N. Roy, "Applications of Artificial Intelligence in Machine Learning: Review and Prospect." International Journal of Computer Applications, vol. 115, no. 9, pp. 31–41, 2015, doi: 10.5120/20182-2402.

Elaine S. and A. Perrig, "Designing Secure Sensor Networks." IEEE Wireless Communications, vol. 11, no. 6, pp. 38–43, 2004, doi: 10.1109/mwc.2004.1368895.

Giri A., S. Dutta, S. Neogy, K. Dahal, and Z. Pervez, "Internet of Things (IoT)." Proceedings of the 1st International Conference on Internet of Things and Machine Learning, 2017, doi: 10.1145/3109761.3109768.

Gupta S. and M. Khattar, "Internet of Things and Artificial Intelligence." Towards Smart World, pp. 99–118, 2020, doi: 10.1201/9781003056751-7.

Hashem I. A. T., I. Yaqoob, N. B. Anuar, S. Mokhtar, A. Gani, and S. Ullah Khan, "The Rise of 'Big Data' on Cloud Computing: Review and Open Research Issues." Information Systems, vol. 47, pp. 98–115, 2015, doi: 10.1016/j.is.2014.07.006.

Hassoun A., "The Fourth Industrial Revolution in the Food Industry—Part II: Emerging Food Trends." Critical Reviews in Food Science and Nutrition, pp. 1–31, 2022, doi: 10.1080/10408398.2022.2106472.

Hooper E., "An Intelligent Intrusion Detection and Response System Using Network Quarantine Channels: Firewalls and Packet Filters." 2007 International Conference on Multimedia and Ubiquitous Engineering (MUE), 2007, doi: 10.1109/mue.2007.81.

Hwang H., G. Jung, K. Sohn, and S. Park, "A Study on MITM (Man in the Middle) Vulnerability in Wireless Network Using 802.1X and EAP." 2008 International Conference on Information Science and Security (ICISS 2008), 2008, doi: 10.1109/iciss.2008.10.

Jaidka H., N. Sharma, and R. Singh, "Evolution of IoT to IIoT: Applications & Challenges." SSRN Electronic Journal, 2020, doi: 10.2139/ssrn.3603739.

Junaid A., A. Nawaz, M. F. Usmani, R. Verma, and N. Dhanda, "Analyzing the Performance of a DAPP Using Blockchain 3.0." 2023 13th International Conference on Cloud Computing, Data Science & Engineering (Confluence), 2023, doi: 10.1109/confluence56041.2023.10048887.

Khang A., Advanced Technologies and AI-Equipped IoT Applications in High-Tech Agriculture (1st Ed.) (2023). IGI Global Press. https://doi.org/10.4018/978-1-6684-9231-4

Khang A., Abdullayev V. A., Hahanov V., Vrushank S., Advanced IoT Technologies and Applications in the Industry 4.0 Digital Economy (1 Ed.) (2024). CRC Press. https://doi.org/10.1201/9781003434269

Khang A., Abdullayev V. A., Hrybiuk, O., Shukla, A. K. Computer Vision and AI-integrated IoT Technologies in Medical Ecosystem. (1 Ed.) (2024). CRC Press. https://doi.org/10.1201/9781003429609

Khang A., Hajimahmud V. A., Gupta S. K., Babasaheb J., Morris G., AI-Centric Modelling and Analytics: Concepts, Designs, Technologies, and Applications. (1 Ed.) (2023). CRC Press. https://doi.org/10.1201/9781003400110

Khang A., Misra A., Gupta S. K., Shah V., AI-aided IoT Technologies and Applications in the Smart Business and Production. (Eds.) (2023). CRC Press. https://doi.org/10.1201/9781003392224

Khang A., Ragimova N. A., Hajimahmud V. A., Alyar V. A., "Advanced Technologies and Data Management in the Smart Healthcare System," *AI-Centric Smart City Ecosystems: Technologies, Design and Implementation* (1st Ed.), 16 (10), (2022). CRC Press. https://doi.org/10.1201/9781003252542-16

Khang A., Rani S., Sivaraman A. K., AI-Centric Smart City Ecosystems: Technologies, Design and Implementation (1st Ed.) (2022). CRC Press. https://doi.org/10.1201/9781003252542

Kumar Y. and R. Singla, "Effectiveness of Machine and Deep Learning in IOT-Enabled Devices for Healthcare System." Internet of Things, pp. 1–19, 2022, doi: 10.1007/978-3-030-81473-1_1.

Lasi H., P. Fettke, H.-G. Kemper, T. Feld, and M. Hoffmann, "Industry 4.0." Business & Information Systems Engineering, vol. 6, no. 4, pp. 239–242, 2014, doi: 10.1007/s12599-014-0334-4.

Li S., L. D. Xu, and S. Zhao, "The Internet of Things: A Survey." Information Systems Frontiers, vol. 17, no. 2, pp. 243–259, 2014, doi: 10.1007/s10796-014-9492-7.

Ma Z., M. Xiao, Y. Xiao, Z. Pang, H. V. Poor, and B. Vucetic, "High-Reliability and Low-Latency Wireless Communication for Internet of Things: Challenges, Fundamentals, and Enabling Technologies." IEEE Internet of Things Journal, vol. 6, no. 5, pp. 7946–7970, 2019, doi: 10.1109/jiot.2019.2907245.

Madhav A. V. S. and A. K. Tyagi, "The World with Future Technologies (Post-COVID-19): Open Issues, Challenges, and the Road Ahead." Intelligent Interactive Multimedia Systems for e-Healthcare Applications, pp. 411–452, 2021, doi: 10.1007/978-981-16-6542-4_22.

Mahmoud R., T. Yousuf, F. Aloul, and I. Zualkernan, "Internet of Things (IoT) Security: Current Status, Challenges and Prospective Measures." 2015 10th International Conference for Internet Technology and Secured Transactions (ICITST), 2015, doi: 10.1109/icitst.2015.7412116.

Maple C., "Security and Privacy in the Internet of Things." Journal of Cyber Policy, vol. 2, no. 2, pp. 155–184, 2017, doi: 10.1080/23738871.2017.1366536.

Merenda M., C. Porcaro, and D. Iero, "Edge Machine Learning for AI-Enabled IoT Devices: A Review." Sensors, vol. 20, no. 9, p. 2533, 2020, doi: 10.3390/s20092533.

Mirkovic J. and P. Reiher, "A taxonomy of DDoS attack and DDoS defense mechanisms." ACM SIGCOMM Computer Communication Review, vol. 34, no. 2, pp. 39–53, 2004, doi: 10.1145/997150.997156.

Mobley R. K., "Predictive Maintenance Techniques." An Introduction to Predictive Maintenance, pp. 99–113, 2002, doi: 10.1016/b978-075067531-4/50006-3.

Munirathinam S., "Industry 4.0: Industrial Internet of Things (IIOT)." Advances in Computers, pp. 129–164, 2020, doi: 10.1016/bs.adcom.2019.10.010.

Muthmainnah, Khang A., Prodhan Mahbub Ibna Seraj, Ahmad Al Yakin, *Ibrahim Oteir, Abdullah Nijr Alotaibi.* "An Innovative Teaching Model—The Potential of Metaverse for English Learning" *AI-Based Technologies and Applications in the Era of the Metaverse.* (1 Ed.) (2023). Page (105–126). IGI Global Press. https://doi.org/10.4018/978-1-6684-8851-5.ch005

Perwej Y., M. Ahmed, B. Kerim, and H. Ali, "An Extended Review on Internet of Things (IoT) and its Promising Applications." Communications on Applied Electronics, vol. 7, no. 26, pp. 8–22, 2019, doi: 10.5120/cae2019652812.

Rana G., Khang A., Sharma R., Goel A. K., Dubey A. K, "Reinventing Manufacturing and Business Processes through Artificial Intelligence", (Eds.) (2021). CRC Press. https://doi.org/10.1201/9781003145011

Rani S., Chauhan M., Kataria A, Khang A., "IoT Equipped Intelligent Distributed Framework for Smart Healthcare Systems," *Networking and Internet Architecture*, (Eds.). Vol.2, p: 30. (2021). https://doi.org/10.48550/arXiv.2110.04997

Sabahi F., "Cloud computing security threats and responses." 2011 IEEE 3rd International Conference on Communication Software and Networks, 2011, doi: 10.1109/iccsn.2011.6014715.

Sakthivel M., Shashi Kant Gupta, Dimitrios A. Karras, Khang A., Chandra Kumar Dixit, Bhadrappa Haralayya. Solving Vehicle Routing Problem for Intelligent Systems using Delaunay Triangulation. *2022 International Conference on Knowledge Engineering and Communication Systems (ICKES).* (2022). https://ieeexplore.ieee.org/abstract/document/10060807/

Shackelford S. J., "Welcome to the Internet of Things." The Internet of Things, 2020, doi: 10.1093/wentk/9780190943813.003.0002.

Shrouf F., J. Ordieres, and G. Miragliotta, "Smart factories in Industry 4.0: A review of the concept and of energy management approached in production based on the Internet of Things paradigm." 2014 IEEE International Conference on Industrial Engineering and Engineering Management, 2014, doi: 10.1109/ieem.2014.7058728.

Shukla, Utkarsh and Dhanda, Namrata and Verma, Rajat, Augmented Reality Product Showcase E-commerce Application (February 16, 2023). Available at SSRN: https://ssrn.com/abstract=4361319 or http://dx.doi.org/10.2139/ssrn.4361319.

Suresh Babu C.V., Bala S. Ganesh, T.K. Kishoor, Khang A., "Automatic Irrigation System Using Solar Tracking Device," Handbook of Research on AI-Equipped IoT Applications in High-Tech Agriculture. Copyright: © 2023 |Page: 239–256. https://doi.org/10.4018/978-1-6684-9231-4.ch013

Verdouw C., A. Beulens, and J. Van der Vorst, "Virtualisation of floricultural supply chains: A review from an Internet of Things perspective." Computers and Electronics in Agriculture, vol. 99, pp. 160–175, 2013, doi: 10.1016/j.compag.2013.09.006.

Verma R. and N. Dhanda, "Application of Supply Chain Management in Blockchain and IoT—A Generic Use Case." 2023 13th International Conference on Cloud Computing, Data Science & Engineering (Confluence), 2023, doi: 10.1109/confluence56041.2023.10048815.

Verma R., N. Dhanda, and V. Nagar, (2021) "Security Concerns in IoT Systems and Its Blockchain Solutions." Cyber Intelligence and Information Retrieval, pp. 485–495, 2021, doi: 10.1007/978-981-16-4284-5_42.

Verma, R., N. Dhanda, and V. Nagar, (2022). "Enhancing & Optimizing Security of IoT Systems using Different Components of Industry 4.0." International Journal of Engineering Trends and Technology, vol. 70(7), pp. 147–157. doi:10.14445/22315381/ijett-v70i7p216.

Vinitha K., R. Ambrose Prabhu, R. Bhaskar, and R. Hariharan, "Review on industrial mathematics and materials at Industry 1.0 to Industry 4.0." Materials Today: Proceedings, vol. 33, pp. 3956–3960, 2020, doi: 10.1016/j.matpr.2020.06.331.

Vrushank S., Khang A., "Internet of Medical Things (IoMT) Driving the Digital Transformation of the Healthcare Sector," *Data-Centric AI Solutions and Emerging Technologies in the Healthcare Ecosystem*. P (1). (1st Ed.) (2023). CRC Press. https://doi.org/10.1201/9781003356189-2

Vrushank S., Vidhi T., Khang A., "Electronic Health Records Security and Privacy Enhancement using Blockchain Technology," *Data-Centric AI Solutions and Emerging Technologies in the Healthcare Ecosystem*. P (1). (1st Ed.) (2023). CRC Press. https://doi.org/10.1201/9781003356189-1

Yarali A., "Intelligent Connectivity." 2021, doi: 10.1002/9781119685265.

# 20 Internet of Things (IoT) Case Studies and Application

*Reena Sharma and Sonam Gour*

## 20.1 INTRODUCTION

Home automation has many applications in areas such as light control, energy management, security systems, door control, and connected entertainment systems. A home can be called smart if there is installation of a number of smart devices that can be controlled remotely by setting them in such a way that you want to automate home maintenance. A smart house is a modern technological experience that will help owners save money, time, and energy spent on everyday life. They can also be connected to a single network. The foundation of an advanced integrated smart home system is made up of IoT, cloud computing, and rule-based event processing. Each element provides its fundamental qualities and technological capabilities to the suggested composition.

Internet connectivity and remote management of mobile devices equipped with different sensors are two ways that IoT contributes. Home equipment like air conditioners, lights, and other environmental gadgets can be connected to sensors. In order to provide the means to measure house conditions and monitor home appliance operation, it incorporates computer intelligence into home equipment. Scalable computing power, storage, and applications are provided via cloud computing for the creation, upkeep, and use of home services and remote access to home appliances.

The complete advanced smart home composition is managed and controlled by a rule-based event processing system (Liam Peters, 2016; Choudhary, 2021). There is an integrated approach to home automation that allows users to control several devices from a single app or dashboard. The following are some examples of applications that can be incorporated into home automation systems:

- Users can grant or reject visitor entry with smart locks and garage door openers. When a resident is nearby, smart locks can also recognize it and unlock the door.
- Residents can keep an eye on their homes when they are away or on vacation, thanks to smart surveillance cameras. Smart motion sensors can distinguish between neighbors, guests, pets, and intruders. When suspect behavior is discovered, these gadgets can notify the authorities.
- There are a variety of kitchen products equipped with IoT technology, such as smart coffee makers that can brew a new cup at a predetermined time.

DOI: 10.1201/9781032686745-20

A smart refrigerator that keeps track of expiration dates, makes shopping lists, and generates recipes using the ingredients it already has on hand.
- Electrical surges that cause appliances to shut down can be detected by home system monitoring, as can water outages.

A smart home is more than just a collection of smart appliances or smart devices that can be controlled remotely but managed by a central home automation system, frequently referred to as a smart home hub. A smart home hub is a piece of hardware that acts as the brain of a smart home system by wirelessly collecting, processing, and communicating data, creating a single smart home app that combines all the other apps and enables remote control for homeowners. Using a Raspberry Pi or another prototyping board, several smart home systems can be created from scratch.

### 20.1.1 History of Home Automation

The X10 communication protocol was created in Scotland in 1970 for home automation businesses. The X10 transmits digital information in bursts of 120 kHz radio frequency (RF) along the house's existing electrical cabling to smart switches. These signals provide instructions to the associated equipment and regulate when and how they work (Norman et al., 2021). For instance, a transmitter may send a signal along a home's electrical wires instructing appliances when to switch on and off. Due to the noise produced when powering equipment linked to the power grid power line, such a system was vulnerable to failure. The X10 system was initially designed as a one-way communication system, allowing smart devices to receive commands but not communicate information back to the central network.

- Nest Labs introduced the Nest Learning Thermostat, its first smart device, in 2010. Since then, the firm has also created smart security cameras and smoke/carbon monoxide detectors. It was bought by Google in 2015 and joined Alphabet Inc. that same year.
- Launching a Kickstarter campaign in 2012, Smart Things Inc. was able to raise $1.2 million to pay for smart home technology. The company went public in August 2013 after receiving further money, and Samsung bought it in 2014.
- At the moment, businesses like Amazon, Apple, and Google are launching their own smart home products like the Amazon Echo, Apple Home Kit, and Google House, as well as house automation (home plus robotics) platforms.

### 20.1.2 Main Components Needed for Home Automation

There are many crucial components that are needed for home automation:

- **Sensor Nodes**: Collect data from various smart home sensors: home entertainment, heating, ventilation, air conditioning, lighting control, presence and population, robotics, security, appliances such as refrigerators, washing machines, and even iKettles.

- **Raspberry Pi and Arduino**: Both are platforms for programming and control for different devices.
- **Data Hub**: It collects data from various sensor nodes within a defined monitored area (Smart Home in this case).
- **Database**: Warehouse for the sensor data.
- **Data Cloud Service**: To collect data from multiple areas in the cloud. HTTP and REST APIs can be used for communication.
- **Data Management Software**: Data point configuration, data rate recording, events and actions, and many more tasks.
- **Data Logging Software**: To collect and process sensor data within the sensor node.
- **Data Monitoring Software**: For monitoring and to trigger alarms, it also handles event-based inputs from multiple sensor nodes.

### 20.1.3 Use Cases of IoT in Home Automation

There are many use cases related to home automation, ranging from security to automation of home appliances, as shown in Figure 20.1.

- Can turn the LED light on/off and monitor the LED status.
- Doors can be monitored and locked/unlocked by servo motors.
- Infrared sensor can monitor whether the door is closed or open.
- You will be notified by email if the door is left open for too long.
- The camera captures an image of the face, emails it to the owner, and notifies the owner who has passed through the door.
- The owner can receive notifications through email if the detector senses smoke. You can surveil your car and monitor your home from anywhere.

The integration of IoT and home automation has made it possible to monitor and control homes in different parts of the world. Some application examples are controlling

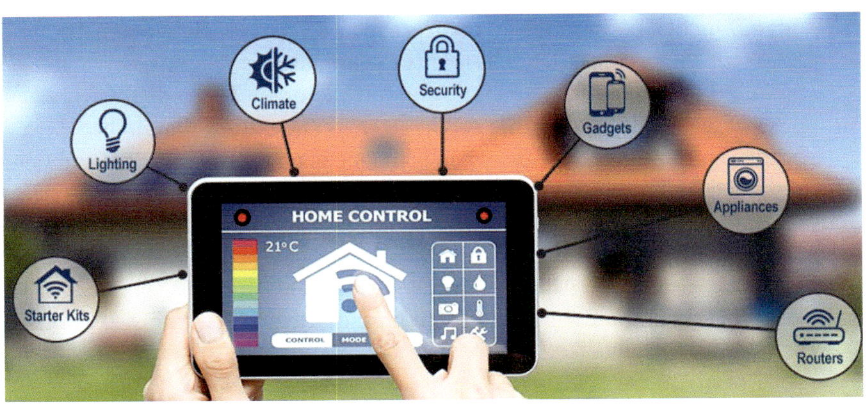


**FIGURE 20.1** Home automation different cases.

and setting the desired temperature in your home before you arrive, turning on/off and adjusting the intensity of lights in the room, starting the washing machine when people are at work, detecting leaks and smoke and alerting, home surveillance with surveillance cameras or cars in the house when people are away, or remote central locking and many other applications.

- **Door Locks:** Since robbery and burglary are unfortunate crimes that can happen to anyone, locking door locks is one of the most often used smart home technologies. The ability of smart door locks to lock your house from anywhere with a smartphone app is one of their main selling advantages. Tired of walking in the rain looking for your keys? Before you even step out of the car, smart locks let you unlock your house. Better access control is provided by internet-connected smart locks, which also enable users to open their houses from the workplace for friends and family or to remember to close them when they leave.
- **Smart Heating:** A smart heating system is a terrific method to avoid wasting money on your home's utility expenses. By tracking usage and notifying users when they may use less heat, many smart heating systems can produce savings in particular areas. After a long day at work, you may quickly and easily return to your toasty flat using the smartphone app. Other more sophisticated smart heating systems, like NEST, can also function as smoke detectors and security cameras, adding still another layer of home security to the mix.
- **Smart Gardening:** In this day of ever-increasing connection, many IoT gadgets are indoors, but the garden is unforgettable. With robotic lawnmowers, automatic remote irrigation systems, and other garden-focused IoT applications already available and more to come, smart gardening is a smart home. It is now a thriving industry. Smart garden systems can automatically decide whether to raise or decrease water delivery with the help of IoT sensors, or they can gather information on upcoming weather patterns to choose the best course of action. Additionally, the user can modify these systems remotely to meet their needs.
- **Video Doorbells:** The video doorbell is one more common Internet of Things gadget for smart homes. Thanks to this feature, users can now receive video calls via the doorbell when someone is at the door. Through smartphone apps, these gadgets also enable people to enter and unlock their houses. The ability to inform homeowners when someone is near their property without pressing a button on the doorbell itself is one of the other security advantages of video doorbells. Some systems allow you to program them to ring at convenient hours or to never ring at all.
- **Personal Assistants:** Although personal assistants for smartphones have been around for some time, they are increasingly more prevalent in homes, and Amazon's Echo features the most recent version of the well-known Alexa personal assistant; the quantity of data that personal assistants can gather is eerily growing as our environment becomes more automated and networked. Using tools like AI and machine learning (Khang & Misra et al.,

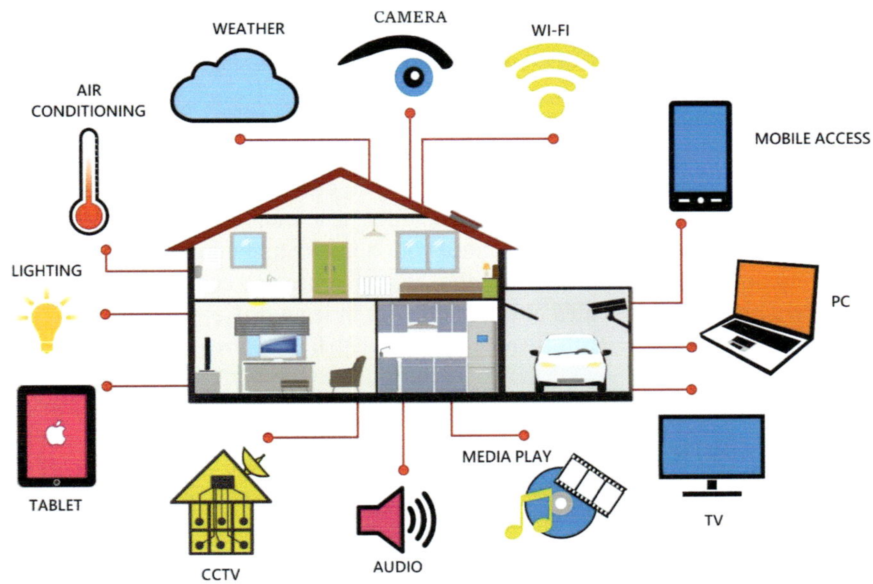


**FIGURE 20.2** Home application using IoT.

2023), it may soon be feasible to exploit this data in ways that go much beyond what is now offered on the market, as shown in Figure 20.2.

### 20.1.4 Benefits of Home Automation

You may add additional features to regular homes by using smart homes. They facilitate life. For instance:

- Smart refrigerators supply your fridge and manage your spreadsheets.
- Smart vacuum cleaners clean the entire house while you are away.
- Smart homes offer peace of mind, security, consistency, and adaptability.

### 20.1.5 Challenges in Smart Home Systems

However, there is no denying that smart homes significantly simplify people's lives. It has the following difficulties:

- When each IoT device is sold by a separate vendor, it is challenging to integrate the system.
- IoT devices frequently are not interoperable with one another. With the exception of connecting to gadgets like Google Assistant (Vishal et al., 2018), all of the devices need to be Wi-Fi-connected.
- Since the cost of installing a smart house is high, users might not want to make such a significant investment when standard homes do not require IoT.

- A significant security risk still exists in smart homes. Strong farewells are required for smart homes in order to avoid system hacking.

Smart homes are not always pricey homes with high-security standards. To protect the city from crimes like theft, personal and public networks must have some level of security. By ensuring the equipment's safety, we guarantee the city's vital expansion. The Internet of Things makes it feasible for us to monitor our own belongings remotely. For instance, thermostats control your home's temperature and your spending, saving time and money. Similar to this, we can reuse and conserve energy much more if we implement this idea at the metropolitan level. IoT-enabled smart homes make for a far more straightforward and practical living environment (Khang & Smart Healthcare, 2023).

## 20.2 IoT APPLICATIONS IN SMART CITIES

The concept of smart cities has caught the attention of policymakers, governments, and industry like never before. The world of sensors, gateways, and cloud applications is reshaping the entire management and control environment available to an organization with assets in remote offices and dispersed regions. Many industries and countries have already benefited tremendously from IoT applications (Khang & Ragimova et al., 2022).

Large cities have thousands of public buildings, each with its own energy patterns, air quality issues, and sensor devices. It can be challenging for managers to identify those who are working effectively (Vishal et al., 2020). What is required is an IoT platform that is flexible and easy to use and generates alerts when something is wrong. It needs to provide user-friendly applications so that building managers can take real-time actions to optimize resource consumption and maintain the safety and comfort of building users. It must be able to connect to any device connected to the Internet, collect data, and manage the device (Khang & Rani et al., 2022). A smart city uses digital technologies to:

- More effectively and actively involve its citizens
- Improve the performance of the city and the wellbeing of citizens
- Reduce operating costs and consumption of urban resources
- Create new business opportunities and increase the attractiveness of the city

### 20.2.1 Applications of IoT in Smart Cities

IoT-compatible services, tools, and technologies are part of smart cities. These provide services that enhance access to water, electricity, roads, public transport, buildings, and digital services like broadband, as shown in Figure 20.3.

### 20.2.2 Smart Traffic Management

Smart traffic management interacts with smart cities to manage traffic in cities. It provides a variety of traffic control routes and promptly dispatches assistance in the

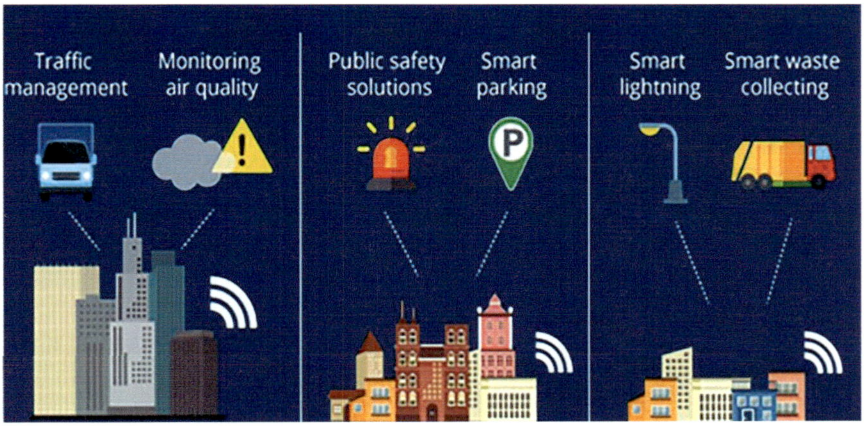
Traffic management
Monitoring air quality
Public safety solutions
Smart parking
Smart lightning
Smart waste collecting

**FIGURE 20.3** Applications of IoT in smart cities.

event of a collision. These technologies communicate continuously with the traffic police and give the control center real-time updates.

By fusing IoT technology with existing infrastructure, intelligent transportation systems can aid in resolving the transportation issue. Think about an IoT-based intelligent traffic signal monitoring system as an illustration (Vishal et al., 2019). It uses a priori data from IoT sensors to change traffic signals so that the time interval is dependent on the volume of traffic on a particular stretch of road. The key benefit of this technology is that it can lower traffic density and downtime in diverse locations.

- **Emergency Routing:** Giving preferential access to police, fire, and emergency services is a fundamental application of an IoT-based smart transportation system.
- **Adaptive Control:** When congestion is detected, systems, including traffic lights, entrance alarms, and express bus lanes, are dynamically adjusted.
- **Interaction with Connected Cars:** Smart Traffic Management can link them to roadside equipment and enable smart cars to talk to junctions directly.
- **Traffic Jam Detection:** From the city's traffic center, technicians can keep an eye on every street in the city thanks to cameras and sensors that continuously monitor intersections.

### 20.2.3 Smart Parking

An IoT-based system that transmits information about available and occupied parking spaces via web/mobile applications is necessary to develop smart parking. Each parking spot has an IoT gadget with sensors and microcontrollers. The user obtains the most recent information on the availability of every parking space and selects the best option. Parking systems are implemented both inside and outside of the structure (Zoughbi et al., 2022) (Asit Behera, 2021). Sensors determine the number of parking spaces available when a car enters a gap. The app delivers this information to the driver's phone. This issue can be resolved by utilizing cutting-edge smart parking technology and IoT connectivity. His Internet of Things (IoT) sensors tell him where the available parking spots are. This IoT data is transmitted wirelessly to the cloud server.

An IoT device with sensors and microcontrollers is installed in each parking space. The user chooses the best alternative after obtaining the most recent information on the availability of each parking place. Parking systems are in place on the outside and inside of the building. When a car drives into a gap, sensors count the number of parking spaces that are still open. The driver's phone receives this information from the app. IoT connectivity and cutting-edge smart parking technology can be used to solve this problem. He is informed of the whereabouts of open parking spaces by his Internet of Things (IoT) sensors. Wireless communication is used to send this IoT data to the cloud server.

### 20.2.4 Smart Waste Management System

A smart city solution called the IoT-based Smart Waste Management System for Smart Cities uses sensors installed in garbage cans and recycling bins to notify the city's collection service providers when it is time to empty the bins. Additionally, it makes public spaces more visually appealing and guarantees that trash cans are removed before they overflow. Even urban regions are willing to undertake smart waste management programs to increase efficiency and produce a cleaner city due to the rise of smart city waste management efforts.

### 20.2.5 Smart Lighting System

The Smart Lighting System (SLS) is a distributed or centralized automatic and intelligent lighting control system that uses a variety of Internet of Things (IoT) communication protocols, devices, and sensors. SLS is a key idea in regulating energy usage in households, workplaces, and public areas using efficient lighting systems. In a smart city environment, IoT-enabled SLS can be utilized as a solution to reduce electricity waste. Three fundamental layers make up the IoT-enabled SLS architecture:

- The layer of perception or sensor
- The layer of communication
- The layer of management

## 20.3 IoT APPLICATIONS IN THE ENVIRONMENT

The IoT application that provides the most value is environmental monitoring. It encourages better sustainability and uses cutting-edge sensor technology to detect the presence of pollutants in the air and water, as shown in Figure 20.4. A clever environmental monitoring solution can make your property safer and cleaner. Maintaining a positive atmosphere is important in enclosed workplaces, such as offices, rooms, or underground mines. Sensors collect air data, which gateways then transmit to the

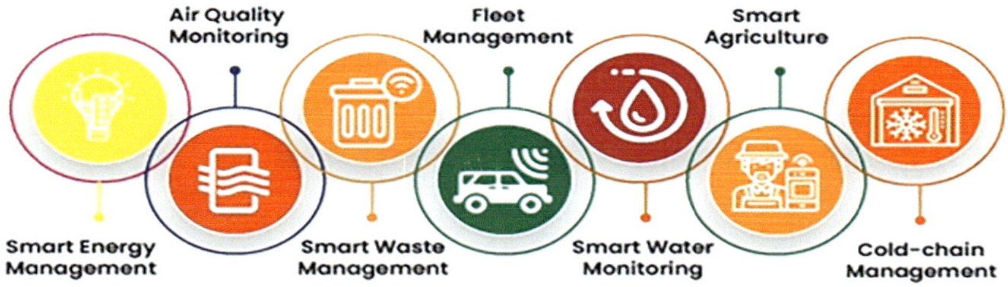


**FIGURE 20.4** Different domains in IoT.

cloud platform. Through a linked dashboard, businesses can simply gather information in an approachable style and analyze it to get improved outcomes.

Using conventional methods to monitor environmental conditions has a lot of drawbacks. Real-time control over people's surroundings has become simpler with the development of technology and intelligent management techniques. IoT has a significant impact on raising environmental standards. It includes clever and cutting-edge methods for water treatment and air quality testing that significantly advance sustainable living. IoT also employs a data-driven methodology that offers actionable insights and predicts outcomes. Your system's ability to measure, monitor, and catalog data will help you better understand your company's operations and provide you with ideas for improvement.

### 20.3.1 Water Quality Monitoring

The most vital resource for survival is water. Effective conservation practices call for ongoing quality control and appropriate management strategies. Smart water meters, sensors, and irrigation systems installed in houses and smart buildings can track water consumption trends in real-time thanks to IoT technology. Additionally, sophisticated sensor equipment is placed to measure the levels of pH, oxygen, and other elements like pollutants that can make the water dangerous to drink. The detection of such factors provides trustworthy use cases that help to advance better human health and raise living standards.

- Air Quality Monitoring
- Energy Monitoring
- Toxic Gas Detection

### 20.3.2 Air Quality Monitoring

To avoid serious health issues, the air quality in the surroundings must be clean and safe to breathe. The air should be pure and fresh, even when working in a small area. When implemented for particular places, IoT-based environmental monitoring systems can be utilized to detect airborne particles and collect information with the use of sensor technology. Data can be moved by organizations to a cloud platform for processing. The user panel is supplied with pertinent information. The entire procedure enables real-time air monitoring, rapid problem-solving, air freshening, and ventilation management for improved air circulation.

### 20.3.3 Energy Monitoring

IoT products are affordable and can be used to enhance the environment. The best solution for reducing energy expenses and increasing worker productivity is sensor-based. It is simpler to cut energy usage using an intelligent environmental monitoring system, which offers complete information on energy consumption trends and places where energy is being consumed unnecessarily. Sensors have supplanted conventional methods of turning lights on and off as technology develops. You may remotely manage energy use and conserve resources by using an IoT-based solution.

### 20.3.4 Toxic Gas Detection

The most practical method of having remote control over your surroundings is through the use of IoT for environmental monitoring. Hazardous gases that can seriously endanger infrastructure and human lives are frequently present in enclosed places. Early detection of these dangerous gases can, however, decrease detrimental effects at a significant cost and provide a clearer picture of future events. The automated real-time identification of these gases is made possible by sensors and gateways, enabling data logging for analysis and predicted results.

IoT now plays a significant role in creating an environment that is safer and cleaner. Better methods for detecting air quality can be provided by installing a smart environment system. It enables businesses to keep up with the most recent smart technology advances that deliver effective industrial advancements

## 20.4 IoT APPLICATION IN THE ENERGY SECTOR

Energy is the main industry that underpins the creation of energy, the movement of products, and numerous other essential daily activities. The energy market's IoT has entered the areas of energy generation and consumption, changing how the industry functions. IoT is a ground-breaking technology that enhances the performance of various industries, including the energy sector. Energy savings are the primary objective of IoT integration with the energy sector. The need for energy use has greatly expanded along with the population growth. IoT makes it feasible to save energy at a high cost and to distribute it equally across all regions, as shown in Figure 20.5.

The Internet of Things, where gadgets are connected through a centralized dashboard and industrial advancements are made everywhere as a result, is where automation is headed in the future. Sensor devices and communication gateways, which make up the full Internet of Things architecture, are included in smart energy systems. Its main goals are to boost industrial value and maintain asset efficiency for improved outcomes.

IoT has a wide range of effects on the energy industry. IoT mostly benefits the energy sector by offering clever strategies to cut back on wasteful energy use. Power

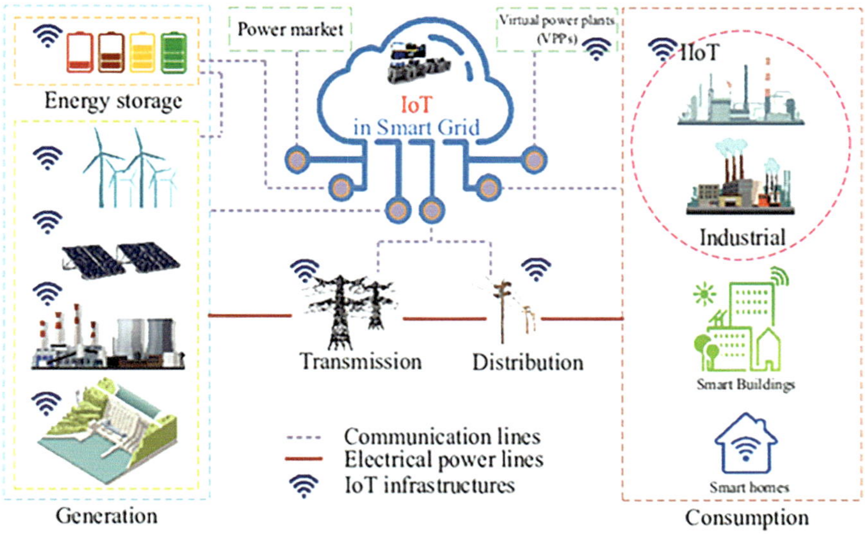


**FIGURE 20.5** Communication between devices in IoT system.

Saving Mode (PSM), extended intermittent reception (eDRX), and wake signals are a few of the low-power IoT approaches that have just entered the market. Many mobile service providers offer the option to turn off mobile data when it is not required to save the device's battery life.

A lot of e-waste will be produced due to significant energy sector developments and the widespread use of embedded devices. This would incorporate a sophisticated mechanism that preserves ecological harmony. These requirements frequently trigger the development of a green IoT. Learn more about green IoT.

## 20.4.1 Optimization of Energy Resources

With the help of the contextual data it gathers, IoT offers improved resource optimization, whether you are talking about a sizable manufacturing facility or a family dwelling. A smart thermostat, for instance, can assist homeowners in maximizing HVAC utilization to reduce energy costs while upholding a suitable indoor atmosphere.

Real estate used for businesses or industries may be subject to the same applications. When no one is present, a smart lighting system will switch itself off to conserve energy and lower electricity costs. Additionally, since they cut down on fuel expenses, energy usage, and even waste, IoT-enabled heavy gear and equipment can benefit from the same advantages.

## 20.4.2 Empowering Micro-Grids

To apply IoT in this industry, however, just lowering the energy footprint is insufficient. Perhaps the implementation of smarter electricity grids is necessary to support the power of the Internet of Things. Smart grids are a network of electrical circuits that facilitate bidirectional power flow and can self-heal when there are maintenance problems. As surplus energy is given back to its source, one feature of smart grids is that they also enable energy customers to participate actively. By reviving it for smart consumption, the end user's circuit is completed in this manner. Smart grids, however, are well ahead of current developments.

Let us use an example to better grasp this. If a residential neighborhood with ten homes is converted into a micro-grid, each home would be wired into the system. These homes can now produce their own electricity for their own purposes thanks to solar panels on their roofs. The quantity of energy a residence generates could, however, be higher than the amount it really consumes. As a result, the remaining energy is wasted. With micro-grids, this is not the case.

When operating in grid mode, homes can transfer energy to grids so that other entities can use it for their own purposes. The Internet of Things can be used to automatically disconnect a home's energy circuits if it decides not to distribute energy.

### 20.4.3 Predictive Protocols for Disasters

One of the largest applications of IoT in the energy sector is its ability to apply disaster prediction protocols and, in a sense, to sound important alarms. Smart sensors that can control energy use, distribution, and management can be installed in the energy sector by leveraging historical data to create predictive patterns and foresee man-made or natural disasters. Energy is a necessary resource for human existence and cannot be eliminated. However, as previous disasters have demonstrated, energy management patterns can be controlled if a warning is given in advance.

### 20.4.4 Smart Meter Technology

Smart meter installation technology can aid in analyzing regions where energy is consumed most heavily and where energy can be significantly saved with regard to the measurement and analysis of energy consumption in a specific home, building, or organization. However, IoT-enabled smart meters can be installed in residences and other structures, which will only benefit customers by allowing them to receive a thorough report on their energy use trends. Additionally, it will assist them in finding legal loopholes, and eventually, smart meter technology will increase the energy sector's operational efficiency and transparency. It provides two-way communication between energy providers and customers, creating a connection between the two parties automatically.

## 20.5 A CASE STUDY OF IoT IN RETAIL

For today's channel-agnostic, mobile-connected consumer, expectations about customer experience, service, speed, and efficiency play a far more significant role. There are numerous other ways that IoT can assist in improving the customer experience, even while logistics can play a significant part in satisfying these needs and

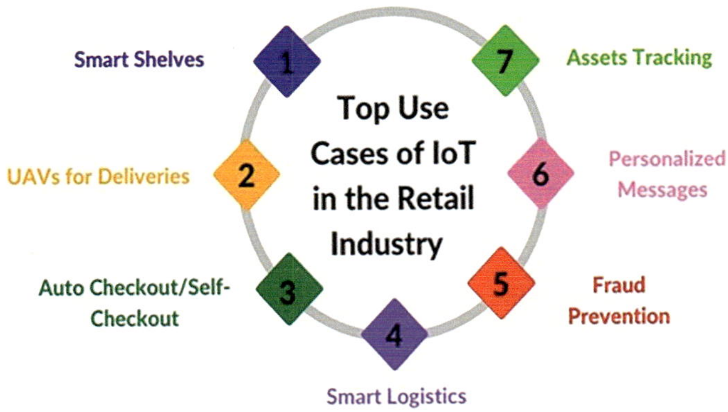


**FIGURE 20.6** Cycle of retail process in IoT.

offering a better customer experience and service (for instance, employing tracking and tracing with full visibility to impatient consumers, as shown in Figure 20.6.

### 20.5.1 Facility Management

Keeping the store environment neat, cozy, secure, and appealing is one of the main daily duties of retailers. Numerous IoT technologies exist that can be used to simplify these processes and lower the expenses involved. To better manage disinfection and cleaning schedules, for instance, presence detection and people computing data can be utilized to distinguish between regularly used locations, such as shop restrooms and locker rooms. In order to effectively manage inventory and restock supplies on schedule, facility managers can use wireless IoT sensors to proactively detect when supplies are running short at entrances and throughout the store.

The most crucial aspect of energy management, which affects customer comfort, operating costs, and sustainability, may now.

### 20.5.2 Supply Chain Management

Retailers can utilize IoT technologies like RFID tags and GPS sensors to get a complete picture of how goods are moved from production to in-store to customer purchase. Real-time analysis of the gathered data (transport duration, product storage temperature, etc.) is possible. When transporting perishables, when storage temperature is crucial, this information is extremely helpful. According to experts, almost 75% of merchants intend to employ IoT technologies to modernize their supply chain management.

### 20.5.3 Better Customer Service

By generating insights into customer data and creating opportunities to use that data, IoT also benefits brick-and-mortar merchants. IoT solutions for businesses, for instance, can combine data from social media, mobile devices, and cameras to help marketers better forecast consumer behavior.

### 20.5.4 Smarter Inventory Management

Inventory management can be a headache. Lack of accurate inventory tracking can lead to out-of-stock and overstocking, costing retailers worldwide billions annually. IoT can solve these problems by automating inventory visibility. By applying intelligent inventory management solutions based on sensors in store shelves, RFID tags, beacons, video monitoring, and digital price tags, retail businesses can improve purchase planning. When product inventory is low, the system will offer to reorder a reasonable amount based on analysis obtained from IoT data.

### 20.5.5 Automated Checkout

Managing inventory can be challenging. Inaccurate inventory tracking can result in out-of-stock and overstocking, which can cost businesses all over the world billions of dollars annually. These issues can be resolved using IoT by automating inventory visibility. Retail businesses can enhance purchase planning by implementing intelligent inventory management solutions based on sensors in shop shelves, RFID tags, beacons, video monitoring, and digital price tags. Based on the analysis of IoT data, the system will offer to place a suitable amount of reorders when product inventory is low.

### 20.5.6 Demand Alert Warehouses

Demand-Aware Warehouse fulfillment refers to warehouse automation that is driven by consumer demand for in-person and online retail. You can track sales and prospects in real time, thanks to IoT. Even tracking missed sales in the business is possible with it. It should be highlighted that RFID is a tried-and-true component of IoT that may be utilized for inventory management and more precise optimization of service levels. The warehouse of the future will be an open area where autonomous pallets will arrange themselves based on demand in real time, thanks to the power of technology.

### 20.5.7 Smart Shelves

Smart shelves are yet another ground-breaking example of IoT in retail. Retailers devote a lot of time and effort to tracking products to ensure they are always in stock and are not misplaced on various shelves. Both of these operations are automated by smart shelves, which also keep an eye out for theft. Smart shelves, which have RFID tags and weight sensors, may scan products on both warehouse and display shelves and alert personnel when supplies are running low or when things are misplaced on the shelf. This not only saves time but also gets rid of the manual mistakes that lead to shortages and overstocking.

## 20.6 IoT IN AGRICULTURE

Smart agriculture is the idea of improving the basic capabilities of traditional agriculture using modern technologies such as the Internet of Things and implementing them into industrial technology that provides real-time information in accordance with ad-hoc sensor networks deployed throughout the agricultural field and maneuvering it through application software systems. Farm equipment is systematically used to increase agricultural production and the quality of production.

Smart agriculture is a low-cost, low-labor implementation method leading to an overall reduction in agricultural costs. It helps to produce higher yield and better quality crops, which leads to higher price and demand, which leads to more profit for the farmers, as shown in Figure 20.7.

To maintain plant health, sensor networks spread across the field monitor growth and water requirements with real-time humidity and temperature data. Farmers can then ensure the correct amount of water with an automatic switch controlled by application software. The data is analyzed with a weekly farmer report that provides a proper record of plant growth with a graphical representation of the data in the app. The use case of IoT in agriculture is discussed in detail in what follows.

### 20.6.1 Monitoring of Climate Conditions

The weather station, which integrates several smart farming sensors, is arguably the most well-liked smart farming tool. While out in the field, they gather and upload various types of environmental data to the cloud. With the help of the measurements, it is possible to map the local climate, choose the best crops, and take the required actions to boost their productivity (such as through precision agriculture).

### 20.6.2 Greenhouse Automation

In order to control the greenhouse environment, farmers often require manual intervention. You may obtain precise real-time information on greenhouse conditions,

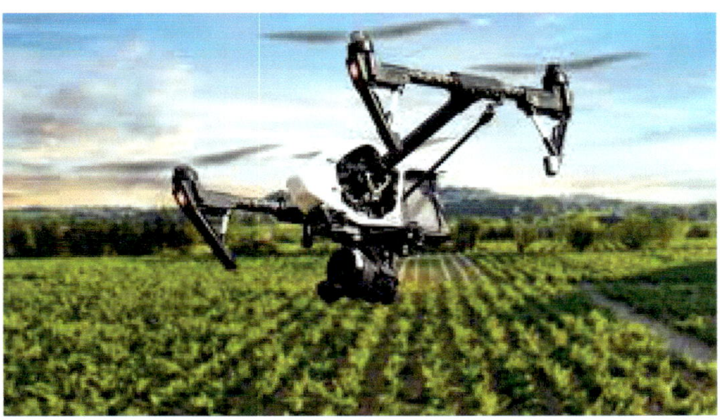

**FIGURE 20.7** Agriculture process using IoT and a drone.

including lighting, temperature, soil quality, and humidity, by using IoT sensors. Weather stations can autonomously modify circumstances to certain parameters in addition to collecting environmental data. Automation systems used in greenhouses, in particular, employ similar ideas.

### 20.6.3 Crop Management

Crop management tools are yet another IoT product category in agriculture and a component of precision farming. It must be deployed onsite, just like meteorological stations, in order to gather information unique to crops, measuring everything from temperature and precipitation to leaf water potential and general plant health. By doing so, you can keep an eye on plant development and abnormalities and successfully ward against illnesses and invaders that could reduce output.

### 20.6.4 Cattle Monitoring and Management

Agricultural IoT sensors can be attached to livestock to track performance and monitor the health of the animals in addition to crops. Data on livestock health, wellbeing, and physical condition are gathered by tracking and monitoring cattle. For instance, these sensors may spot unwell animals, allowing farmers to remove them from the herd and prevent contamination. Drones used for real-time livestock monitoring assist farmers in cutting labor expenditures. It functions as an IoT gadget for animal care.

### 20.6.5 Precision Farming

Precision farming, also known as data-driven efficiency and precise decision-making, is a growing industry. Additionally, it is among the most popular and successful IoT applications in agriculture. The microclimate of the field and all components of the ecosystem, including illumination, temperature, soil composition, humidity, CO2 levels, and pest outbreaks, may be measured using IoT sensors. Using this information, farmers may determine how much water, fertilizer, and pesticides are necessary for their crops, cutting expenses and resulting in the growth of better and healthier harvests.

### 20.6.6 Agricultural Drones

The use of agricultural drones in smart agriculture is arguably one of the most promising developments in agricultural technology. Drones, commonly referred to as UAVs (Unmanned Aerial Vehicles), are more capable of gathering agricultural data than satellites and aircraft. Drones are capable of a variety of formerly labor-intensive functions in addition to surveillance. Crop cultivation, pest and disease control, agricultural spraying, and crop monitoring are a few examples.

### 20.6.7 Predictive Analytics for Smart Farming

Forecast data analysis and precision agriculture go hand in hand. The Internet of Things (IoT) and smart sensor technologies offer a gold mine of pertinent real-time data, but with data analysis, farmers can comprehend it and make crucial predictions about harvest time, the likelihood of illness and epidemics, yield levels, and more (Asit Behera, 2021). Tools for data analysis assist agriculture. What is naturally heavy is more under your control, predictable, and is dependent on the weather.

### 20.6.8 Requirements of Smart Farming

If you are considering investing in smart farming, there are certain issues you need to be aware of. Some values of requirement are given in what follows.

#### 20.6.8.1 Hardware

You must pick (or create your own) sensors for your gadgets to construct an IoT solution for agriculture. The decision you make will rely on the kind of data you gather and the overall goal of your solution. In every case, the success of the product depends on the sensor's quality. It depends on how reliable and accurate the data that was gathered is.

#### 20.6.8.2 Data Analytics

Any smart farming system should be built around data analytics. If the information gathered cannot be interpreted, it is of no use. They must, therefore, possess good data analytics skills and utilize machine learning and predictive algorithms to extract useful information from the data they gather (Rani & Bhambri et al., 2023).

#### 20.6.8.3 Maintenance

The biggest problem for agricultural IoT products is hardware maintenance because sensors are frequently utilized in the field and are easily broken. As a result, you must ensure that your hardware is robust and simple to maintain. If not, you will have to replace the sensor more frequently than is necessary.

#### 20.6.8.4 Mobility

Intelligent agricultural applications need to be adapted for field use. Business owners or operations managers must be able to access information onsite or remotely using their smartphones or desktop computers. In addition, each connected device must be autonomous and have sufficient wireless range to communicate with other devices and send data to the central server.

#### 20.6.8.5 Infrastructure

Intelligent agricultural apps must be modified for use in the field. Using their cell phones or desktop computers, business owners or operations managers must be able to access information locally or remotely. Each linked device must also be independent and have a long enough wireless range to talk with other devices and relay information to the main server.

#### 20.6.8.6 Connectivity

The adoption of smart farming continues to be hampered by the requirement to transport data between several agricultural devices. Naturally, the connections between these components must be strong enough to survive bad weather and guarantee continuous operation. IoT devices now employ a number of different connectivity protocols, but efforts are being made to create a single standard in this area. Hopefully, new technologies like 5G and space internet will make it easier to solve this issue.

#### 20.6.8.7 Data Collection Frequency

Choosing the right frequency for data collection can be challenging because there are so many different types of data in agriculture. Restrictions and limitations may apply to data from fields, air and environmental sensors, applications, machines and equipment, and processed analytical data. One of the major problems of intelligent agriculture is providing and conveying this data in a timely and safe manner.

#### 20.6.8.8 Data Security

Working with huge datasets is necessary for IoT and precision agriculture technologies, which raises the risk of security weaknesses that can be used by hackers to steal data. Unfortunately, nothing is known about data security in agriculture. For instance, several farms relay data to their agricultural gear using drones (Aswani et al., 2022). Although it has an Internet connection, this gadget has minimal security features like password user authentication or remote access. Basic IoT security advice includes traffic monitoring, the use of cryptographic techniques to safeguard critical data, and the use of AI-based security technologies to find real-time indicators of suspicious activity.

Farmers must comprehend the notion of data security, establish internal security standards, and uphold them in order to benefit from the IoT fully.

## 20.7 INTERNET OF THINGS IN INDUSTRY

The fourth industrial revolution, or Industry 4.0, is a global reorganization of manufacturing, as shown in Figure 20.8. The manufacturing sector's efficiency is impacted

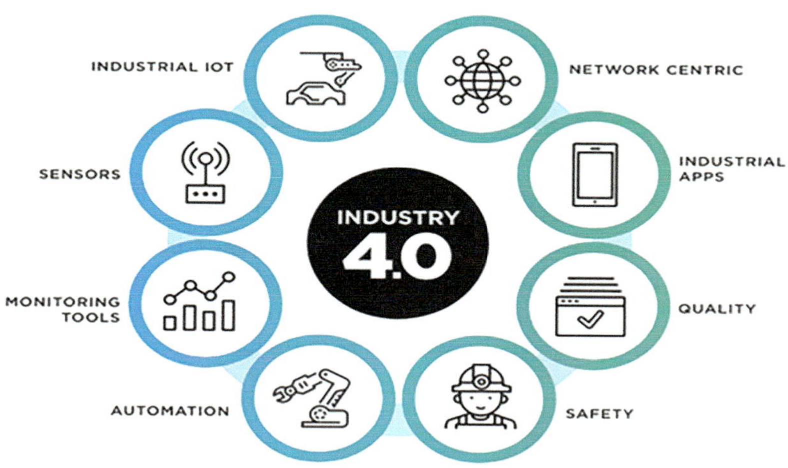


**FIGURE 20.8** IoT in Industry 4.0.

by new information technology, which also allows organizations to find more efficient working practices. Early adopters have shown that networked factories and industrial organizations benefit from higher capacity, quicker communication, and visibility into manufacturing operations (Banerjee et al., 2022).

IoT use cases come in a variety of forms. Because virtually anything can be made "smart" by adding IoT sensors, a world of possibility opens up. The number of systems, gadgets, and people that can be linked together to form a network is unfathomable.

### 20.7.1 Remote Monitoring

You may monitor device usage and health with IoT-connected assets and IoT sensors on the Industrial Internet to assess performance and deploy service in case of any concerns. Additionally, you can better understand your device's performance to enhance product design and guarantee client happiness if you have access to device data. Not to mention, it might create a brand-new business opportunity for device-as-a-service.

### 20.7.2 Supply Chain Management and Optimization

Imagine if the whole supply chain for manufacturing was interconnected. Consider how data could be accessed and utilized by every part of supply chain operations to guarantee the highest levels of productivity. The supply chain will enjoy a number of key benefits with the Internet of Things. Assets and products can be tracked in real-time. Warehouse chores can be automated. Paperwork can be managed digitally. Forecasting accuracy can be improved. Inventory can be controlled more tightly.

### 20.7.3 Digital Twins

A digital twin is a representation of a real-world idea, item, or location that is virtual or simulative in nature. They serve as an intriguing and effective illustration of how the industrial Internet of Things is being used. Even a 3D model of every physical asset, operating system, and building's architecture may be included. Without making any actual physical changes, this can assist manufacturers in testing modifications and simulating the impact.

### 20.7.4 Real-Time Machine Monitoring

Imagine a manufacturing technology that provides managers and operators with a real-time evaluation of the efficiency of the machines. All the information they require to address issues promptly and guarantee that production schedules are met would be available to them. It offers real-time machine monitoring, which delivers a stream of precise data straight from the machine, enabling quick decision-making or in-depth study.

### 20.7.5 Predictive Maintenance

Manufacturers can utilize a variety of maintenance techniques on their machinery. They can implement more sophisticated types of data-driven predictive maintenance as they develop. Advanced IoT tools, such as machine learning algorithms, can "learn" from IoT devices in digital factories and deliver helpful information. The maintenance crews can more clearly determine when equipment needs to be fixed thanks to the data's insights into the functionality and condition of the equipment (Chelsea et al., 2020). Manufacturers can switch from a calendar-based maintenance program to a condition-based strategy using IoT-connected equipment. They can carefully monitor the variables and set a threshold to foresee impending machine failure if they gather enough information on the functionality and state of the equipment (Khang & Hajimahmud et al., 2023).

### 20.7.6 Production Visibility

For the majority of producers, going out onto the work floor is the only way to find out what is going on there. Even then, it could take some time to watch the workers and the equipment in order to grasp where performance stands fully. They might have to talk to supervisors, examine part counts on a whiteboard, etc. Manufacturing executives, plant managers, and operators now have access to connected equipment through a machine monitoring solution, and visual dashboards measuring the performance against production targets provide them with insight into all of their machines. This makes a variety of use cases for improving equipment performance possible, such as process optimization, preventative maintenance, and quality.

### 20.7.7 Automation

One of the main promises of Industry 4.0 is industrial automation using the Industrial Internet. Manufacturers can decrease downtime, ensure predictable maintenance, and enhance decision-making as they progressively enable automation in their plants (Chivarov et al., 2021). Although we frequently picture automation as a warehouse full of robots, it actually has more uses. Think about how manually gathering components and downtime numbers differs from automatically gathering data from equipment. IoT-connected shop floors offer more options for automation than ever before.

## 20.8 IoT IN HEALTH AND LIFESTYLE

The rise of the Internet of Things into almost every business area, from medical devices and healthcare applications to the Industrial Internet of Things (IIoT), is amazing. There are a number of IoT use cases illustrating how IoT products and services are being deployed around the world by industry (Khang & Abdullayev et al., 2024).

### 20.8.1 ECG Monitoring

The electrical activity of the heart is represented by the electrocardiogram (ECG). The ECG serves as a tool for diagnosing various cardiac abnormalities and offers details about the fundamental rhythm of the heart muscle. The early diagnosis of heart problems by ECG monitoring can be utilized via IoT technology. A wireless data gathering system and a receiving processor make up an Internet of Things-based ECG monitoring system. We employed an automated search technique for real-time cardiac abnormality detection. The end user received recorded data via Bluetooth. A smartphone app can display recorded ECG data. Real-time monitoring of IoT systems may be feasible after merging IoT systems with big data analytics to manage large-scale data storage.

### 20.8.2 Glucose Level Monitoring

Recent developments in IoT technology have been leveraged to develop a variety of wearable blood glucose monitoring devices that are non-invasive, comfortable, convenient, and safe. In the IoT, non-invasive blood glucose meters have been developed to monitor blood glucose levels in real-time as shown in Figure 20.9. The wearable sensor and healthcare provider were connected by a suitable communication line (Choudhary et al., 2022). A blood glucose glove is also integrated with a Raspberry Pi camera and a visible laser beam. A series of fingertip images were used to determine a patient's diabetic status. Optical sensors such as infrared LEDs and near-infrared photodiodes are also used to measure glucose levels. The optical signal reflected by the human body is used to calculate the level of glucose in the human body.

### 20.8.3 Temperature Monitoring

Change in body temperature can be a warning sign for some illnesses, such as trauma and sepsis. Tracking temperature changes over time helps doctors make inferences about the health of patients with many illnesses. The traditional way to measure temperature is to use a thermometer attached to the mouth or the ear. However, the problem with these methods is that the patient's level of comfort is always low, and the likelihood of infection is high (Pooja & Babasaheb et al., 2023).

However, recent developments in IoT-based technologies have proposed a variety of solutions to this problem. 3D-printed wearable IoT devices that could be worn on the ear and monitor body temperature using infrared sensors are available. The device was integrated with a wireless sensor module and a data processing unit. The measured temperature is not affected by the environment or other physical activity (Kumar et al., 2016). An IoT-based temperature monitoring system using Arduino and Raspberry Pi is also possible. Temperature data can be stored in a database and displayed on a web page accessible from a computer or mobile phone. Portable, lightweight sensors are also available for real-time temperature measurements in infants. It can also alert parents when temperatures exceed dangerous levels (Samanta et al., 2023).

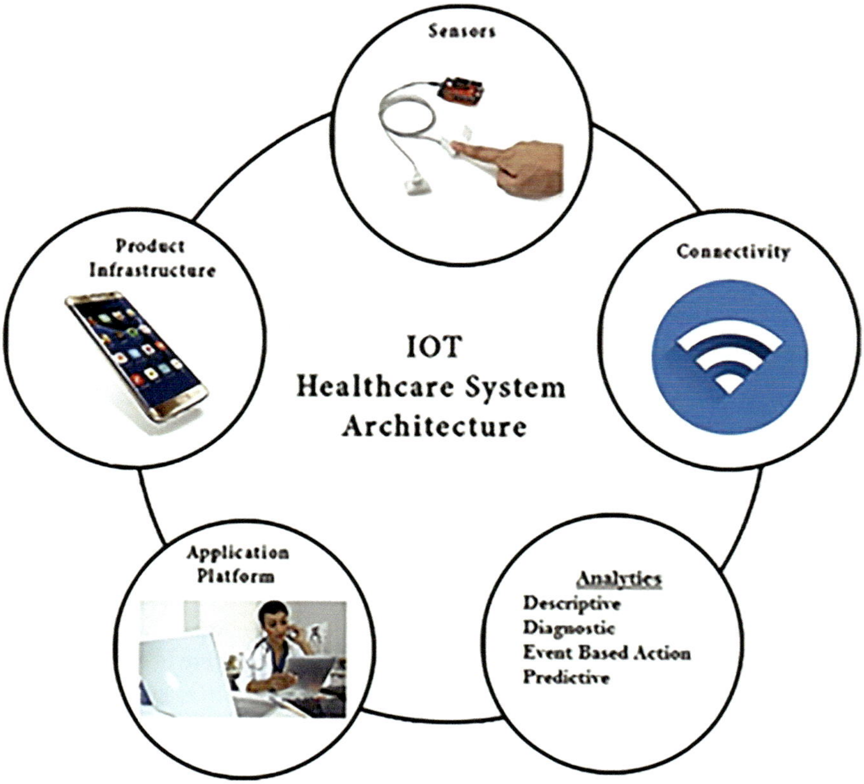


**FIGURE 20.9** IoT in the healthcare system.

### 20.8.4 Blood Pressure Monitoring

One of the essential steps in any diagnostic process is blood pressure (BP) measurement. The most common method of measuring blood pressure requires at least one person to record the blood pressure. However, the integration of IoT and other sensor technologies has changed the way BPs were previously monitored. Wearable and coffles devices that could measure both systolic and diastolic pressure are available. The recorded information can be saved in the cloud. You can also measure blood pressure with ECG signals recorded from your fingertips. This technique uses a connected microcontroller module to calculate blood pressure and send the recorded data to cloud storage.

### 20.8.5 Oxygen Saturation Monitoring

A pulse oxy-meter is a non-invasive measure of oxygen saturation and can be used as a vital sign for medical analysis. Non-invasive methods eliminate problems associated with traditional approaches and provide real-time monitoring. Advances in pulse oxy-meters with the integration of IoT-based technologies have revealed potential applications in the healthcare industry (Khang & Rana et al., 2023). Non-invasive tissue oxy-meters that can measure blood oxygen saturation levels along with heart rate and pulse parameters are available. The recorded information can also be transmitted to our servers using various communication technologies such as ZigBee and Wi-Fi. Medical intervention was decided based on the data collected. An alarm system is also possible that can warn the patient when oxygen saturation reaches a critical level (Anh & Vladimir et al., 2024).

### 20.8.6 IoT-Based Wheelchairs

Wheelchairs are an integral part of the lives of disabled patients. Provide physical and psychological support. An IoT-based control system integrated with a real-time obstacle avoidance system was developed. The steering system can detect obstacles in real time using image processing techniques on recorded video (Langer et al., 2021). The use of mobile computers has made wheelchair management more interactive and easier for patients. Smart wheelchairs include the integration of various sensors, mobile technology, and cloud computing. The system includes a mobile application that can assist patients in interacting with their wheelchairs and caregivers.

## 20.9 CONCLUSION

The Internet of Things (IoT) has revolutionized the way we interact with technology and the environment around us, and it is becoming more and more common in our daily lives. Applications for the Internet of Things (IoT) have impacted many areas of our lives, providing ease, efficiency, and improved experiences. Smart houses are one key area where IoT has had an influence. Smart thermostats, lighting controls, security cameras, and home assistants are just a few examples of connected devices that have improved the comfort, security, and energy efficiency of our homes (Khang & Hahanov et al., 2022). Greater convenience and peace of mind are provided by the ability to remotely monitor and control our houses, change settings, and receive alerts. Healthcare has changed due to IoT (Vrushank et al., 2023).

Wearable technology, like fitness trackers and smartwatches, may track activity levels, monitor vital signs, and give consumers and medical professionals access to important health information. Continuous health tracking and early identification of potential health issues are made possible through remote patient monitoring, which enhances patient care and lowers healthcare expenses (Khang & Vladimir et al., 2023). IoT applications have also revolutionized the transportation industry. Road safety and efficiency can be improved by connected vehicles by collecting and transmitting data about their performance, traffic patterns, and maintenance requirements. Intelligent traffic management systems can improve circulation, ease congestion, and cut back on carbon emissions. Thus the IoT can be used for different applications (Vrushank et al., 2023).

## REFERENCES

Anh, P. T. N., Hahanov, V., Triwiyanto, Ragimova, N. A., Rashad, İ., Abdullayev, V., Abuzarova, V. A. (2024). AI Models for Disease Diagnosis and Prediction of Heart Disease with Artificial Neural Networks. In *Computer Vision and AI-Integrated IoT Technologies in Medical Ecosystem* (1st Ed.). CRC Press. https://doi.org/10.1201/9781003429609-9

Asit Behera, J. P. (2021). Temperature Nanosensors for Smart Manufacturing. In *Nanosensors for Smart Manufacturing* (pp. 249–272). Science Direct. www.sciencedirect.com/science/article/pii/B9780128233580000137

Aswani, D., Aguru, E. S. (2022). Integrated Industrial Reference Architecture for Smart Healthcare in Internet of Things: A Systematic Investigation. *Algorithms*, 300–309. www.mdpi.com/1999-4893/15/9/309

Banerjee, A. (2022). A Comparative Study on IoT-Aided Smart Grids Using Blockchain Platform. In S. K. Rajiv Pandey, ed., *Artificial Intelligence and Machine Learning for EDGE Computing* (pp. 443–467). Academic Press. www.sciencedirect.com/science/article/pii/B978012824054000006X

Chelsea Nauta, C. J. (2020). Techgenics' Data Security Compliance. *Muma Case Review*, 001–027. www.informingscience.org/Publications/4563?Type=conferenceproceedings&ConferenceID=47

Chivarov, S., Chivarov, N., Chikurtev, D., Pleva, M. (2021). Cost Oriented Software System for Animal Husbandry Smart Automation. In *International Conference Automatics and Informatics (ICAI)* (pp. 256–261). IEEE. https://ieeexplore.ieee.org/abstract/document/9639708/

Choudhary, V. S. A. (2021). An Intrusion Detection Technique Using Frequency Analysis for Wireless Sensor Network. In *International Conference on Computing, Communication, and Intelligent Systems (ICCCIS)* (pp. 206–210). IEEE. https://journals.sagepub.com/doi/abs/10.1177/15501329221077922

Choudhary, V. S. A. (2022). Comparative Analysis of Security Issues and Trends in IoT and WSN. *A Journal of Physical Sciences, Engineering and Technology*, 216–222. www.smsjournals.com/index.php/SAMRIDDHI/article/view/2731

Khang, A., Abdullayev, V. A., Hrybiuk, O., Shukla, A. K. (2024). *Computer Vision and AI-Integrated IoT Technologies in Medical Ecosystem* (1st Ed.). CRC Press. https://doi.org/10.1201/9781003429609

Khang, A., Hahanov, V., Abbas, G. L., Hajimahmud, V. A. (2022). Cyber-Physical-Social System and İncident Management. In *AI-Centric Smart City Ecosystems: Technologies, Design and Implementation* (1st Ed., Vol. 2, p. 15). CRC Press. https://doi.org/10.1201/9781003252542-2

Khang, A., Hahanov, V., Litvinova, E., Chumachenko, S., Triwiyanto, Hajimahmud, V. A., Ragimova, N. A., Abuzarova, V. A., Anh, P. T. N. (2023). The Analytics of Hospitality of Hospitals in Healthcare Ecosystem. In *Data-Centric AI Solutions and Emerging Technologies in the Healthcare Ecosystem* (p. 4). CRC Press. https://doi.org/10.1201/9781003356189-4

Khang, A., Hajimahmud, V. A., Gupta, S. K., Babasaheb, J., Morris, G. (2023). *AI-Centric Modelling and Analytics: Concepts, Designs, Technologies, and Applications* (1st Ed.). CRC Press. https://doi.org/10.1201/9781003400110

Khang, A., Misra, A., Gupta, S. K., Shah, V. (2023). *AI-Aided IoT Technologies and Applications in the Smart Business and Production*. CRC Press. https://doi.org/10.1201/9781003392224

Khang, A., Ragimova, N. A., Hajimahmud, V. A., Alyar, V. A. (2022). Advanced Technologies and Data Management in the Smart Healthcare System. In *AI-Centric Smart City Ecosystems: Technologies, Design and Implementation* (1st Ed., Vol. 16, p. 10). CRC Press. https://doi.org/10.1201/9781003252542-16

Khang, A., Rana, G., Tailor, R. K., Hajimahmud, V. A. (2023). *Data-Centric AI Solutions and Emerging Technologies in the Healthcare Ecosystem*. CRC Press. https://doi.org/10.1201/9781003356189

Khang, A., Rani, S., Sivaraman, A. K. (2022). *AI-Centric Smart City Ecosystems: Technologies, Design and Implementation* (1st Ed.). CRC Press. https://doi.org/10.1201/9781003252542

Kumar, N. H., Baskaran, S., Hariraj, S., Krishnan, V. (2016). An Autonomous Aquaponics System Using 6LoWPAN Based WSN. In *4th International Conference on Future Internet of Things and Cloud Workshops (FiCloudW)* (pp. 125–132). IEEE. https://ieeexplore.ieee.org/abstract/document/7592711/

Langer, D. A. (2021). *Analysis and Design of Next-Generation Software Architectures: 5G, IoT, Blockchain, and Quantum Computing*. Springer. https://link.springer.com/content/pdf/10.1007/978-3-030-36899-9.pdf

Liam Peters, C. B. (2016). Designing an Automatic Beacon Ejection System for Aircraft. In *16th AIAA Aviation Technology, Integration, and Operations Conference* (pp. 1–10). American Institute of Aeronautics and Astronautics. https://arc.aiaa.org/doi/pdf/10.2514/6.2016-3918

Norman Gwangwava, T. B. (2021). Design and Simulation of IoT Systems Using the Cisco Packet Tracer. *Advances in Internet of Things*, 59–76. www.scirp.org/html/1-4000279_108495.htm

Pooja, K., Jadhav, B., Kulkarni, A., Khang, A., Kulkarni, S. (2023). The Role of Blockchain Technology in Metaverse Ecosystem. In *AI-Based Technologies and Applications in the Era of the Metaverse* (1st Ed., pp. 228–236). IGI Global Press. https://doi.org/10.4018/978-1-6684-8851-5.ch011

Rani, S., Bhambri, P., Kataria, A., Khang, A., Sivaraman, A. K. (2023). *Big Data, Cloud Computing and IoT: Tools and Applications* (1st Ed.). Chapman and Hall/CRC. https://doi.org/10.1201/9781003298335

Samanta, D. P. S., Patnaik, B. C. M., Satpathy, I., Khang, A. (2023). Revolutionizing Agriculture Through Blockchain: A Bibliometric Analysis of Emerging Trends and Applications. In *Handbook of Research on AI-Equipped IoT Applications in High-Tech Agriculture* (pp. 295–312). IGI Global. https://doi.org/10.4018/978-1-6684-9231-4.ch016

Vishal, S. T. (2019). An Efficient Quantum Key Management Scheme. In *4th International Conference on Internet of Things and Connected Technologies (ICIoTCT)* (pp. 269–277). Springer. https://link.springer.com/chapter/10.1007/978-3-030-39875-0_29

Vishal Choudhary, S. (2018). *A Distributed Key Management Protocol for Wireless Sensor Network: Advanced Informatics for Computing Research, ICAICR 2018*. Springer. https://link.springer.com/chapter/10.1007/978-981-13-3143-5_21

Vishal Choudhary, S. (2020). The Highly Secure Polynomial Pool-Based Key Pre-Distribution Scheme for Wireless Sensor Network. *Journal of Discrete Mathematical Sciences and Cryptography*, 95–114. www.tandfonline.com/doi/abs/10.1080/09720529.2020.1721880

Vrushank, S., Khang, A. (2023). Metaverse-Enabling IoT Technology for a Futuristic Healthcare System. In *AI-Based Technologies and Applications in the Era of the Metaverse* (1st Ed.). IGI Global Press. https://doi.org/10.4018/978-1-6684-8851-5.ch008

Vrushank, S., Vidhi, T., Khang, A. (2023). Electronic Health Records Security and Privacy Enhancement Using Blockchain Technology. In *Data-Centric AI Solutions and Emerging Technologies in the Healthcare Ecosystem* (1st Ed.). CRC Press. https://doi.org/10.1201/9781003356189-1

Zoughbi, S. G. (2022). Significant Trends of Smart Technologies. In S. G. Zoughbi, ed., *Planning and Designing Smart Cities in Developing Nations*. IGI Global. www.google.com/books?hl=en&lr=&id=gm9bEAAAQBAJ&oi=fnd&pg=PR1&dq=Significant+trends+of+smart+Technologies.+In+S.+G.+Zoughbi,+Planning+and+Designing+Smart+Cities+in+Developing+Nations.+IGI+&ots=Ec64en5a_e&sig=KAIQms4l-1BewJozYgCNs2hEl1rE

# 21 Cybersecurity Infrastructure and Solutions for Healthcare Systems

*Abhishek Vaghela and Vrushank Shah*

## 21.1 INTRODUCTION

There have been many positive effects that technological progress has had on society, one of which is in the medical field. It is anticipated that the increased usage of electronic health records (EHR) will lower the cost of healthcare by enhancing the overall quality of healthcare services and the timely delivery of those services. In light of these advantages, the Health Information Technology for Economic and Clinical Health Act (HITECH Act) was passed with the intention of encouraging a greater number of healthcare institutions to implement Health Information Technology (HIT). Integrating healthcare with technology has resulted in an increase in the possibility of breaches of patient records, despite the fact that HIT has a considerable number of positive effects (Rani & Chauhan et al., 2021).

A breach of information is described as data that is lost, stolen, displaced, hacked, or disclosed to unofficial recipients. This disruption in data information is regarded to be an act of cyber-attack. It is estimated that approximately 94% of healthcare companies have been victims of at least one of these types of cyber-attacks. Between the years 2009 and 2014, an estimated 150 million patient health records were stolen or otherwise compromised. According to the findings of a study that was carried out by McCue (2023), insiders rather than outsiders are responsible for 70% of the data fraud that occurs in businesses. One of the key reasons that healthcare is vulnerable to high levels of data breach and financial risk is the richness of data that is kept by healthcare institutions. Typically, healthcare institutions have access to a substantial volume of private information (Kavita et al., 2023).

Records kept by hospitals and insurance companies typically include a wealth of personal information, including patients' names, dates of birth, social security numbers, addresses, and credit card numbers. In addition, hackers choose to concentrate their efforts on healthcare firms since, on the dark web, data from healthcare organizations is more valuable than data from other industries. On the dark web, for example, an electronic health record (EHR) is valued anywhere from ten to one hundred times as much as credit card information. The healthcare industry already


DOI: 10.1201/9781032686745-21

faces the challenge of high expenses and low profit margins in comparison to many other industries (Khang & Hahanov et al., 2022).

Cyber breaches add to the financial strain that this industry already bears. At the moment, the typical cost of losing data is far more expensive for healthcare businesses than it is for organizations operating in other industries. Although they provide an incentive for businesses to improve their cyber security, the penalties and fines imposed by organizations such as the Office for Civil Rights of the Department of Health and Human Services further compound the financial burden that healthcare organizations already bear. It is anticipated that breaches in data security will result in a revenue loss of 309 billion dollars by the year 2019.

The issue of cyber security not only endangers the patients' right to privacy and places a financial strain on the sector, but it also poses a risk to the well-being of patients. For instance, the usage of wireless medical devices may put patients at risk of being victimized by cybercriminals. Cybercriminals may be able to harm a patient by taking advantage of a vulnerability in a cardiac device's cyber security, such as the one that was just discovered by the United States Department of Homeland Security (Anh et al., 2024).

Implementing safeguards such as encryption, shredding documents, locking doors, and employing passwords should be done in order to limit exposures, eliminate unintended disclosures, protect sensitive information related to healthcare, and reduce the number of cyber-attacks. In spite of the growing danger posed by cyber-attacks on the healthcare industry, the study on this subject is in its infancy, and there are significant holes in the relevant literature. This chapter highlights new concerns faced by cyber-attacks in healthcare, as well as crucial stakeholders involved in cyber security, in an effort to raise awareness of the issue and stimulate additional research on the subject.

In addition to that, this chapter investigates the cyber security rules that are already in place at both the federal and state levels of government, and it provides recommendations for policymakers to improve healthcare cyber security. In conclusion, it outlines potential lines of inquiry for additional study on healthcare cyber security.

## 21.2 ELECTRONIC HEALTH RECORD (EHR)

The EHR stores all of the information that has been provided about the patient. This pertains to the patients' Personally Identifiable Information (PII), Protected Health Information (PHI), and any other Financial Information. EHR is essential not only for the purposes of accounting or billing but also because it maintains up-to-date information about patients' medical histories and demographics, medications, comprehensive lists of patients' allergic reactions, electronic prescriptions, physician clinical notes, monitoring patients' progress toward better health, and conducting research. The use of electronic health records makes the exchange of information between hospitals, healthcare practitioners, and public health authorities more effective and more easily managed, as shown in Figure 21.1.

The use of an electronic health record (EHR) not only raises the standard of medical care but also lowers associated costs and makes more effective use of clinicians' time, as shown in Figure 21.2.

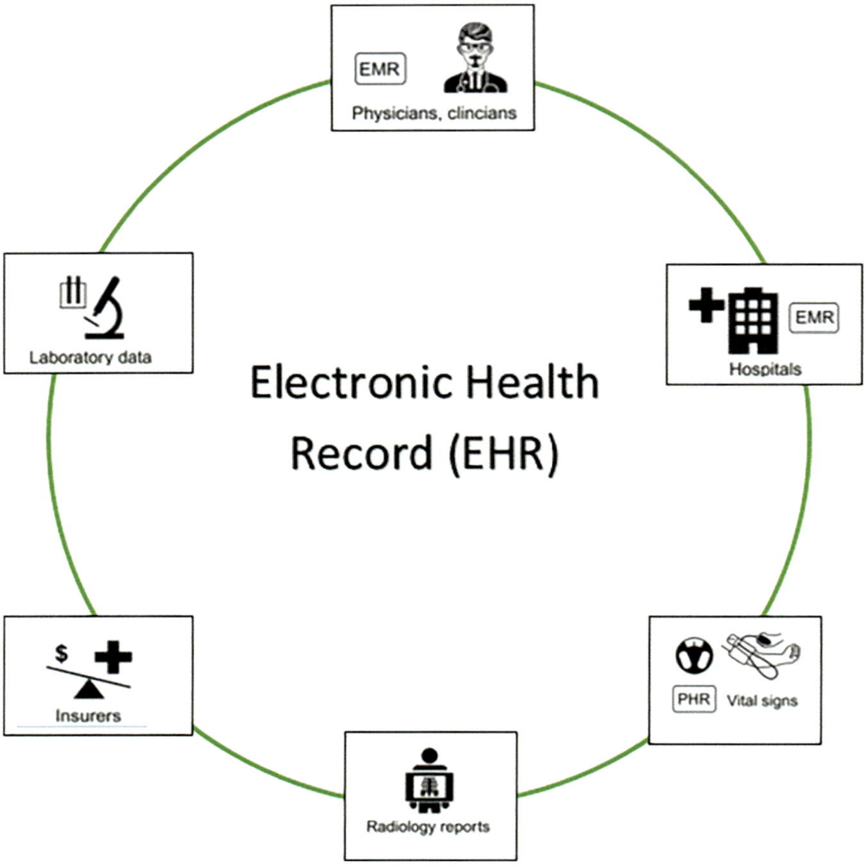


**FIGURE 21.1** Electronic health record system.

**Source: Author.**

## 21.3 TYPES OF CYBER ATTACKS IN HEALTHCARE SYSTEMS

Attempts have been made to categorize cyber risks. The goal, severity, extent, and legitimacy of cyber-attacks have all been considered by these studies, but they have all used different criteria to categorize cyber security. We go over the most common forms of cyber-attacks, and the thought processes that go into them.

### 21.3.1 Denial-of-Services (DoS)

A denial-of-service (DoS) attack is an attempt to disrupt service and prevent users from accessing network resources by overwhelming the targeted network with traffic. A healthcare organization's network could come to a complete halt or experience considerable delays if attacked in this way. An example of a distributed denial-of-service (DoS) assault used by "hacktivists" to disrupt a number of networks at once is

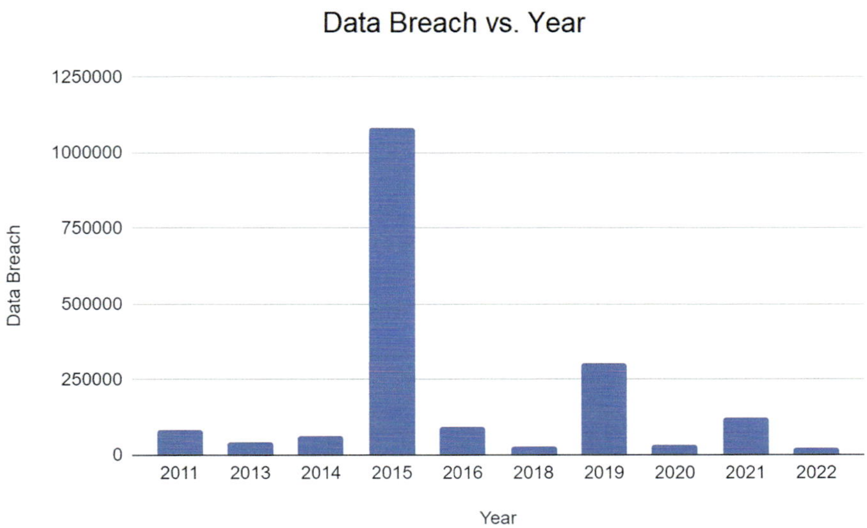


**FIGURE 21.2** Health data breach incident disclosures from 2011 to 2022 according to the HHS Breach Notification data.

**Source: Author.**

the 2014 attack on Boston Children's Hospital. In the healthcare industry, a denial of service assault poses a particularly grave threat since it prevents providers from gaining access to or transmitting life-saving data.

### 21.3.2 Privilege Escalation

The end goal of a privilege escalation attack is to gain access to resources that would otherwise be inaccessible. Superior privileges within a system have often been carried out by taking advantage of flaws in software or a system. This is made possible by hackers with the heightened ability to compromise the system. They do things like alter a patient's chat information, protecting the health of the patient.

Both vertical and horizontal privilege escalation attacks are common. However, malware can also be used in "multi-layered attacks" to get administrative access to a system and do a lot of damage to it.

### 21.3.3 Man-in-the-Middle (MITM) or Eavesdropping

In the context of attacks, eavesdropping falls under the category of reconnaissance. It happens when an unauthorized third party listens to a conversation between two people. An attacker can eavesdrop on a conversation by posing as a third party during a conversation. Since the intruder can change the data before sending it to the other party or parties, the integrity of the conveyed data is easily compromised. An eavesdropper in the healthcare industry could potentially blackmail patients by gaining access to private information. Similar to Man-in-the-Middle (MITM) attacks,

Man-in-the-Browsers (MITB) attacks rely on remote access to browsers to carry out their malicious deeds. The most advanced MITB attacks employ Trojan malware that can hide from security software.

### 21.3.4 Structured Query Language Injections Exploit

The Structured Programming Language is used by a number of popular websites nowadays, and databases use Structured Query Language (SQL). SQL injection vulnerabilities allow hackers to potentially execute arbitrary code. Dangerous SQL statements (payloads) trick data servers into disclosing sensitive information. When hackers perform a SQL injection attack, they might change data in the database, impacting the database's availability, confidentiality, and integrity.

### 21.3.5 Malicious Software

The term "malware" refers to a collection of programs that are designed to do harm. These are created with the intention of doing damage to or compromising a computer system, providing unauthorized access without the user's consent. These programs are responsible for carrying out a variety of functions, including modifying, harming, spying, and or deleting user information. Malware can be distributed in two ways: physically through the use of an external drive or digitally through internet downloads, such as emails used for "phishing." A few examples of widespread malware are worms, bots, viruses, adware, Trojans, spyware, adware, backdoors, ransomware, and rootkits.

### 21.3.6 Virus

The most common form of malware, a virus, can replicate itself and infect other systems without the user's knowledge or permission. The malicious intent of most viruses means that they can destroy or corrupt data. While viruses can replicate independently, they have little power unless someone actually uses them. Users must initiate virus infection since the vast majority of viruses are executable files that are bound to the host file. After a virus crippled the computer system at the Erie County Medical Center in upstate New York in 2017, the hospital had to provide laptops to staff so they could access patients' backed-up records, which slowed down operations (Khang, 2024).

### 21.3.7 Trojans

This virus, similar to the fabled Trojan horse, conceals itself as a piece of software that appears to have no malicious intent. Trojan horses, in contrast to viruses and worms, do not have the ability to replicate themselves and do not need a host file in order to carry out their malicious activities. Hackers have the potential to get into a system by employing a "backdoor" that is supplied by a Trojan. Trojan malware was found to be present on two of the computers that are part of the Alaska Department of Health and Social Services. This information has only recently come to light. It is possible that the Trojan horse has already opened a backdoor, exposing private patient information in the process.

### 21.3.8 Spyware

"Spyware" is defined as software that is installed on a computer without the knowledge of the user and broadcasts information about the user's computer activities across the Internet. Spyware is a derogatory word for "malware." Spyware is software that runs undetected on a computer system and allows the attacker the opportunity to monitor and collect personal information about the computer system's target. Spyware is a type of program that functions invisibly. There is a chance that a piece of malware may pose as a Trojan horse in order to carry out man-in-the-middle (MITM) assaults. Spyware may also slow down a computer's performance, typically because it requires the operating system to perform more tasks.

### 21.3.9 Ransomware

Recent years have seen ransomware attacks become commonplace in news coverage. Essential to this type of malware attack is the demand for a ransom in exchange for the decryption of data. However, ransomware can use a wide variety of other software to gain access to a system and encrypt its victims' data. Information is often encrypted, and if the ransom is not paid, the hackers threaten to sell or leak the data to the public. This takes place when the victim's data is encrypted. WannaCry (sometimes called WannaCrypt) ransomware played a significant role in the 2017 attack on the United Kingdom's National Health Service (NHS). Patients' access to care was hampered throughout the healthcare system as a result of this attack.

### 21.3.10 Phishing

Phishing is utilizing social engineering to trick an individual or organization into disclosing information or performing an action that is harmful to their computer. Phishing is also known as spear phishing and email phishing. The term "phishing" more accurately refers to a method or vector than it does an actual attack. In fact, this is one of the most common ways that malicious software is disseminated. Emails are frequently used by attackers because they may quickly and simply send a target to a website designed to steal information or force the installation of malicious software. This makes emails a popular tool for cybercriminals. Spear-phishing is a specialized form of phishing that targets specific individuals or organizations to commit fraud against them. At Kaleida Health, New York's largest provider, two spear phishing assaults in 2017 compromised more than 3,000 patient records.

### 21.3.11 Worms

Worms, in contrast to viruses, do not need a host file in order to execute, replicate themselves, or spread. In most cases, the spread of worms is dependent on the existence of vulnerabilities inside the target system or on the utilization of social engineering. The WannaCry ransomware that caused disruptions in the NHS in the United Kingdom is a worm.

## 21.4 INTRUSION DETECTION SYSTEMS FOR HEALTHCARE

As a combination of the words "intrusion" and "detection system," "IDS" is an abbreviation commonly used in the field. Intruding into a computer or network system compromises the security of the information contained inside. On the other side, the detection system is a precautionary step meant to reveal such illegal activity. In conclusion, an IDS is a tool for ensuring the safety of a system by monitoring all host and network activity for signs of intrusion that could compromise its confidentiality, integrity, or availability. The IDS will alert the host or network administrators of any suspicious activity it detects. In order to monitor network traffic for intrusions, all incoming and outgoing packets must be mirrored to the NIDS. NIDS can be positioned between a firewall and a network switch, allowing for a comprehensive inspection of data before it reaches either component, as shown in Figure 21.3.

### 21.4.1 Types of Intrusion Detection Systems

A number of different types of IDSs exist, each catering to a specific deployment or detection strategy.

#### 21.4.1.1 Intrusion Detection System (IDS) Based on Deployment Method

Based on where it is installed, intrusion detection systems (IDS) can be further broken down into two subsets: host-based IDS (HIDS) and network-based IDS (NIDS). HIDS has been implemented on exactly one data host. Its purpose is to monitor the system for any unusual behavior or security issues. A major drawback is that it must be installed on all hosts that require intrusion protection, which increases

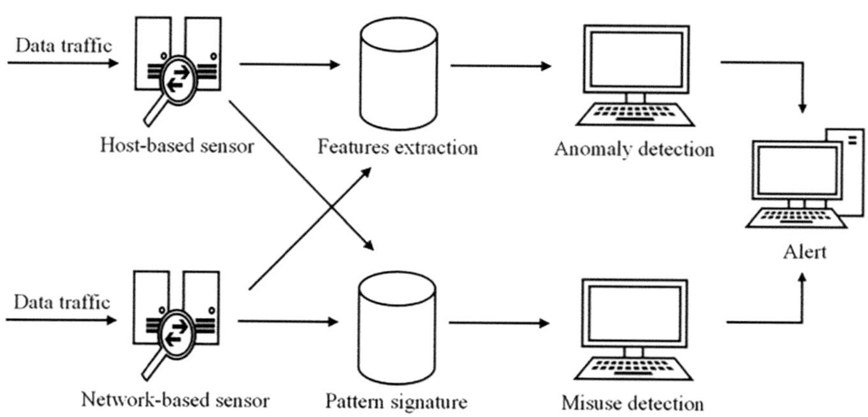


**FIGURE 21.3** Intrusion Detection System.

**Source: Author.**

the workload on each node and, hence, slows down the IDS. However, NIDSs are deployed across the network to protect each and every device and the infrastructure as a whole. The NIDS will routinely perform scans of all network traffic to detect security holes and vulnerabilities.

#### 21.4.1.2 Intrusion Detection Systems Based on Detection Methods

Subcategories of IDS that emphasize detection include signature-based intrusion detection (SIDS) and anomaly-based intrusion detection (AIDS). In order to identify specific sorts of attacks, signature-based intrusion detection systems (SIDS), also known as "misuse intrusion detection" or "knowledge-based intrusion detection," use a database of known malicious code. Data patterns are compared to these signatures, stored in a signature database, to identify attacks. The availability of a signature for known assaults allows for their efficient identification, which is a major benefit. However, this method is insufficient for detecting novel threats because it does not leverage signature patterns.

Keeping a big signature database and comparing it to data packets to find vulnerabilities is also laborious. The AIDS system, also called the "behavior-based IDS," is based on the idea of defining a normative pattern of behavior in advance. Assume abnormality for any behavior that deviates from this standard. The key advantages of AIDS are in its ability to detect undiscovered and new attacks and in the ability to tailor the normal activity profile. However, the high false accept rate needed for intrusion detection is a big drawback because it is hard to tell where regular and anomalous profiles begin and end.

Recent years have seen an uptick in the use of machine learning methods for intrusion detection, with the goal of reducing the frequency and severity of security incidents and protecting networks against malicious entry. Today, the healthcare industry makes use of cutting-edge technology like robotics, computer vision, and Artificial Intelligence (AI). In recent years, the healthcare sector has relied on machine learning methods to address healthcare security issues. However, Intrusion Detection Systems (IDS) that rely on machine learning can be implemented in a number of different ways.

The ever-expanding variety of machine learning techniques, as well as their capacity to achieve a high rate of false-positive traffic with a low computing cost, justify their deployment. The field of cyber security relies heavily on machine learning techniques. Intrusion detection systems have included machine learning algorithms, including Convolutional Neural Networks (CNN), Decision Trees (DT), K-Nearest Neighbors (K-NN), and Support Vector Machines (SVM) to improve categorization results. Healthcare systems contain sensitive and life-critical medical data, so while they present a number of opportunities, they also present a number of challenges, such as privacy problems and major security difficulties.

According to studies conducted in this area, the healthcare business is currently one of the most at-risk sectors when it comes to cyber-attacks. Healthcare facilities benefit greatly from the efficiency and convenience of the Intrusion Detection System (IDS). Authorized individuals are given easier access to data. When an IDS detects suspicious activity, it notifies the administrator. Since the detecting process is now automated, the likelihood of human error has decreased. The machine has been given proper training with effective algorithms, allowing it to perform at a higher level of efficiency (Sihare & Khang, 2023; Khang & Gadirova et al., 2023).

### 21.4.2 Machine Learning-Based Intrusion Detection Systems for Healthcare Systems

A medical server stores all of the collected sensor data, making it easily accessible to the medical team. There are two main categories of information kept here: electronic medical records (EMR) and electronic health records (EHR). Electronic medical records (EMR) centralize a patient's health and treatment information so it may be accessed from any facility that uses the system. Although the primary concern of an electronic health record is the patient's overall health, information about the patient's health, including medical history, prescriptions, lab results, and personal details, can be stored and transmitted. Protecting the privacy of patients, maintaining the secrecy of medical records, and ensuring the availability and integrity of these data are all crucial to providing a correct diagnosis.

From this aspect, Boxwala et al. (2011) proposed utilizing statistics and ML to detect anomalous activity in electronic health record (EHR) access logs. The authors implemented linear regression (LR) and SVM to rank suspicious new access for classification as potentially harmful. Initially, privacy officers looked into the incident with the highest score. Using an iterative refining process, the authors of the paper employed the privacy agent to classify the selected events as suspicious or appropriate and then used that information to develop a model based on LR and SVM. They used 10-fold cross-validation to train the model.

Using sensitivity and AUC, as well as a comparison to the rule-based technique, the authors analyzed the efficacy of their model. As a result of their extensive testing, the authors achieved an AUC of more than 0.90 and a sensitivity of greater than 0.75. They conclude that it is possible to detect suspect access in EHR using a strategy based on statistics and ML and that this method is superior to a rule-based approach. For a similar goal of identifying privacy breaches caused by unauthorized access to electronic health records, Menon et al. (2014) present a different method. To identify cases of unauthorized access, the authors adopt a collaborative filtering-inspired method, in which they attempt to anticipate a label based on the characteristics of an interaction between two entities.

Incorporating both overt and covert characteristics, their system generates a fingerprint customizer based on a user's unique access patterns, making it ideal for both medical professionals and patients. The model was tested on two datasets, "hospital" and "amazon," and its performance was measured using root-mean-squared error, area under the curve, and precision-recall curves. The authors then compared their findings with those of three machine learning (ML) algorithms: linear regression (LR), support vector machine (SVM), and logistic regression. After running all of the experiments, the authors saw a significant improvement in performance compared to competing methods, and they were able to identify instances of improper access.

In addition, (Malin & Bradley, 2014) proposed a community-based anomaly detection system, an unsupervised learning model for detecting insider threats in a collaborative setting by analyzing access records. The authors offer a hybrid method, first using singular value decomposition (SVD), a special instance of principal component analysis (PCA), to infer communities from user relational networks, then KNN to generate a set of nearest neighbors. In order to identify users whose communication habits have deviated from the norm, the developed model looks for statistical outliers. The scientists employed two datasets—one containing access records from a real-world EMR over the course of six months and the other containing editorial board composition data for a group of journals over five years—to test and refine their model. After a battery of testing, it became clear that their model outperformed the competition in identifying the simulated user.

Marwan et al. (2018) developed an alternative, ML-based method for processing images safely in the cloud. Using Fuzzy C-Means Clustering (FCM) and SVM, they divide the image into four sections based on the intensity of the pixels in each. The FCM is used to get pixel-level color characteristics. This information is then used by the SVM to categorize the image into distinct areas before being uploaded to the cloud for long-term storage. By adding a CloudSec module that supports in-transit encryption through the HTTPS/Secure Socket Layer, the authors suggest a three-layer architecture in place of the conventional two-layer model. Data access can be limited, and cloud resource abuse can be uncovered with the help of the CloudSec module.

Sicuranza and Paragliola (2020) presented a hybrid IDS to identify cyber-attacks against EHR. The proposed approach uses agents stationed throughout the IT infrastructure under surveillance. Local logs are their responsibility, and they must be gathered, normalized, and analyzed for security. Then, the events produced by these agents are relayed to the IDS for further investigation. The IDS has a module for finding abuse as well as one for finding anomalies. Since it is rule-based, the module for detecting abuse can accurately identify the typical pattern of an attack. Anomaly detection software can spot new security holes that zero-day exploits exploit. DT, Neural Network, and k-means are the three classifiers used in anomaly detection. Voting on the findings from these classifiers helps to increase their overall precision.

If the abuse detection module and the anomaly detection voting system come to opposite conclusions about the presence or lack of attacks, an expert system module will mediate the disagreement. A dataset was collected by keeping tabs on the Italian EHR system to put the suggested approach to the test. The abuse and anomaly detection modules were put through their paces using three distinct attacks on EHR systems. The outcomes prove the effectiveness of the strategy. In addition, a paradigm was proposed to identify privacy and availability vulnerabilities in EMR systems in a paper by (McGlade & Scott-Hayward, 2019). The SVM is used to detect privacy-related issues, and the Exponential Moving Average (EMA) is used to detect irregularities in message flow that could lead to a denial of service, all of which are based on machine learning (Khang & Abdullayev et al., 2024).

The authors have used simulated patient data created using the Synthea program to validate the system. The dataset has been put through the paces using three different ML algorithms, including SVM, KNN, and multinomial NB, for detecting abnormalities related to the privacy of the EMR system and EMA for detecting anomalies related to the accessibility of the EMR system. After running a battery of experiments, the authors settled on SVM as the method with the highest accuracy and recall. They also confirm that EMA is capable of identifying message spikes that can cause a denial of service (Khang & Abdullayev et al., 2024).

The majority of the contributions of the examined publications centered on methods for identifying illegal access to electronic health records. Only one study looked at the privacy and accessibility of electronic medical record data. However, there is no proposed method utilizing ML to guarantee the accuracy of medical records in either the form of electronic medical records or electronic health records (EHR), which is an area where further study is recommended (Vrushank & Khang et al., 2023).

## 21.5 CONCLUSION

There are various restrictions and difficulties with the way IDS is envisioned on a healthcare server. It is difficult to generalize a machine learning model from one medical server (EHR) to another since each server's training data has a unique structure and composition. Because of the sensitive nature of the information housed on these medical servers, the labeling procedure is quite meticulous (Vrushank et al., 2023).

As such, intrusion detection at the level of medical servers is not fully automated, and the correct tagging of data necessitates an interview with the patient. Therefore, more research into unsupervised or semi-supervised ML techniques, with a focus on false-positive rate reduction, should be conducted at this level. If an attacker only needs to alter the value of one characteristic in an EMR for one patient, it can be difficult for a machine learning (ML)-based model trained on patterns observed in a vast body of medical data to detect the change. However, because of the sensitive nature of the data, collecting public medical data in the form of an electronic medical record (EMR) or electronic health record (EHR) is challenging (Khang & Rana et al., 2023).

## REFERENCES

Anh, P. T. N., Hahanov, V., Triwiyanto, Ragimova, N. A., Rashad, İ., Abdullayev, V., Abuzarova, V. A. AI Models for Disease Diagnosis and Prediction of Heart Disease with Artificial Neural Networks. *Computer Vision and AI-Integrated IoT Technologies in Medical Ecosystem* (1st Ed.) (2024). CRC Press. https://doi.org/10.1201/9781003429609-9

Boxwala, A. A., Kim, J., Grillo, J. M., Ohno-Machado, L. Using Statistical and Machine Learning to Help Institutions Detect Suspicious Access to Electronic Health Records. *Journal of the American Medical Informatics Association* 18 (2011) 498–505. DOI: https://doi.org/10.1136/amiajnl-2011-000217

Kavita, M., Khang, A. Hospital 4.0: Capitalization of Health and Healthcare in Industry 4.0 Economy. *Data-Centric AI Solutions and Emerging Technologies in the Healthcare Ecosystem* (p. 14, 1st Ed.) (2023). CRC Press. https://doi.org/10.1201/9781003356189-19

Khang, A. *AI and IoT-Based Technologies for Precision Medicine* (2024). IGI Global Press. ISBN: 9798369308769. https://doi.org/10.4018/979-8-3693-0876-9

Khang, A., Abdullayev, V. A., Hrybiuk, O., Shukla, A. K. *Computer Vision and AI-integrated IoT Technologies in Medical Ecosystem* (1st Ed.) (2024). CRC Press. https://doi.org/10.1201/9781003429609

Khang, A., Hahanov, V., Abbas, G. L., Hajimahmud, V. A. Cyber-Physical-Social System and İncident Management. *AI-Centric Smart City Ecosystems: Technologies, Design and Implementation* (1st Ed., vol. 2, p. 15) (2022). CRC Press. https://doi.org/10.1201/9781003252542-2

Khang, A., Musrat, G. E., Abdullayev, V. Role of Photochemical Reactions in the Treatment of Water used in the High-Tech Agriculture. *Advanced Technologies and AI-Equipped IoT Applications in High-Tech Agriculture* (1st Ed., pp. 326–325) (2023). IGI Global Press. https://doi.org/10.4018/978-1-6684-9231-4.ch018

Khang, A., Rana, G., Tailor, R. K., Hajimahmud, V. A. *Data-Centric AI Solutions and Emerging Technologies in the Healthcare Ecosystem* (2023). CRC Press. https://doi.org/10.1201/9781003356189

Malin, Y., Bradley, C. Detection of Anomalous Insiders in Collaborative Environments via Relational Analysis of Access Logs. *Bone* 23 (2014) 1–7. DOI: https://doi.org/10.1145/1943513.1943524

Marwan, M., Kartit, A., Ouahmane, H. Security Enhancement in Healthcare Cloud Using Machine Learning. *Procedia Computer Science* 127 (2018) 388–397. DOI: https://doi.org/10.1016/j.procs.2018.01.136

McCue. Your World. Protected by McCue (2023). https://www.mccue.com/

McGlade, D., Scott-Hayward, S. ML-Based Cyber Incident Detection for Electronic Medical Record (EMR) Systems. *Smart Health* 12 (2019) 3–23. DOI: https://doi.org/10.1016/j.smhl.2018.05.001

Menon, A. K., Jiang, X., Kim, J., Vaidya, J., Ohno-Machado, L. Detecting Inappropriate Access to Electronic Health Records Using Collaborative Filtering. *Machine Learning* 95 (2014) 87–101. Amazon access data competition, 2022. DOI: https://doi.org/10.1007/s10994-013-5376-1

Rani, S., Chauhan, M., Kataria, A., Khang, A. IoT Equipped Intelligent Distributed Framework for Smart Healthcare Systems. *Networking and Internet Architecture* (Vol. 2, p. 30) (2021). https://doi.org/10.48550/arXiv.2110.04997

Sicuranza, M., Paragliola, G. *Ensuring Electronic Health Record Cyber-Security Through a Hybrid Intrusion Detection System* (2020). Consiglio Nazionale delle Ricerche, Istituto di Calcolo e Reti ad Alte Prestazioni (ICAR), RT-ICAR-NA-2020-01. https://intranet.icar.cnr.it/wp-content/uploads/2020/05/RT-ICAR-NA-2020-01.pdf

Sihare, S. R., Khang, A. Effects of Quantum Technology on Metaverse. *AI-Based Technologies and Applications in the Era of the Metaverse* (1st Ed., pp. 104–203) (2023). IGI Global Press. https://doi.org/10.4018/978-1-6684-8851-5.ch009

Vrushank, S., Khang, A. Internet of Medical Things (IoMT) Driving the Digital Transformation of the Healthcare Sector. *Data-Centric AI Solutions and Emerging Technologies in the Healthcare Ecosystem* (p. 1, 1st Ed.) (2023). CRC Press. https://doi.org/10.1201/9781003356189-2

Vrushank, S., Vidhi, T., Khang, A. Electronic Health Records Security and Privacy Enhancement Using Blockchain Technology. *Data-Centric AI Solutions and Emerging Technologies in the Healthcare Ecosystem* (p. 1, 1st Ed.) (2023). CRC Press. https://doi.org/10.1201/9781003356189-1

# 22 Securing the Internet of Things (IoT) Environment Using Bio-Inspired Meta-Heuristic Methodologies

*Harikrishna P., Kaviarasan R. and Kalaiyarasan R.*

## 22.1 INTRODUCTION

In 1999, Kevin Ashton, a computer scientist at Proctor and Gamble, coined the term "Internet of Things," often abbreviated as IoT (Baskoro et al., 2023). IoT consists of computers and devices that can either transmit or receive data, like an animal in the forest that has a biochip embedded in it to track its location, a human who has an implant that can monitor his/her heart rate per second or in real-time or a set of sensors that are present in the wheels of a car that relays the tire pressure to the driver via an application. So, if a device needs to connect to IoT (Vipul et al., 2023), it should be a web-based smart device. These smart devices have sensors to collect the data, processors to act on the data collected from sensors and communication capabilities to transmit them to others in the network. Several organizations make use of IoT in order to increase brand value and revenue as well as revamp the user's experience. IoT is used in several applications like home automation, healthcare, energy harvesting (Sherali et al., 2020) and other industries (Adam et al., 2023).

With the use of several networking technologies, IoT devices can communicate with other IoT devices in their network and run their services on the cloud. Bluetooth technology is at the lower end of the stack of technologies on which the network is built. There are several protocols present in the IoT that are helpful in creating, managing and maintaining the network, along with the data being transmitted across these networks. IoT has a three-tier architecture, as shown in Figure 22.1, consisting of Application Layer, Network Layer and Perception Layer.

The Perception Layer, also considered the physical layer, is made up of sensors that are helpful in collecting information regarding the environment. This layer is also helpful in identifying the other smart objects present in its environment (Khang & Vugar et al., 2024). Most researchers in the field of IoT feel that this three-layer architecture is insufficient, so they have proposed a five-layer architecture, shown in Figure 22.2, which has additional business and processing layers.


DOI: 10.1201/9781032686745-22

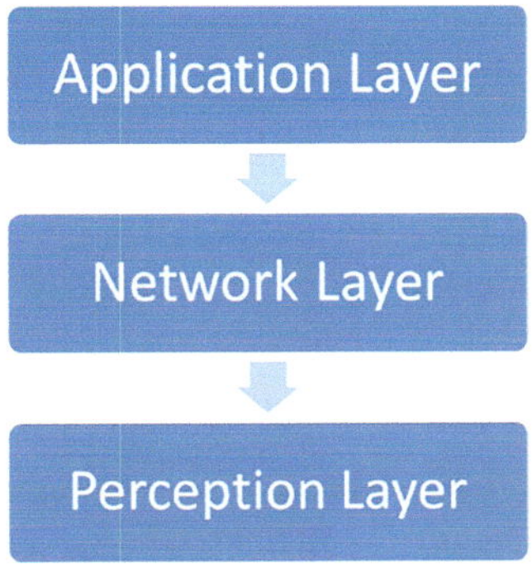


**FIGURE 22.1** Application Layer, Network Layer and Perception Layer (Khang, 2021).

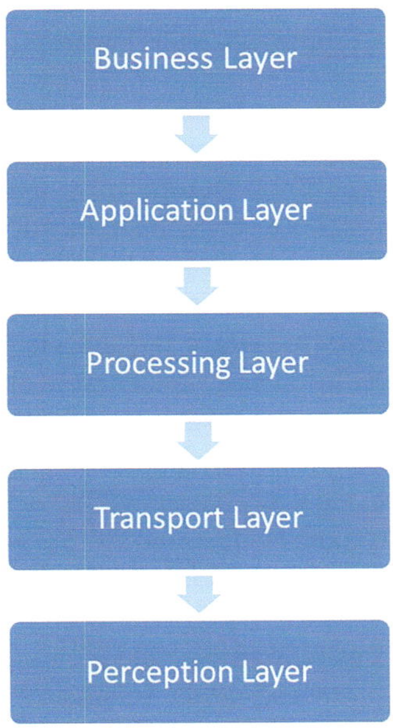


**FIGURE 22.2** Five Layer IoT Architecture (Khang, 2021).

## 22.2 SECURITY ISSUES IN IoT

Even though IoT has several advantages like automation, proper resource utilization and accessibility, which makes the work of its user simple, it is constantly plagued with several drawbacks like lack of international standards, complexity, dependence and security concerns (Vijayakumar et al., 2022; Pillutla et al., 2018). Out of these, security (Apostolos et al., 2023) is an important concern in IoT. Some security issues with the IoT are poor testing, outdated software, open-source code vulnerabilities, malware risk, weak passwords and lack of privacy and encryption (Padmalaya et al., 2023). In poor testing, the developers of IoT concentrated on the effectiveness of the devices and their ability to communicate but were not worried about identifying the weakness of IoT from a security point of view. Similar to that of other software, there is a need to ensure that the software that runs IoT devices is kept up to date to ensure that new vulnerabilities do not penetrate the system. A stark feature of the IoT system is its ability to work efficiently on open-source software, but this feature is also an issue since most of the open-source software has unknown vulnerabilities (Jesús et al., 2023) and bugs.

An attacker can use malware to gain access to IoT devices and damage it. Prowli and Mira are some of the malware that affect the performance of IoT devices. Cyberattacks (Yusuf et al., 2023) commonly occur in IoT due to weak passwords, outdated software and a lack of encryption. Denial of Service (DoS) attacks (Pillutla et al., 2021), spoofing, data theft and DNS poisoning are the most commonly occurring cyberattacks that confront the IoT system. A DoS attack is a type of cyberattack that ensures that a particular computing resource is unavailable to the authentic user at any given time.

A Distributed Denial of Service (DDoS) is a powerful variant wherein the attacker, with the help of other infected computers, namely bots, attacks the victim. In IoT, spoofing (Haixia et al., 2023) attacks are simple cyberattacks wherein the attacker acts as a legitimate user but steals the authentic user's IP or MAC address. The legitimate user's credentials can be stolen by the attacker by sending some fake messages, which are very hard to differentiate from normal messages. In Mid-2022, a DNS (Chris et al., 2015) poisoning attack was detected in IoT, which affected millions of devices connected via IoT. These attacks were due to uClibe and UClibc-ng, which were popular C libraries that had allowed attackers to perform DNS attacks on victim IoT devices. After successfully performing the attack, the attackers had full control of the IoT device and deceived the victim device into accepting a forged response. So, from these, it is quite evident that there is a scope in research to pursue mechanisms that can be deployed to prevent unauthorized users from gaining access to the IoT network.

This chapter is organized as follows: Section 22.3 includes the literature survey, Section 22.4 highlights the proposed work, Section 22.5 depicts the experimental results highlighting the significance of the proposed work compared to its benchmarks and is followed by the conclusion in Section 22.6.

## 22.3 LITERATURE SURVEY

As mentioned in the previous paragraphs, there are several security issues in IoT that need to be addressed. The best methods to address these issues are by using meta-heuristic algorithms like Ant Colony Optimization (ACO) (Sreeja et al., 2023), Particle Swarm Optimization (PSO) (Amuthan et al., 2018), Grey Wolf Optimization (GWO) (Jesús et al., 2023), etc. This section sheds light on how researchers have devised different security mechanisms to thwart security issues in IoT and recent security issues that were prevented using different meta-heuristics algorithms (Absalom et al., 2021; Zhongqiang et al., 2023).

Vuk et al. (2022) presented security-aware modeling and verification techniques that can be used on Control Interpreted Petri Nets (CIPN)-based sequential control applications. They have also demonstrated how to transform CIPN-based models for a network industrial controller into Time PetriNet (TPN)-based models. They also discussed steps to design a channel-specific attack model to capture the anomaly behavior with the help of non-determinism.

IoTGuard (Berkay et al., 2019) is used in IoT as a policy-based enforcement system that is dynamic in nature. IoTGuard has three distinct phases. The first phase deals with the code instrument implementation that can be used to add additional logic to the application's code, which is used to collect its information during runtime. The second phase has a dynamic model that stores the app's information. The model helps represent the app's runtime execution behavior. The final phase identifies the different safety and security policies along with their enforcement on the individual app's dynamic model. The main goal of this system is to protect the user from insecure and unsafe device states, which can be achieved by constantly monitoring the behavior of the IoT (Kali & Khang et al., 2024).

Wenbo et al. (2021) proposed IoTSAFE, which can be used as an enforcement system to protect the safety and security of the system. The IoTSAFE system helps envisage the risky situation and blocks any hazardous device states by generating the device's physical model. This system had been implemented on the SmartThings platform. The IoTSAFE system was around 96% accurate and could prevent around 53 highly risky conditions for 36 user policies.

Othmane et al. (2022) proposed FELIDS (Federated Learning-based Intrusion Detection System) to thwart attacks on agriculture-based IoT. This system makes use of three deep learning-based classifiers, namely CNN (Convolutional Neural Networks), RNN (Recurrent Neural Networks) and DNN (Deep Neural Networks). This system effectively preserves privacy and provides a higher accuracy level in detecting attacks in IoT.

Simon et al. (2019) designed Peeves to automatically verify all the smart home events by considering the event's physical signature. These events can be detected with the help of different sensors that are already present in the smart home or can be purchased off the shelf. Different events like opening a door, fridge and window can be spoofed in real-time, but because the detection rate of Peeves is high, the probability of the attack occurring is very low. Hussain et al. (2021) generated a DDoS dataset with the help of 33 types of scans and as many as 60 types of DDoS attacks. They combined the generated dataset with three publicly available datasets to maximize the attack coverage and train the Machine Learning (ML) algorithms (Khang & Misra et al., 2023). They proposed a twofold ML approach to detect and prevent IoT-based botnet attacks.

Yuan et al. (2017) proposed SmartAuth, which can be used to gather security-related information from an IoT app's description and code and generate a user interface for authorization. This system can be used to dodge apps that are being over-privileged. Murillo et al. (2018) proposed a novel approach that can be compared to the two-factor authentication used worldwide today. This approach uses an operational authority that can provide a real-time two-factor authorization for the requests made by the service provider on behalf of the pervasive user.

RF-IoT (Anil et al., 2019) was proposed by the authors to prevent different attacks in IoT-based networking environments. RF-IoT has been designed as a security framework that provides a balancing act between security and network latency. This framework can be used in various applications, like health and environment monitoring, and in smart transportation. The authors Pengfei et al. (2017) proposed a framework to transmit sensitive data like personal information and face identifiers in fog and cloud. They also ensure that the CIA (confidentiality, integrity and availability) properties are well preserved by developing a data encryption scheme, authentication and key agreement scheme to check the integrity. By this proposed framework, the security of the system is increased, but there is also a slight increase in the communication overhead (Khang & Gupta et al., 2023).

ITACS (IP Traceback Ant Colony System) (Chen et al., 2010) can identify the source of the network attacks in specific DoS attacks. The main goal of this system is to pursue the attack path. This is achieved by considering the traffic flow and time as metrics. The efficiency and the effectiveness are calculated at each phase. Roshni et al. (2017) proposed an efficient ABC algorithm to improve the security and QoS-aware scheduling in a cloud-based platform. Here, the algorithm assigns a task to an optimal VM (Virtual Machine) depending on the QoS policy and the security level of the user.

Qusay et al. (2022) used hybrid-modified bPSO (Binary Particle Swarm Optimizer) and bGWO (Binary Gray Wolf Optimization) to make improvements in Intrusion Detection Systems. There are different feature selection techniques to provide an effective classification and attack detection in an IDS. The proposed hybrid IDS technique uses benchmark datasets like UNSW-NB15 and NSL KDD'99. The system is effective in detection accuracy and reduction in false alarm rates. Patrizia et al. (2022) proposed a novel decentralized cybersecurity model for securing data in the healthcare sector. There are two types of agents, namely primary agents and supervisor agents. Primary agents are lightweight agents designed to monitor a certain space of the healthcare system, and supervisor agents protect the whole healthcare system. It is achieved by cybersecurity awareness and activating cooperative intelligence (Khang & Hahanov et al., 2022).

SFLA-QIM (Shuffled Frog Leaping Algorithm-Quantization Index Modulation) (Xia et al., 2013) watermarks images. SFLA is used to find the right position to embed, and QIM is used as a fitness function based on SNR (Signal to Noise Ratio). Using the proposed SFLA-QIM, the authors proved they could prevent attacks like noise addition, cropping, amplitude scaling, etc.

## 22.4 OVERVIEW OF THE PROPOSED WORK

This section conveys the proposed method for detecting the attack (see Figure 22.3). The IoT-23 dataset is used in the proposed method, as the datasets are yardsticks for IoT traffic and possess 20 internments of malware in IoT devices. This dataset is a collection of 500 hours of network traffic and contains 760 million packets in additional. The dataset is pre-processed, and the feature extraction will be carried out using Recursive Feature Elimination. Once the data are extracted, the proposed methodology is used to detect the attacks.

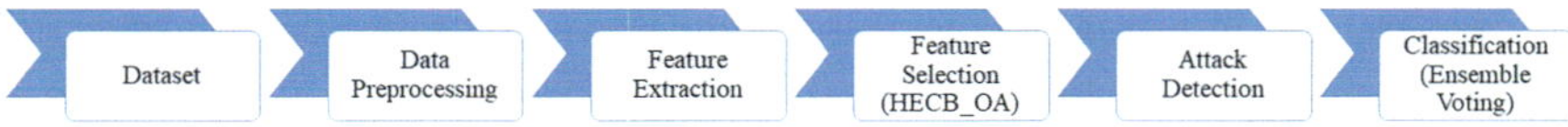


**FIGURE 22.3** Block diagram of the proposed work in detecting the attack (Khang, 2021).

### 22.4.1 Data Pre-Processing

Data pre-processing is an activity done after the input has been collected. It is the process of identifying and removing unwanted noise and eliminating the missing data from the dataset.

- **Data Cleaning**: This is an approach to identifying the incorrect and corrupt data from the datasets and removing incorrect and corrupt data found within the dataset. The missing data is handled by dropping the observations.
- **Normalization**: This is the pre-processing stage where a new range is attained from the present range. It is quite evident that data sets will contain incomplete, irrelevant and missing data. These kinds of data have to be removed to enhance the quality. The min-max algorithm will do integration and normalization activity. The normalization approach predicts the new range based on the forecasted and the predicted range. Normalization is the process of scaling the data such that the values are normalized to fall between the range of 0 and 1. The effects of variation can be eliminated by comparing with the values from more than two datasets.
- **Data Transformation**: This is a technique to convert the raw dataset into a specific format used to retrieve the data efficiently. The raw data has to be converted into a suitable format before retrieving the data. Data transformation is vital to provide patterns that make it easy to understand the strategy used in data conversion. Various transformation methods include smoothing, aggregation and generalization.
- **Data Integration**: It is one of the pre-processing approaches that combines the data from different sources and gives the user a unique view of the data. Data are collected from databases or flat files. The data received from different sources is stored in a heterogeneous database used by the client to access the files.

### 22.4.2 Recursive Feature Elimination

Feature selection is an approach that selects the most relevant features from the dataset. When a minimal number of features are present, it makes the machine learning algorithm run more efficiently. If the input features are irrelevant, it may mislead the machine learning algorithm, resulting in the worst predictive performance (Khang & Hajimahmud et al., 2023). Recursive Feature Elimination (RFE) is a feature selection algorithm. It is a completely different machine learning algorithm used in the fundamentals of the method wrapped by Recursive Feature Elimination, which helps select the features. It completely contrasts with filter-based selection as it selects the features based on the score, whatever score is the largest.

RFE tries to eliminate the weakest features from the dataset till the needed feature is obtained. It eradicates the collinearity and the dependencies found prevalent in the proposed method and keeps a specified number of features. After the extraction of the feature, it is not possible to determine how many numbers of features are valid and invalid. Cross-validation is used, with RFE using a scoring method to identify which features have the best score to determine the valid features. The RFE trains the entire system with an entire set of identified features to find the cause for the least decrement that designates the reason for stopping.

### 22.4.3 Feature Selection

The meta-heuristic algorithm is used in feature selection, which improves the rate of detecting attacks. The unselected features, identified and extracted using RFE, are not used for the classification of the attack. The meta-heuristic approach selects the appropriate features in the search space. The proposed work is created by hybridizing two bio-inspired meta-heuristic approaches (Vrushank & Khang, 2023).

### 22.4.4 Elephant Search Optimization

This algorithm (Mrutyunjaya et al., 2020) mimics the behavior of elephants when searching for food. The female elephant matriarch will lead a clan of female and baby elephants toward the food source. The matriarch is responsible for finding the food source outside the group, and the clan will do a local search nearer to the matriarch.

There are some predefined assumptions to consider based on the biological behavior of the elephants: A) every elephant has a visual range identifying other elephants that might threaten them when they are in search of food. The visibility of the elephant is calculated using Euclidean distance. The visibility range of the male elephant is higher compared to the female elephant present in the clan. B) In case the two elephants come into visual contact with each other, the fitness value of the two male elephants is calculated. Based on the calculated fitness, the elephant with the lowest fitness value will leave the territory, and the elephant with the highest fitness value will take over the clan. The weakest elephant will abscond in a random direction. C) Every elephant in the group has a maximum lifetime. After the death of an elephant, a newborn elephant will proceed to take the gender of the dead elephant. The matriarch is the elephant that leads the clan and is considered the eldest with the best fitness value, directing the clan during the food search and protecting the clan, represented using Equation 22.1.

$$MT_{best,clan} = \alpha.MT_{center,clan} \tag{22.1}$$

Where $MT_{best.clan}$ denotes the matriarch of the clan who has the best fitness value and $\alpha$ is a parameter that controls the movement, which ranges between 0 to 1, keeping the matriarch at the center of the clan using Equation 22.2.

$$MT_{center,clan,d} = \frac{1}{n_{clan}} \sum_{i=1}^{n_{clan}} MT_{center,clan,d} \tag{22.2}$$

Where d is the dimension in the total dimension Dn, $n_{clan}$ highlights the total number of elephants in the clan. The center is the average of all the present solutions obtained in the clan.

The female elephants present in the clan always follow the rules levied by the matriarch. They carry out a local search to fetch food and add more details to the matriarch of the clan. The movement of the female elephants is given by Equation 22.3.

$$FE_{new,clan,j} = FE_{clan,j} + \beta\left(FE_{best,clan} - FE_{clan,j}\right).r \tag{22.3}$$

Where $FE_{new,clan,j}$ is the new position of the female elephant j in clan and $FE_{clan,j}$ denotes the previous position of the elephant, $FE_{best,clan}$ is the best solution of the female elephant and $r$ indicates the influence of the leader in determining the best solution and the value of r ranges between 0 to 1.

The male elephants are responsible for exploring the search space during food search. The male elephant with the worst fitness value is moved in a random direction using Equation 22.4. This will happen when two male elephants come within close visibility range, and the elephant with the best fitness value will take over the clan, and the defeated male will flee from the territory.

$$MT_{worst,clan} = MT_{min}\left(MT_{max} - MT_{min}\right).ran \tag{22.4}$$

Where $MT_{max}$ & $MT_{min}$ represents the lower and upper bound of the solution and running is the number that changes randomly between 0 and 1.

### 22.4.5 Chaotic Map Bat Optimization Algorithm

This algorithm is created based on the prey-hunting behavior of bats (Liang et al., 2017) using echolocation. In nature, there are many categories of bats that are different in size and weight. But all of them possess similar characteristics during navigation and hunting their prey. Bats, when hunting prey, emit higher ultrasonic waves and decrease loudness when the prey is in close proximity.

The velocity vector of the bats is updated using Equation 22.5.

$$Vel_i\left(t+1\right) = Vel_i\left(t\right) + \left(X_i\left(t\right) - G_{best}\right) Freq_i \tag{22.5}$$

$$X_i\left(t+1\right) = X_i\left(t\right) + Vel\left(t+1\right) \tag{22.6}$$

The position vector is updated with respect to the velocity of the bat over a period of time t, which is obtained from equ.6 and $G_{best}$ is the best solution obtained for the bat i.

The frequency of the bat is determined with Equation 22.7.

$$Freq_i = Freq_{min} + \left(Freq_{max} - Freq_{min}\right)\beta \tag{22.7}$$

Where $\beta$ is a random number for uniform distribution, its value falls in the range [0, 1].

With the help of Equations 22.1–22.3, a better exploration of the food source in the search space and the best solution can be obtained.

To perform better exploration, a random walk has to be carried out to attain the global optima using Equation 22.8. Thus, the bat starts to increase the loudness emitted and starts to perform exploration instead of performing the exploitation process.

$$X_n = X_o + \varepsilon Å \tag{22.8}$$

Where $\varepsilon$ is the random number between 0 and 1 and Å tells about the loudness emitted by the bat.

The balancing of the equations is well-ordered by two factors: loudness (Å) and pulse rate (r), using Equations 22.9 and 22.10.

$$Å_i\left(t+1\right) = \alpha Å_i\left(t\right) \tag{22.9}$$

$$r_i = \left(t+1\right) = r_i\left(0\right)\left[1-\exp\left(-\gamma t\right)\right] \tag{22.10}$$

The constant $\alpha$ and $\gamma$ are the cooling factors used in simulated annealing. The simulated annealing, adapted from the physics annealing process, is suitable in situations where there is a lot of local optima where the algorithms may strike into it, and the simulated annealing is used to attain global optima. The value of loudness and pulse rate will be updated and improved over a period of time, which indicates the bats are obtaining the best solution for predicting the prey.

In the traditional Bat algorithm, the randomness can be replaced with a chaotic map because of its better properties (statistics and dynamics). The chaotic map replaces the random variables, and it is called a chaotic optimization. The chaotic maps can increase the iterative steps at a higher speed when compared with a standard probability distribution.

### 22.4.6 Hybrid Elephant and Chaotic Bat Optimization Algorithm (HECB_OA)

In this algorithm, the populations are randomly initialized in the search space. The velocity vector and frequency associated with the Chaotic Bat algorithm are used in the Elephant Algorithm Objective Function. The frequency and velocity of the elephants vary with respect to the distance of the prey. The rest of the elephant population is randomly divided into clans led by a matriarch. Every clan consists of female elephants led by a male elephant. During the food search, the matriarch will lead the clan in search of food, followed by the clan. The clan does a local search, and the matriarch does a global search in a larger search space. The position of the food source is updated over a period of time by varying the velocity and frequency. The best position of the food source is obtained. When the matriarch comes in close contact with another male elephant within the same territory, the male elephant with the best fitness value will lead the clan, and the defeated elephant will flee in a random direction (Vrushank et al., 2023; Lakshmi et al., 2023).

### 22.4.7 Ensemble Voting Classifier

The voting classifier algorithm classifies the attacks present in the dataset. The voting classifier algorithm predicts the result based on the highest probability as the algorithm trains on numerous ensemble models. This model works based on the prediction of other models. It aggregates the findings of classifiers like Random Forest and Decision Tree algorithms and predicts based on the highest voting. There are two types of voting: hard voting and soft voting.

#### 22.4.7.1 Hard Voting

In hard voting, the output is based on the highest vote that has been obtained from other classifiers. Let us consider two classifiers: a Random Forest classifier and a Decision Tree algorithm. If the Random Forest algorithm is the highest, then the Random Forest output will be the final prediction. A weighted majority vote can be computed using Equation 22.11.

$$y = \arg max_i = \sum_{n=1}^{m} w_n x_a \left(C_n\left(x\right) = i\right) \tag{22.11}$$

$x_a$ is the characteristics function and $C_n\left(x\right) = i \in A$, where A is class labels.

#### 22.4.7.2 Soft Voting

In this type, the output is based on the average of probabilities given to the class. The average of the Random Forest is computed, the average of the Decision Tree is computed and the highest average is the final output obtained. The class labels is predicted based on the probabilities p and $w_j$ is the weight assigned to the jth classifier using Equation 22.12.

$$y = \arg max_i \sum_{j=1}^{m} w_j p_{ij} \tag{22.12}$$

## 22.5 EXPERIMENTAL RESULTS

The proposed HECB_OA is carried out against the IoT 23 dataset (Jeelani et al., 2022; Sebastian et al., 2020) and analyzed using the benchmarks identified during the literature, and it is evaluated against the performance metrics. The metrics such as recall, precision, bandwidth, lifetime of devices, drop rate and detection rate have been used to evaluate the proposed work. From the results, it is inferred that the proposed work HECB_OA is found to have par excelled when compared with the benchmarks identified, as shown in Figure 22.4.

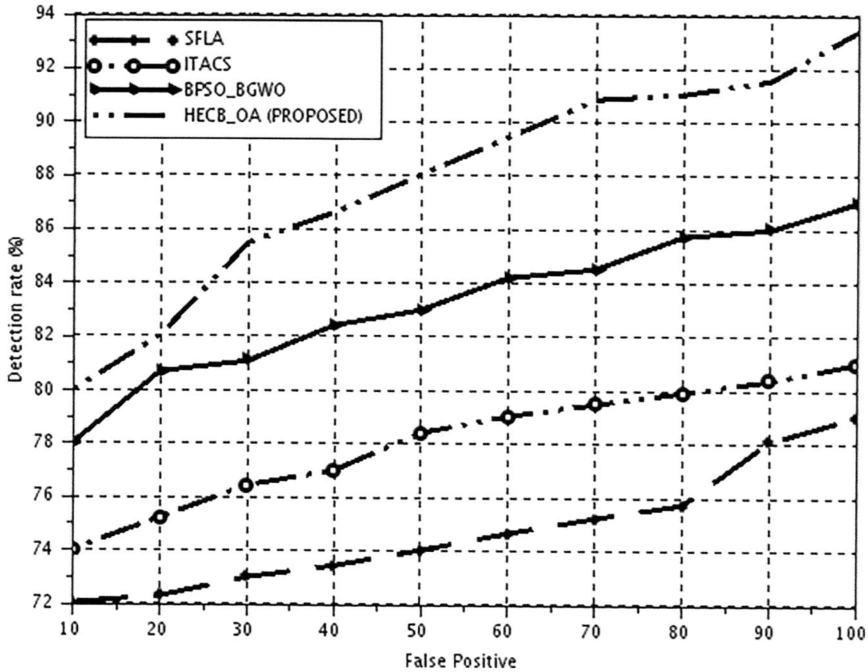


**FIGURE 22.4** False positive against detection rate.

During communication, packet drop is quite common in IoT devices. When more packet drops happen, it is hard to reconstruct the messages sent from the IoT devices. The graph in Figure 22.5 highlights the drop rate found to a minimum for HECB_OA when compared to other existing works SFLA, ITACS and BPSO_BGWO by 13%, 7% and 3%.

The bandwidth is being depleted by the attacker nodes, and it decreases the lifetime of the IoT devices. The graph portrays effective utilization of bandwidth despite the presence of attacks. The proposed HECB_OA utilized minimal bandwidth when compared to the existing works SFLA, ITACS and BPSO_BGWO by 120 mb/s, 100 mb/s and 35 mb/s at an average, as shown in Figure 22.6.

The lifetime may be depleted when attacks happen in the network, as many attacks target draining the energy level of the nodes. The proposed work HECB_OA has an improved lifetime even in the presence of attacks when compared to SFLA, ITACS and BPSO_BGWO by 270 mAh, 220 mAh, 80 mAh at an average, as shown in Figure 22.7.

The proposed work HECB_OA has a better performance when compared to SFLA, ITACS and BPSO_BGWO by 17%, 15% and 12%, as shown in Figure 22.8.

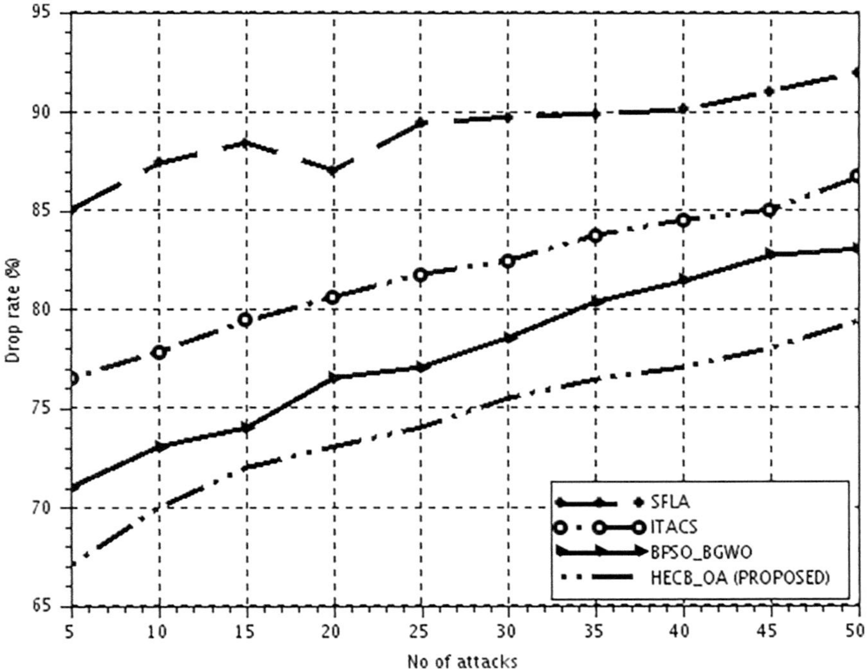


**FIGURE 22.5** Drop rate vs. number of attacks.

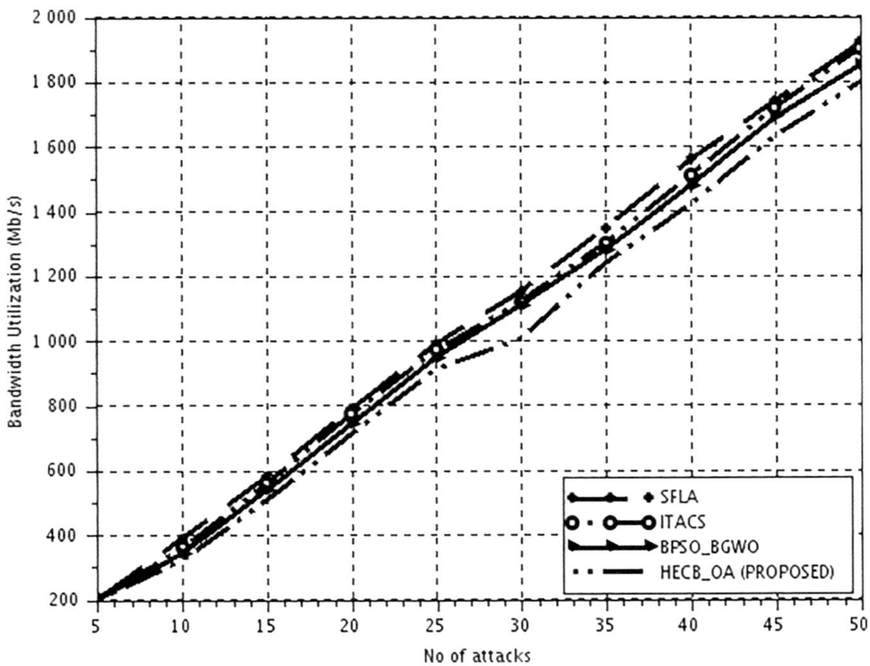


**FIGURE 22.6** Bandwidth utilization vs. number of attacks.

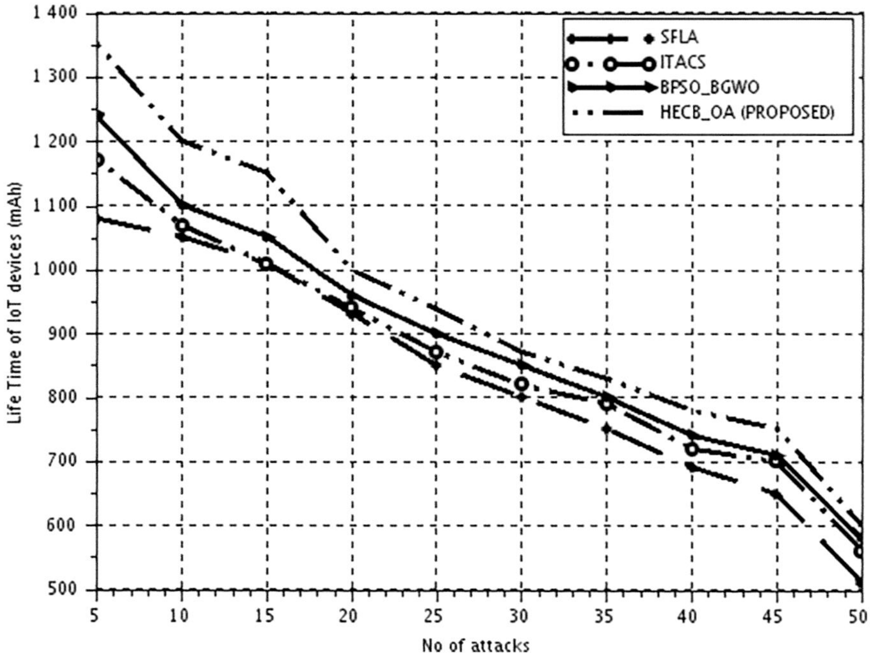


**FIGURE 22.7** Lifetime of IoT devices vs. number of attacks.

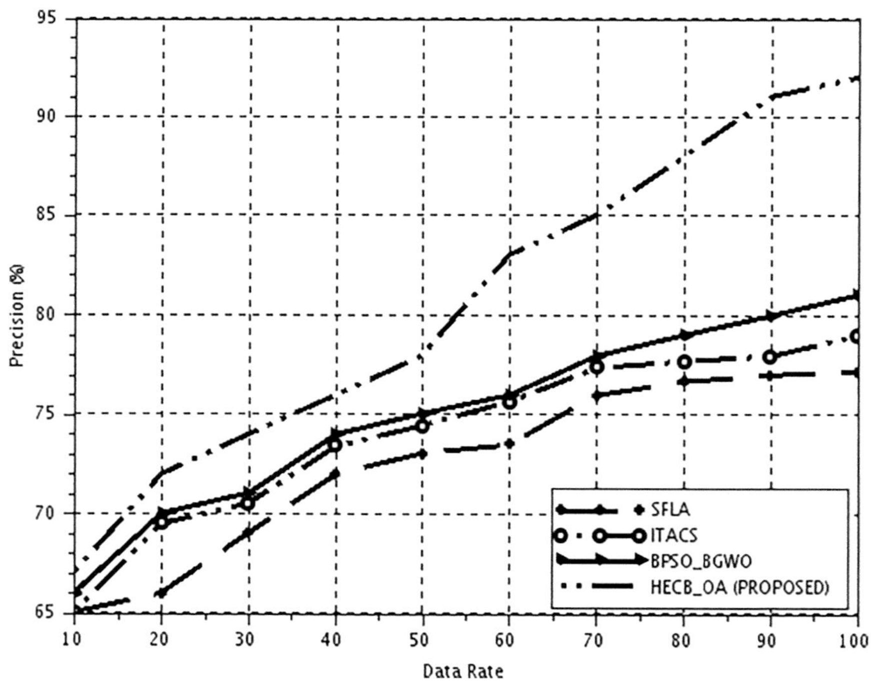


**FIGURE 22.8** Precision vs. data rate.

## 22.6 CONCLUSION

IoT consists of several physical entities like humans, devices and sensors and is used in different domains like medicine, agriculture and traffic monitoring systems. In the last decade, there has been a substantial rise in the use of IoT networks because of its several advantages in the previously mentioned domains. However, there have been several concerns regarding the robustness of the IoT Network; hence, we have proposed a novel meta-heuristics algorithm, namely HECB_OA, which makes use of the Elephant Search Optimization and Chaotic Map Bat Optimization algorithm (Mohamed et al., 2024).

The proposed algorithm HECB_OA was compared with several existing benchmark techniques like SFLA, ITACS and BPSO_BGWO in order to test the efficiency of the proposed system with metrics like false positive, drop rate, bandwidth utilization, etc. In drop rate, the proposed system was found to be 13%, 7% and 3% better when compared with SFLA, ITACS and BPSO_BGWO, respectively. In the future, different types of metaheuristic algorithms can be incorporated to increase the efficiency of our system (Ushaa & Khang, 2024).

## REFERENCES

Absalom E. Ezugwu et al., "Metaheuristics: a comprehensive overview and classification along with bibliometric analysis," Artificial Intelligence Review, Vol. 54, pp. 4237–4316, Mar. 2021. https://link.springer.com/article/10.1007/s10462-020-09952-0

Adam Trendowicz et al, "User experience key performance indicators for industrial IoT systems: A multivocal literature review," Digital Business, Vol.3, Issue 1, June 2023. www.sciencedirect.com/science/article/pii/S2666954423000054

Amuthan A. and R. Kaviarasan, "Weighted inertia-based dynamic virtual bat algorithm to detect NLOS nodes for reliable data dissemination in VANETs," Journal of Ambient Intelligence and Humanized Computing, Vol.10, Issue 11, Nov. 2018. https://link.springer.com/article/10.1007/s12652-018-1145-0

Anil G. N., "RF-IoT: A robust framework to optimize internet of things (IoT) security performance," Software Engineering Methods in Intelligent Algorithms, May 2019. https://link.springer.com/chapter/10.1007/978-3-030-19807-7_21

Apostolos Gerodimos, Leandros Maglaras, Mohamed Amine Ferrag, Nick Ayres, Ioanna Kantzavelou, "IoT: Communication Protocols and Security Threats," Internet of Things and Cyber-Physical Systems, Vol. 3, 2023. https://doi.org/10.1201/9781003434269

Baskoro Azis et al, "IoT Human Needs Inside Compact House," Journal of Open Innovation: Technology, Market, and Complexity, Vol. 9, Mar. 2023. www.sciencedirect.com/science/article/pii/S2199853123000033

Berkay Celik Z., Gang Tan, and Patrick McDaniel, "IOTGUARD: Dynamic Enforcement of Security and Safety Policy in Commodity IoT," Proceedings 2019 Network and Distributed System Security Symposium, Feb 2019. https://cs.uwaterloo.ca/~yaafer/teaching/papers/ndss2019_07A-1_Celik_paper.pdf

Chen H. -H. and W. Yang, "The Design and Implementation of a Practical Meta-Heuristic for the Detection and Identification of Denial-of-Service Attack Using Hybrid Approach," 2010 Second International Conference on Machine Learning and Computing, May 2010. https://ieeexplore.ieee.org/abstract/document/5460692/

Chris M, "Understanding the Threats to DNS and How to Secure It," Network Security, Vol. 2015, Issue 10, Pages 8–10, Oct. 2015. www.sciencedirect.com/science/article/pii/S1353485815300908

Hahanov V., Khang A., E Litvinova, S Chumachenko, Hajimahmud V. A., Alyar V. A., "The Key Assistant of Smart City—Sensors and Tools," *AI-Centric Smart City Ecosystems: Technologies, Design and Implementation* (1st ed.), 17 (10), (2022). CRC Press. https://doi.org/10.1201/9781003252542-17

Haixia W. et al., "Anti-Spoofing Study on Palm Biometric Features," Expert Systems with Applications, Vol. 218, May 2023. www.sciencedirect.com/science/article/pii/S0957417423000477

Hussain F. et al., "A Two-Fold Machine Learning Approach to Prevent and Detect IoT Botnet Attacks," IEEE Access, vol. 9, pp. 163412–163430, Nov. 2021. https://ieeexplore.ieee.org/abstract/document/9627657/

Jeelani F., D. S. Rai, A. Maithani and S. Gupta, "The Detection of IoT Botnet using Machine Learning on IoT-23 Dataset," 2nd International Conference on Innovative Practices in Technology and Management (ICIPTM), Pp. 634–639, April 2022. https://ieeexplore.ieee.org/abstract/document/9754187/

Jesús E. Díaz-Verdejo, Rafael Estepa Alonso, Antonio Estepa Alonso, German Madinabeitia, "A critical review of the techniques used for anomaly detection of HTTP-based attacks: taxonomy, limitations and open challenges," Computers & Security, Vol. 124, Jan. 2023. www.sciencedirect.com/science/article/pii/S0167404822003893

Khang A. (2021). "Material4Studies," *Material of Computer Science, Artificial Intelligence, Data Science, IoT, Blockchain, Cloud, Metaverse, Cybersecurity for Studies*. Retrieved from www.researchgate.net/publication/370156102_Material4Studies

Khang A., Gupta S. K., Rani S., D. A. Karras, Smart Cities: IoT Technologies, Big Data Solutions, Cloud Platforms, and Cybersecurity Techniques. (Eds.) (2023). CRC Press. https://doi.org/10.1201/9781003376064

Khang A., Hahanov V., Abbas G. L., Hajimahmud V. A., "Cyber-Physical-Social System and İncident Management," *AI-Centric Smart City Ecosystems: Technologies, Design and Implementation* (1st Ed.), 2 (15), (2022). CRC Press. https://doi.org/10.1201/9781003252542-2

Khang A., Hajimahmud V. A., Gupta S. K., Babasaheb J., Morris G., AI-Centric Modelling and Analytics: Concepts, Designs, Technologies, and Applications. (1 Ed.) (2023). CRC Press. https://doi.org/10.1201/9781003400110

Khang A., Misra A., Gupta S. K., Shah V., AI-aided IoT Technologies and Applications in the Smart Business and Production. (Eds.) (2023). CRC Press. https://doi.org/10.1201/9781003392224

Khang A., Vugar Abdullayev, Vladimir Hahanov, Vrushank Shah, Advanced IoT Technologies and Applications in the Industry 4.0 Digital Economy (1 Ed.) (2024). CRC Press. https://doi.org/10.1201/9781003434269

Lakshmi Haritha Medida, Kumar G.L.N.V.S., Khang A., "*Predictive Analytics for High-tech Agriculture*" Advanced Technologies and AI-Equipped IoT Applications in High-Tech Agriculture (1st Ed.). Page: 336–346. (2023). IGI Global Press. https://doi.org/10.4018/978-1-6684-9231-4.ch019

Liang H., Y. Liu, Y. Shen and F. Li, "A multiobjective chaotic bat algorithm for economic and emission dispatch," 2017 Chinese Automation Congress, Pp. 4684–4689, Oct. 2017. https://ieeexplore.ieee.org/abstract/document/8243606/

Mohamed N., Khang A., "Applications of Internet of Things (IoT) in Smart Cities," *Advanced IoT Technologies and Applications in the Industry 4.0 Digital Economy* (1 Ed.) (2024). CRC Press. https://doi.org/10.1201/9781003434269-6

Mrutyunjaya P, "Elephant Search Optimization Combined with Deep Neural Network for Microarray Data Analysis," Journal of King Saud University—Computer and Information Sciences, Vol. 32, Issue 8, Pp. 940–948, Oct. 2020. www.sciencedirect.com/science/article/pii/S1319157817302112

Murillo M.J., "A Two-Factor Authorization Approach for Increasing the Resiliency of IoT-Based Autonomous Consumer-Oriented Systems," IEEE Internet of Things Journal, Vol. 5, Issue 5, pp. 4132–4141, Oct.2018. https://ieeexplore.ieee.org/abstract/document/8480630/

Othmane Friha et al., "FELIDS: Federated learning-based intrusion detection system for agricultural Internet of Things," Journal of Parallel and Distributed Computing, Vol. 165, Pp. 17–31, Jul. 2022. www.sciencedirect.com/science/article/pii/S0743731522000570

Padmalaya N., G. Swapna, "Security issues in IoT Applications Using Certificateless Aggregate Signcryption Schemes: An Overview," Internet of Things, Vol.21, Apr. 2023. www.sciencedirect.com/science/article/pii/S2542660522001226

Patrizia Ribino, Mario Ciampi, Shareeful Islam and Spyridon Papastergiou, "Swarm Intelligence Model for Securing Healthcare Ecosystem," Procedia Computer Science, Vol. 210, Pages 149–156, Nov.2022. www.sciencedirect.com/science/article/pii/S1877050922015885

Pengfei Hu et al., "Security and Privacy Preservation Scheme of Face Identification and Resolution Framework Using Fog Computing in Internet of Things," IEEE Internet of Things, Vol. 4, Issue. 5, Oct. 2017. https://ieeexplore.ieee.org/abstract/document/7835115/

Pillutla H., A. Arjunan, "A Survey of Security Concerns, Mechanisms and Testing in Cloud Environment," 2018 Second International Conference on Electronics, Communication and Aerospace Technology (ICECA), pp. 1519–1524, Sept.2018. https://ieeexplore.ieee.org/abstract/document/8474855/

Pillutla Harikrishna and A. Amuthan, "Rival-Model Penalized Self-Organizing Map enforced DDoS attack prevention mechanism for software defined network-based cloud computing environment," Journal of Parallel and Distributed Computing, Vol. 154, Pp. 142–152, Aug. 2021. www.sciencedirect.com/science/article/pii/S0743731521000587

Qusay M Alzubi et al., "Intrusion detection system based on hybridizing a modified binary grey wolf optimization and particle swarm optimization," Expert Systems with Applications, Vol. 204, Oct. 2022. www.sciencedirect.com/science/article/pii/S0957417422009095

Rani S., Chauhan M., Kataria A, Khang A., "IoT Equipped Intelligent Distributed Framework for Smart Healthcare Systems," *Networking and Internet Architecture*, (Eds.). Vol.2, p: 30. (2021). https://doi.org/10.48550/arXiv.2110.04997

Rath, K. C., Khang A., Debanik Roy, "The Role of Internet of Things (IoT) Technology in Industry 4.0," *Advanced IoT Technologies and Applications in the Industry 4.0 Digital Economy* (1 Ed.) (2024). CRC Press. https://doi.org/10.1201/9781003434269-1

Roshni Thanka M., P. Uma Maheswari and E. Bijolin Edwin, "An improved efficient: Artificial Bee Colony algorithm for security and QoS aware scheduling in cloud computing environment," Cluster Computing, Vol.22, Issue. S5, pp. 10905–10913, Oct. 2017. https://link.springer.com/article/10.1007/s10586-017-1223-7

Sebastian Garcia, Agustin Parmisano, & Maria Jose Erquiaga. (2020). IoT-23: A labeled dataset with malicious and benign IoT network traffic (Version 1.0.0) [Data set]. 623–634. https://essay.utwente.nl/81979/

Sherali Zeadally, Faisal Karim Shaikh, Anum Talpur, Quan Z. Sheng, "Design architectures for energy harvesting in the Internet of Things," Renewable and Sustainable Energy Reviews, Vol. 128, Aug. 2020. www.sciencedirect.com/science/article/pii/S136403212030188X

Simon Birnbach, Simon Eberz and Ivan Martinovic, "Peeves: Physical Event Verification in Smart Homes," ACM SIGSAC Conference on Computer and Communications Security, Nov. 2019. https://ora.ox.ac.uk/objects/uuid:75726ff7-fee1-420d-8a17-de9572324c7d

Sreeja N.K., "A hierarchical heterogeneous ant colony optimization based fingerprint recognition system," Intelligent Systems with Applications, Vol.17, Feb. 2023. www.sciencedirect.com/science/article/pii/S2667305323000054

Ushaa Eswaran, Khang A., "Application of Internet of Things (IoT) and Sensors Technologies for Agriculture," *Advanced IoT Technologies and Applications in the Industry 4.0 Digital Economy* (1 Ed.) (2024). CRC Press. https://doi.org/10.1201/9781003434269-8

Vijayakumar M. & T. S. Shiny Angel, "A Survey on IoT Security: Security Threads and Analysis of Botnet Attacks Over IoT and Avoidance," Lecture Notes in Networks and Systems, Vol.370, May 2022. https://link.springer.com/chapter/10.1007/978-981-16-8664-1_13

Vipul Moudgil, Kasun Hewage, Syed Asad Hussain, Rehan Sadiq, "Integration of IoT in building energy infrastructure: A critical review on challenges and solutions," Renewable and

Sustainable Energy Reviews, Vol. 174, Mar. 2023. www.sciencedirect.com/science/article/pii/S1364032122010024

Vrushank Shah, Khang A., "Metaverse-Enabling IoT Technology for a Futuristic Healthcare System," *AI-Based Technologies and Applications in the Era of the Metaverse*. (1 Ed.) (2023). P (1). IGI Global Press. https://doi.org/10.4018/978-1-6684-8851-5.ch008

Vrushank Shah, Khang A., "Metaverse-Enabling IoT Technology for a Futuristic Healthcare System," *AI-Based Technologies and Applications in the Era of the Metaverse*. (1 Ed.) (2023). Page (165–173). IGI Global Press. https://doi.org/10.4018/978-1-6684-8851-5.ch008

Vuk Lesi, Zivana Jakovljevic and Miroslav Pajic, "Security Analysis for Distributed IoT-Based Industrial Automation," IEEE Transactions on Automation Science and Engineering, vol. 19, no. 4, pp. 3093–3108, Oct. 2022. https://ieeexplore.ieee.org/abstract/document/9528498/

Wenbo Ding, Hongxin Hu and Long Cheng, "IOTSAFE: Enforcing Safety and Security Policy with Real IoT Physical Interaction Discovery," Network and Distributed System Security Symposium, Feb.2021. https://par.nsf.gov/servlets/purl/10399983

Xia Li, Lingjun Liu, Na Wang and Jeng-Shyang Pan, "A New Robust Watermarhing Scheme Based on Shuffled Frog Leaping Algorithm," Intelligent Automation & Soft Computing, Vol. 17, 2011, Issue 2, Mar. 2013. www.tandfonline.com/doi/abs/10.1080/10798587.2011.10643144

Yuan Tian et al., "SmartAuth: User-Centered Authorization for the Internet of Things," 26th USENIX Security Symposium, Aug.2017. www.usenix.org/conference/usenixsecurity17/technical-sessions/presentation/tian

Yusuf Alaca and Yüksel Çelik, "Cyber-attack detection with QR code images using lightweight deep learning models," Computers & Security, Vol.126, Mar. 2023. www.sciencedirect.com/science/article/pii/S0167404822004576

Zhongqiang Ma et al., "Performance assessment and exhaustive listing of 500+ nature-inspired metaheuristic algorithms," Swarm and Evolutionary Computation, Vol. 77, Mar. 2023. www.sciencedirect.com/science/article/pii/S2210650223000226

# 23 Internet of Things (IoT)-Based Technologies for Reliability Evaluation with Artificial Intelligence (AI)

*Khushwant Singh, Yudhvir Singh, Alex Khang, Dheerdhwaj Barak, and Mohit Yadav*

## 23.1 INTRODUCTION

IoT-based technology has provided the globe with a greater degree of accessibility, integrity, availability, scalability, secrecy, and interoperability in terms of device connection. IoTs, on the other hand, lack security rules given criteria and are thus susceptible to attacks due to a combination of different attack surfaces and their youth. Attackers may employ a wide variety of cyber-attacks on IoTs, depending on which part of the system they are targeting and what they want to achieve from the assault. As a consequence, much research has been conducted on cyber security concerning IoT, as discussed by Chetna et al. (2022) and Mustafa and Shaikh (2021). It involves the integration of Artificial Intelligence (AI) techniques to protect Internet of Things (IoT) systems against attackers, which mainly includes spotting unusual activity that can point to an attack.

While cyber security experts must safeguard several targets, cyber-attacks always have the upper hand when it comes to IoT since they only need to find one vulnerability (Vrushank & Vidhi et al., 2023). Cyber-attackers increasingly use AI to circumvent the complex algorithms that identify anomalous behavior and let it go undetected. With the growth of IoT technology, AI has received a lot of attention during the past few decades. IoT plays a key role in various sectors, such as the healthcare sector, as analyzed by Aghdam et al. (2021) and Asghari et al. (2019). Khan et al. (2021), Azari and Abbasi (2020), and Kim et al. (2022) investigate the various challenges involved in reliable IoT, as shown in Figure 23.1.

An AI-based control approach for identifying, assessing, managing, and mitigating cyber hazards in industrial IoT systems has been discussed by various researchers in the past few decades. To deliver reliable ubiquitous detection for IoT environments, the researchers build a variety of adversarial strategies and defensive mechanisms. They then assess their methodology using datasets including MNIST, CIFAR-10, and

DOI: 10.1201/9781032686745-23

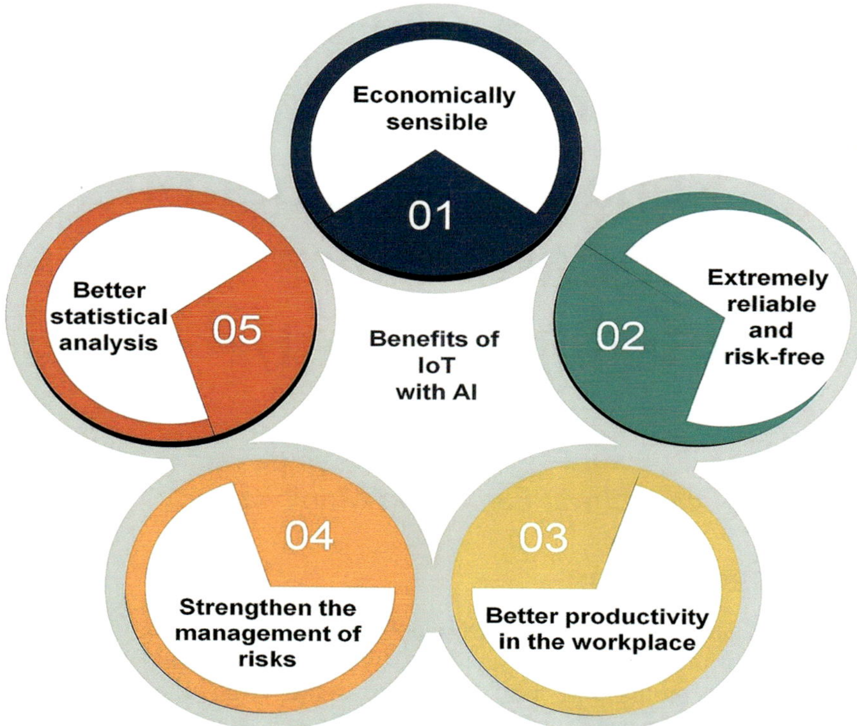
Economically sensible
01
Extremely reliable and risk-free
02
Better productivity in the workplace
03
Strengthen the management of risks
04
Better statistical analysis
05
Benefits of IoT with AI

**FIGURE 23.1** Benefits of the Internet of Things (IoT) with artificial intelligence (AI).

SVHN. Many researchers analyze the most recent evolution of AI decision-making in cyber-physical systems and conclude that this evolution is almost entirely autonomous as a result of the growing integration of IoT devices in cyber-physical systems. It has been concluded that the value of AI decision-making because of its speed and efficiency in handling large amounts of data will almost certainly make this evolution inevitable. A cutting-edge method for AI and machine learning-based risk analyses, with an emphasis on IoT networks in commercial settings, has been discussed.

To standardize these procedures, a method for figuring out and assessing cyber security hazards related to IoT devices. To more effectively identify and manage risk in IoT systems. Gao et al. (2021) examined the various critical applications of AI. The main application of AI focuses on anomaly detection. Prompt detection allows for rapid response and mitigation. By analyzing data from IoT devices, AI models provide insights, recommendations, and predictions to aid operators and decision-makers. This enables proactive actions to prevent failures or address reliability issues. In conclusion, integrating AI and IoT offers significant potential for improving reliability evaluation techniques (Anh et al., 2024).

By leveraging AI's capabilities, IoT systems can become more reliable, efficient, and secure, improving performance and user satisfaction. As a result of this increase,

IoT cyber security apps have started to use AI technologies, including decision trees, linear regression, machine learning, support vector machines, and neural networks, to detect threats and possible attacks. A comparison of IoT technologies in terms of resilience, self-organization, access control, anonymity, confidentiality, and privacy has been done (Khang & Hahanov et al., 2022).

Barak et al. (2020) provide a thorough analysis of the security risks posed by IoT applications and workable mitigation strategies. The authors provide deep learning models with a high accuracy of 97.16 percent for detecting DDoS attacks in IoT (Internet of Things) cyber security. Artificial Neural Networks (ANN) are tested in a gateway device by the authors to see whether they can identify abnormalities in data coming from edge devices. The results demonstrate that the suggested strategy may improve IoT system security. Singh et al. (2023), Yadav et al. (2022) have analyzed the various modeling, optimization, and evaluation-based techniques for various parameters for assessing the reliability of Internet of Things (IoT) technologies.

The current research addresses a range of subjects connected to cyber security and the Internet of Things (IoT), including Artificial Intelligence (AI), as well as how they all relate to one another in three survey-style parts. Additionally, it offers a thorough analysis of assaults on IoT devices and suggests AI-based defenses against them. This report's main goal is to link relevant articles that address different aspects of these concerns and summarize them to serve as a resource for persons who are researching these frequent problems. The rest of the paper contains the reviews of the extant literature, various machine learning models, evaluation for the classification of the model, result discussion, and conclusion.

## 23.2 LITERATURE REVIEW

In the past few decades, various techniques and methodologies based on the IoT have been developed by various researchers, which shows how this area has grown, as shown in Table 23.1.

## 23.3 MACHINE LEARNING MODEL

Various machine learning models have been developed by various scientists depending upon the needs of the modern era. Some of the important key models, such as SVM, RF, and K-Nearest Neighbor are explained in a concise way in what follows.

### 23.3.1 Support Vector Machine (SVM)

As there is no knowledge of the underlying joint probabilities functions, all that is accessible is a training set; one must undertake distribution-less learning procedures. SVMs are called "non-parametric" models; this is not because their model contains no parameters at all, but unlike classical statistics, the parameter is not pre-defined, and its number depends on the training data used. In other words, the model's capabilities are matched to the complexity of the data by the parameters, which are driven by the data. This is the fundamental paradigm for structural risk reduction that advocates facilitating the discovery of a novel algorithm. There are two primary

**TABLE 23.1**
**The Literature Summary of the Integration of IoT-Based Technologies with AI by Various Researchers**

| Year | Author's Name | Research Title | Proposed Work/Future Scope |
|---|---|---|---|
| 2021 | Iwendi and Rehman et al. | Sustainable Security for the Internet of Things Using Artificial Intelligence Architectures | A deep learning methodology for detecting cyber-attacks on the Internet of Things using a Long Short Term Networks classifier, which was better than other state-of-the-art models in detecting cyber-attacks with proficiency. |
| 2021 | Mustafa and Shaikh | Aspects of Security for Accelerating Artificial Intelligence Inside Internet of Things Centric Distributed Storage Network | Deep learning technologies that are already in use in IoT contexts cannot assign and compute tasks reasonably, which leads to resource waste. |
| 2020 | Moore and Nugent et al. | IoT reliability: a review leading to five key research directions | Quantifies dependability in the IoT, highlighting the many difficulties involved in this job. Several important research objectives for IoT have been used. |
| 2020 | Lyu and Yin et al. | Internet of Things transmission and network reliability in the complex environment | Investigation of the effect of a new communication connection on the mobile node's network capacity for future work and research. |
| 2018 | Mo and Xing et al. | Reliability Analysis of IoT Networks with Community Structures | The suggested ordering heuristics outperform the conventional ordering heuristics in terms of model complexity via extensive trials. |

constructive methods for developing a model with excellent generalization properties. The training error (i.e., empirical risk) is reduced by preserving the estimated error (interval of confidence or sometimes known as the variance of the model) and using a suitable framework of the model (order of polynomials, the number of neurons HL, and number of regulations in the fuzzy logic model).

SVM helps to minimize the confidence interval and keep the value of the confidence interval stable (equal to zero or equal to a particular acceptable amount). An SVM creates a hyperplane that divides the input points and maximizes the margin m between the classes in this space. After the first mapping, the input points to a higher-dimensional feature space (if the input points are in R2, the SVM transfers them to R3). The goal of SVM is to produce a model (based on the training data) that predicts the objective values of the test data, given only the test data attributes. Given a training set of, for instance, label pairs, support vector machines require the solution of the optimization problem. Searching for the best separator field with the addition of the variable i is often called a soft margin hyperplane. Reliability measures how well a model's behavior can be described in terms of human behavior, considering both the outcome and the full decision-making process. Explaining the data utilized, how the findings are achieved, how the inputs impact the outputs, and how the system intends to affect the persons involved are all included in this. As a result, reliability may be considered a more expansive term than interpretability with a more ambitious goal.

### 23.3.2 Random Forest (RF)

The optimum split is determined by comparing all potential predictors in this subsample and all potential cutoffs based on their capacity to reduce the residual sum of squares for the resultant tree. The trees that make up the random forest often grow entirely and are not trimmed unless a minimum number of observations are met at a particular node. We do certainly acquire these K trees by constructing them K function estimators f(h1,h2, . . . . . hk). The average of these individual estimators is calculated with the help of Random Forest.

The process description makes it evident that three parameters must have values established before random pruning development can occur. These three parameters are the number of cultivated trees, the size of the node, and the number of randomly picked variables in each division. They each regulate one part of the randomness inside the tree, the size of the forest, and the size of each tree. Although certain default settings have been recommended following empirical research on different datasets, the best default values for the particular dataset under investigation may be chosen using an optimization-fit technique for prediction performance (Khang, 2024).

### 23.3.3 k-Nearest Neighbor (kNN)

The basic implementation of kNN for classification problems is to calculate the distance between a query and each of the objects in the set of training (i.e., database) to obtain the neighborhood formed by the k nearest objects and assign the most repeated class in the neighborhood to the query. The kNN algorithm needs to store the entire training set, and learning needs to read the stored data without needing to do any processing on them. In addition, for its implementation, the data does not need to be linearly separable, nor do we know the distribution of the data in general. These characteristics make it very simple and widely used.

The kNN algorithm is illustrated where we have, as an example, a value of $k = 3$ in a two-class classification problem with two-dimensional data (x1 and x2). In the example, the decision for q1 is made directly because all its neighbors are of class 1, so q1 is also of class 1. On the other hand, for q2, there is one neighbor of class 1 and two neighbors of class 2, for which a rule to decide which class to assign to the query q2. This case can be solved with a simple majority rule, which would assign q2 class 2 or a rule that adds weights to the distances to give greater influence to the closer neighbors. To use the kNN classifier, it is necessary to have a distance measure that compares the stored examples with the queries to classify. Since, in most cases, the data is represented by vectors in a multidimensional space, a training set X is assumed to be made up of $(x_i) \in [1,n]$ training examples (where $n = |D|$). The Training vectors o examples are described by a set of F features that equal the number of

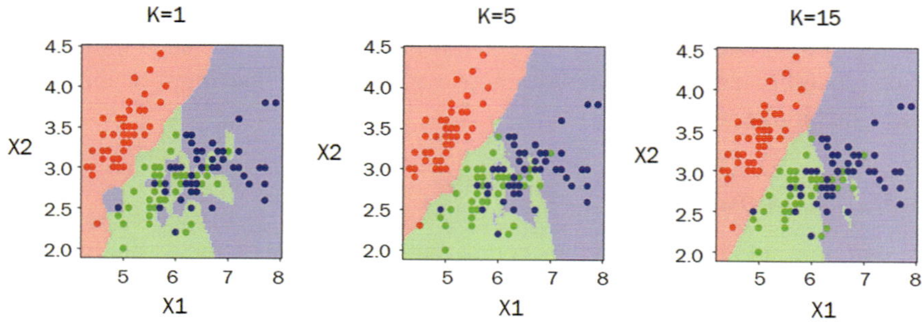


**FIGURE 23.2** Effect of the choice of k.

dimensions. Each example is classified with the label $yj \in Y$. The goal is to classify the unknown example q. For each $xi \in X$, the distance between q and xi has been shown in the equation. With this function, there is a sum over all the characteristics F with weight wf for each characteristic.

Finally, in addition to the distance function used to define the closeness or similarity between two objects, the performance of kNN crucially depends on the size of the neighborhood defined by the hyperparameter k. The selection of the optimal value of k is a particularly difficult task. A small value typically results in very noise-sensitive decision boundaries, while a large value produces a noise-robust neighborhood likely to include many neighbors of other classes, as shown in Figure 23.2. Usually, a balance is sought between both cases. There is an optimal k for each distribution of the data, but it is not possible to know it since it would be necessary to know the label of the query, which is tautological. For these reasons, many methods have been proposed to find good values for k, which, despite being effective, increase the overall complexity of the algorithm.

## 23.4 EVALUATION OF CLASSIFICATION MODELS

### 23.4.1 Recall

Also known as sensitivity (although it is more common to find it as recall in the literature of any language), recall is the number of true positives relative to the number of true positives and false negatives. The recall allows us to know how successful the classifier is in predicting positive cases.

### 23.4.2 Scope or Sensitivity

Scope or sensitivity determines whether the fraction of positive cases is correctly classified or not. It has been classified into two parts: false-positive ratio and false-negative ratio. The false-positive ratio is the percentage of negative cases erroneously classified as positive, while the false-negative ratio is the proportion of positive cases erroneously classified as negative.

### 23.4.3 Area under Curve (AUROC)

The area under the curve actually refers to the area under the receiver operating characteristic curve (AUROC). This is obtained from the graph where the vertical axis contains the recall and on the horizontal axis the rate of classified positive examples erroneously as such, as the decision threshold for the classifier varies. Note that, for this reason, the metric cannot be used with classifiers in which its exit is not a probability.

In this way, you have a vision of how it affects the ability of the model to classify examples correctly when the threshold of decision. This curve is expected to be steep, regardless of the value. The chosen model performs well. One of the benefits of using this metric is that the bias that can induce the choice of the value for the threshold is removed. It is a graphical representation of the relationship between the true positive and false positive ratios of the classifier. As pointed out, the area under the ROC curve (AUC) provides an approach to assess which model is better on average. If the model is perfect, then its AUC would be equal to 1. If the model is random, its AUC would be equal to 0.5.

### 23.4.4 F-Measure/Score

F-Measure/Score is a metric that unifies precision and recalls. F-Score, commonly referred to as the F1-Score, is a metric that combines accuracy and recall. By itself, it does not have a relevant interpretation, but it is generally used to compare the overall performance of various predictive models. It is calculated as Equation 23.1:

$$F\text{-}Score = 2 * \left\{ \frac{(Precision * Recall)}{(Precision + Recall)} \right\} \quad (23.1).$$

## 23.5 CONCLUSION

AI's role in fault diagnosis assists in identifying the root causes of failures in IoT systems. By analyzing historical data and leveraging machine learning algorithms, AI models can identify patterns associated with specific failure modes. This knowledge enables targeted troubleshooting and remediation, improving system reliability and minimizing disruptions. Anomaly detection powered by AI algorithms helps identify abnormal behavior in IoT data streams, enabling the rapid detection and mitigation of failures or cyber-attacks. By establishing baseline patterns and continuously monitoring sensor data, AI models can detect deviations and trigger appropriate responses to maintain system reliability (Khang, 2023).

Adaptive control and optimization of IoT systems using AI algorithms ensure that the system operates within safe and reliable limits. By continuously analyzing sensor data, AI models can adapt system parameters and configurations in real-time, minimizing the risk of failures or performance degradation and maintaining system reliability. Finally, AI serves as a decision support system in IoT environments by analyzing data from IoT devices and providing insights, recommendations, and predictions. This empowers operators and decision-makers to proactively prevent failures or address reliability issues, improving overall system performance (Khang & Abdullayev et al., 2024).

## REFERENCES

Amin Azari, Abbasi M., "Reliability and Battery Lifetime Improvement for Iot Networks: Challenges and AI-Powered Solutions," *arXiv Preprint*, 2008. P: 01414, (2020). https://doi.org/10.48550/arXiv.2008.01414

Anh P. T. N., Vladimir Hahanov, Triwiyanto, Ragimova Nazila Ali, Rashad İsmibeyli, Vugar Abdullayev, Abuzarova Vusala Alyar. "AI Models for Disease Diagnosis and Prediction of Heart Disease with Artificial Neural Networks," *Computer Vision and AI-integrated IoT Technologies in Medical Ecosystem*. (1 Ed.) (2024). CRC Press. https://doi.org/10.1201/9781003429609-9

Barak Dheer Dhwaz, Kushwant Singh, Prashant Ahlawat Hitesh Kumar Sharma, "Real Time Tracking System: An IoT Based Application," In 5th International Conference on Next Generation Computing Technologies (NGCT-2019), (2020). https://dx.doi.org/10.2139/ssrn.3545226

Celestine Iwendi, Rehman, S. U., Abdul Rehman Javed, Suleman Khan, Gautam Srivastava, "Sustainable Security for the Internet of Things Using Artificial Intelligence Architectures," *ACM Transactions on Internet Technology (TOIT)* Vol. 21, No. 3, P: 1–22, (2021). https://doi.org/10.1145/3448614

Chetna Vaid Kwatra, Jain, A., Angelina Royappa, Susama Bagchi, SBG Tilak Babu, Harish Chowdhary, "Artificial Intelligence Application for Security Issues and Challenges in IoT " In 2022 5th International Conference on Contemporary Computing and Informatics (IC3I), pp. 2100–2104. IEEE, (2022), https://doi.org/10.1109/IC3I56241.2022.10072808

Dong-Seong Kim, Hoa, T. D., Huynh-The Thien "On the Reliability of Industrial Internet of Things from Systematic Perspectives: Evaluation Approaches, Challenges, and Open Issues," *IETE Technical Review* Vol. 39, No. 6, P: 1277–1308, (2022). https://doi.org/10.1080/02564602.2022.2028586

Fawad Mustafa, Shaikh, M. H., "Aspects of Security for Accelerating Artificial Intelligence inside Internet of Things Centric Distributed Storage Network," 2021 6th International Multi-Topic ICT Conference (IMTIC). IEEE, (2021). https://doi.org/10.1109/IMTIC53841.2021.9719866

Khang A. *AI and IoT Technology and Applications for Smart Healthcare Systems*. Taylor and Francis Group, CRC Press, (2024). HBK: 9781032684901. PBK: 9781032679648 EBK: 9781032686745. https://doi.org/10.1201/9781032686745

Khang A., Abdullayev V. A., Olena Hrybiuk, Arvind Kumar Shukla. *Computer Vision and AI-integrated IoT Technologies in Medical Ecosystem*. (1 Ed.) (2024). CRC Press. https://doi.org/10.1201/9781003429609

Khang A., Hahanov V., Abbas G. L., Hajimahmud V. A., "Cyber-Physical-Social System and İncident Management," *AI-Centric Smart City Ecosystems: Technologies, Design and Implementation* (1st Ed., vol. 2, p. 15), (2022). CRC Press. https://doi.org/10.1201/9781003252542-2

Mohammad Zubair Khan, Alhazmi O. H., Muhammad Awais Javed, Hamza Ghandorh, Khalid S. Aloufi, "Reliable Internet of Things: Challenges and future trends," *Electronics*, Vol. 10, No. 19, P: 2377, (2021). https://doi.org/10.3390/electronics10192377

Mohit Yadav, Kumar, S., Ashish Kaushik, Deepak Chhabra, "Piezo-beam structure in a pipe with turbulent flow as energy harvester: mathematical modeling and simulation," *Journal of The Institution of Engineers (India): Series D*, P: 1–14, (2022). https://doi.org/10.1007/s40033-022-00440-z

Parvaneh Asghari, Rahmani, A. M., Hamid Haj Seyyed Javadi, "Internet of Things applications: A systematic review," *Computer Networks*, Vol. 148, P: 241–261, (2019). https://doi.org/10.1016/j.comnet.2018.12.008

Moore S. J., Nugent, C. D., Zhang, S., Cleland, I., "IoT reliability: a review leading to 5 key research directions," *CCF Transactions on Pervasive Computing and Interaction*, Vol. 2, P: 147–163, (2020). https://doi.org/10.1007/s42486-020-00037-z

Singh K., Singh, Y., Barak, D., Yadav, M., "Comparative Performance Analysis and Evaluation of Novel Techniques in Reliability for Internet of Things with RSM," *International Journal of Intelligent Systems and Applications in Engineering* Vol. 11, No. 9s, P: 330–341, (2023). www.ijisae.org/index.php/IJISAE/article/view/3123

Upinder Kaur, Manjit Kaur, Khang A., "*Futuristic Technologies in Agriculture Challenges and Future Prospects*." Advanced Technologies and AI-Equipped IoT Applications in High-Tech Agriculture (1st Ed.). Page: 347–364. (2023). IGI Global Press. https://doi.org/10.4018/978-1-6684-9231-4.ch020

Vineeta S. Chauhan, Jaydeep Chakravorty, Khang A., "Smart Cities Data Indicator-Based Cyber Threats Detection Using Bio-Inspired Artificial Algae Algorithm," Handbook of Research on AI-Based Technologies and Applications in the Era of the Metaverse". Copyright: © 2023 | Page (436–447). https://doi.org/10.4018/978-1-6684-8851-5.ch024

Vrushank S., Vidhi T., Khang A., "Electronic Health Records Security and Privacy Enhancement using Blockchain Technology," *Data-Centric AI Solutions and Emerging Technologies in the Healthcare Ecosystem*. P (1). (1st Ed.) (2023). CRC Press. https://doi.org/10.1201/9781003356189-1

Xiang Gao, Li, Q. and Fengrui Liu, "Research on the new normal technology and application of artificial intelligence in the internet of things," *Journal of Physics: Conference Series*, Vol. 1865, No. 4, IOP Publishing, (2021). doi:10.1088/1742-6596/1865/4/042062

Yi Lyu, Yin, P., "Internet of Things transmission and network reliability in complex environment,"*Computer Communications*, Vol. 150, P: 757–763, (2020). https://doi.org/10.1016/j.comcom.2019.11.054

Yuchang Mo, Xing, L., Wenzhong Guo, Shaobin Cai, Zhao Zhang, and Jianhui Jiang, "Reliability analysis of IoT networks with community structures," *IEEE Transactions on Network Science and Engineering*, Vol. 7, No. 1, P: 304–315, (2018). https://doi.org/10.1109/TNSE.2018.2869167

Zahra Nasiri Aghdam, Rahmani, A. M., Mehdi Hosseinzadeh, "The Role of the Internet of Things in Healthcare: Future Trends and Challenges," *Computer Methods and Programs in Biomedicine*, Vol. 199, P: 105903, (2021). https://doi.org/10.1016/j.cmpb.2020.105903

# Index